MECHANICS OF THE CIRCULATION

DEVELOPMENTS IN CARDIOVASCULAR MEDICINE

Recent volumes

Hanrath P, Bleifeld W, Souquet, J. eds: Cardiovascular diagnosis by ultrasound. Transesophageal, computerized, contrast, Doppler echocardiography. 1982. ISBN 90-247-2692-1.

Roelandt J, ed: The practice of M-mode and two-dimensional echocardiography. 1983. ISBN 90-247-2745-6.

Meyer J, Schweizer P, Erbel R, eds: Advances in noninvasive cardiology. 1983. ISBN 0-89838-576-8.

Morganroth J, Moore EN, eds: Sudden cardiac death and congestive heart failure: Diagnosis and treatment. 1983. ISBN 0-89838-580-6.

Perry HM, ed: Lifelong management of hypertension. 1983. ISBN 0-89838-582-2.

Jaffe EA, ed: Biology of endothelial cells. 1984. ISBN 0-89838-587-3.

Surawicz B, Reddy CP, Prystowsky EN, eds: Tachycardias. 1984. ISBN 0-89838-588-1.

Spencer MP, ed: Cardiac Doppler diagnosis. 1983. ISBN 0-89838-591-1.

Villarreal H, Sambhi MP, eds: Topics in pathophysiology of hypertension. 1984. ISBN 0-89838-595-4.

Messerli FH, ed: Cardiovascular disease in the elderly. 1984. ISBN 0-89838-596-2.

Simoons ML, Reiber JHC, eds: Nuclear imaging in clinical cardiology. 1984. ISBN 0-89838-599-7.

Ter Keurs HEDJ, Schipperheyn JJ, eds: Cardiac left ventricular hypertrophy. 1983. ISBN 0-89838-612-8.

Sperelakis N, ed: Physiology and pathophysiology of the heart. 1984. ISBN 0-89838-615-2.

Messerli FH, ed: Kidney in essential hypertension. 1984. ISBN 0-89838-616-0.

Sambhi MP, ed: Fundamental fault in hypertension. 1984. ISBN 0-89838-638-1.

Marchesi C, ed: Ambulatory monitoring: Cardiovascular system and allied applications. 1984. ISBN 0-89838-642-X.

Kupper W, MacAlpin RN, Bleifeld W, eds: Coronary tone in ischemic heart disease. 1984. ISBN 0-89838-646-2.

Sperelakis N, Caulfield JB, eds: Calcium antagonists: Mechanisms of action on cardiac muscle and vascular smooth muscle. 1984. ISBN 0-89838-655-1.

Godfraind T, Herman AS, Wellens D, eds: Calcium entry blockers in cardiovascular and cerebral dysfunctions. 1984. ISBN 0-89838-658-6.

Morganroth J, Moore EN, eds: Interventions in the acute phase of myocardial infarction. 1984. ISBN 0-89838-659-4.

Abel FL, Newman WH, eds: Functional aspects of the normal, hypertrophied, and failing heart. 1984. ISBN 0-89838-665-9.

Sideman S, Beyar R, eds: Simulation and imaging of the cardiac system. 1985. ISBN 0-89838-687-X.

Van der Wall E, Lie KI, eds: Recent views on hypertrophic cardiomyopathy. 1985. ISBN 0-89838-694-2.

Beamish RE, Singal PK, Dhalla NS, eds: Stress and heart disease. 1985. ISBN 0-89838-709-4.

Beamish RE, Panagio V, Dhalla NS, eds: Pathogenesis of stress-induced heart disease. 1985. ISBN 0-89838-710-8.

Morganroth J, Moore EN, eds: Cardiac arrhythmias. 1985. ISBN 0-89838-716-7.

Mathes E, ed: Secondary prevention in coronary artery disease and myocardial infarction. 1985. ISBN 0-89838-736-1.

Lowell Stone H, Weglicki WB, eds: Pathology of cardiovascular injury. 1985. ISBN 0-89838-743-4.

Meyer J, Erbel R, Rupprecht HJ, eds: Improvement of myocardial perfusion. 1985. ISBN 0-89838-748-5.

Reiber JHC, Serruys PW, Slager CJ: Quantitative coronary and left ventricular cineangiography. 1986. ISBN 0-89838-760-4.

Fagard RH, Bekaert IE, eds: Sports cardiology. 1986. ISBN 0-89838-782-5.

Reiber JHC, Serruys PW, eds: State of the art in quantitative coronary arteriography. 1986. ISBN 0-89838-804-X.

Roelandt J, ed: Color Doppler Flow Imaging. 1986. ISBN 0-89838-806-6.

Van der Wall EE, ed: Noninvasive imaging of cardiac metabolism. 1986. ISBN 0-89838-812-0.

Liebman J, Plonsey R, Rudy Y, eds: Pediatric and fundamental electrocardiography. 1986. ISBN 0-89838-815-5.

Hilger HH, Hombach V, Rashkind WJ, eds: Invasive cardiovascular therapy. 1987. ISBN 0-89838-818-X

Serruys PW, Meester GT, eds: Coronary angioplasty: a controlled model for ischemia. 1986. ISBN 0-89838-819-8.

Tooke JE, Smaje LH: Clinical investigation of the microcirculation. 1986. ISBN 0-89838-819-8.

Van Dam RTh, Van Oosterom A, eds: Electrocardiographic body surface mapping. 1986. ISBN 0-89838-834-1.

Spencer MP, ed: Ultrasonic diagnosis of cerebrovascular disease. 1987. ISBN 0-89838-836-8.

Legato MJ, ed: The stressed heart. 1987. ISBN 0-89838-849-X.

Roelandt J, ed: Digital techniques in echocardiography. 1987. ISBN 0-89838-861-9.

Sideman S, Beyar R, eds: Activation, metabolism and perfusion of the heart. 1987. ISBN 0-89838-871-6.

Safar ME et al., eds: Arterial and venous systems in essential hypertension. 1987. ISBN 0-89838-857-0.

Ter Keurs HEDJ, Tyberg JV, eds: Mechanics of the circulation. 1987. ISBN 0-89838-870-8

MECHANICS OF THE CIRCULATION

edited by

H.E.D.J. TER KEURS MD, PhD and
J.V. TYBERG MD, PhD

1987 **MARTINUS NIJHOFF PUBLISHERS**
a member of the KLUWER ACADEMIC PUBLISHERS GROUP
DORDRECHT / BOSTON / LANCASTER

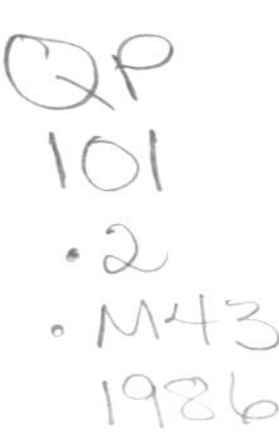

Distributors

for the United States and Canada: Kluwer Academic Publishers, P.O. Box 358, Accord Station, Hingham, MA 02018-0358, USA
for the UK and Ireland: Kluwer Academic Publishers, MTP Press Limited, Falcon House, Queen Square, Lancaster LA1 1RN, UK
for all other countries: Kluwer Academic Publishers Group, Distribution Center, P.O. Box 322, 3300 AH Dordrecht, The Netherlands

Library of Congress Cataloging in Publication Data

```
Mechanics of the circulation.

  (Developments in cardiovascular medicine)
  Proceedings of a satellite symposium of the XXXth
Congress of the International Union of Physiological
Sciences, held in Banff, Alberta, 7/9-11/86.
  Includes index.
  1. Blood--Circulation--Congresses.  2. Heart--Muscle--
Congresses.  I. Keurs, H. E. D. J. ter.  II. Tyberg,
J. V.  III. International Congress of Physiological
Sciences (30th : 1986 : Banff, Alta.)  IV. Series.
QP101.2.M43  1987      612'.1              86-33331
```

ISBN 0-89838-870-8

Copyright

© 1987 by Martinus Nijhoff Publishers, Dordrecht.

All rights reserved. No part of this publication may be reproduced, stored in a retrieval system, or transmitted in any form or by any means, mechanical, photocopying, recording, or otherwise, without the prior written permission of the publishers,
Martinus Nijhoff Publishers, P.O. Box 163, 3300 AD Dordrecht,
The Netherlands.

PRINTED IN THE NETHERLANDS

Preface

This volume constitutes the proceedings of a satellite symposium of the XXXth congress of the International Union of Physiological Sciences. The symposium has been held in Banff, Alberta Canada July 9–11 1986. The program was organized to provide a selective overview of current developments in cardiac biophysics, biochemistry, and physiology. In order to highlight areas of developing ideas and to stimulate the participants' inquisitiveness into the nature and complexity of the integrated cardiovascular system, lectures and discussions were presented that emphasized evolving and sometimes provocative concepts in the field. With the same goal in mind we have, for the readers of this volume, briefly summarized the general discussions.

We would like to thank several individuals whose dedication made this symposium and publication of the proceedings possible. Mrs. Lois Kokoski and Mrs. Madeleine Aldridge of the Conference Office of the University of Calgary seemingly effortlessly handled the details of the symposium. Peter de Tombe, Dr. Peter Backx and Dr. Jeroen Bucx transcribed the general discussions. Finally, we appreciate the extra effort of our secretaries, Lenore Doell and Gregory Douglas, and the work of Anna Tyberg who prepared the final manuscripts for publication.

Henk E.D.J. ter Keurs, M.D. Ph.D.
John V. Tyberg, M.D. Ph.D.
Calgary, Alberta, Canada
September, 1986

'As an animal body consists not only of a wonderful texture of solid parts but also of a large proportion of fluids which are continually circulating and flowing thro' an inimitable embroidery of blood vessels and other inconceivably minute canals; and as the healthy state of an animal principally consists in the maintaining of a due equilibrium between those solids and fluids; it has ever since the important discovery of the circulation of the blood been looked upon as a matter well worth enquiring into to find the force and velocity with which these fluids are impelled; as a likely means to give a considerable insight into the animal oeconomy.'

Stephen Hales 1769

Contents

1. How do crossbridges produce the sliding force between actin and myosin filaments in muscle

HUGH E. HUXLEY

Introduction

I will discuss in this chapter the mechanism of muscular contraction in general, and focus on current work concerned with the central question of discovering how the crossbridges produce the sliding force between the actin and myosin filaments.

There have been a number of very important advances in the last two or three years involving quite novel kinds of experiment and I think it might be interesting to mention one or two of these before I describe some of the structural studies we have been carrying out to explore the dynamics of the corssbridge cycle and how it is switched on and off.

Motion of cross bridges

These new types of experiment are, in a way, all trying to do the same thing but they sometimes have unexpected biproducts and bonuses. Essentially, they involve finding more direct ways to relate what goes on in individual protein molecules in solution in a biochemical or kinetic experiment to what goes on when the proteins are part of a movement producing system. Perhaps the most spectacular of these are the in vitro motile systems of Spudich and his colleagues in which a number of individual myosin molecules are attached to small plastic beads, which will then slide their way for long distances along either natural or synthetic bundles of actin filaments in the presence of ATP, providing the actin filaments all have the same structural polarity [1, 2]. This is a very useful essay system, for one is able to measure, for instance, the sliding velocity of the beads with myosins from different muscles, and to find that the bead velocity is approximately the same as the sliding velocity of the actin and myosin filaments past each other during unloaded shortening of the muscle from which the myosin was derived – typically a few microns per second for vertebrate striated muscle. These systems enable one to show that the myosin does not have to be organized into filaments for the bead movement to occur – it just has to be attached, with a spacer, to the surface of the bead – and it doesn't even have to be an intact myosin molecule. Short heavy meromyosin will work, i.e. the fragment lacking both LMM and the lower melting point helical region on the HMM side of the HMM/ LMM junction. Even single headed HMM will work, and the system will also work on actin in the absence of tropomyosin. Moreover, since the beads move distances very large compared with their diameters, it is clear that the myosin molecules attached to them, i.e. the crossbridges, must be working repetitively. So here we have sliding reduced to very simple terms.

There are also reconstructed systems in which individual actin and myosin filaments are made visible by fluorescent labels and can be seen actively sliding past each other in the presence of MgATP.

Energy conversion

Another type of study involves mechanical measurements on single muscle fibres in which ATP is suddenly released by a laser flash from 'caged' ATP previously diffused into the fibre. This enables one to do enzyme kinetic type experiments on the myosin in situ in the crossbridges, and compare the rate constants and substrate concentration dependence of various steps in the crossbridge cycle – for instance, the dissociation step – with the value measured in solution. The mechanical and biochemical rate constants in the fibre agree very well with the biochemical rate constants in solution, and this is enabling people such as Yale Goldman [3] and David Trentham [4], to trace out an increasingly detailed correspondence between the multiple steps that have been worked out largely by Eisenberg and Taylor and their colleagues in kinetic studies on solutions [5, 6], and steps that can be picked up in the crossbridge cycle in skinned muscle fibres. For example, there is now very good evidence that it is at the inorganic phosphate release step (during product release) that tension is developed by the attached crossbridge.

I mention these studies because they are very interesting and elegant and also to make the point that there is now very extensive documentation that the force producing elements in a muscle behave both physically and biochemically, to a considerable degree of detail, in precisely the same way the actin and myosin do when they interact with ATP in vitro. That means that the crossbridges are acting cyclically all the time the muscle is shortening, and that all the cross-bridges in the region of filament overlap are involved in tension production and energy release. It is therefore pertinent to enquire what enzyme kinetic studies tell us about the nature of this process, since it has been studied very intensively by a number of groups during the past 15 years, since the publication of the original Lymn and Taylor model [7].

It had been recognized since the 1950's that the ATPase of myosin on its own was very low under physiological ionic conditions, but that enzyme activity was greatly activated when actin was present, under conditions where actin and myosin could combine. Using a variety of kinetic methods, Lymn and Taylor showed that when ATP was added to the actomyosin complex, the first thing that happened was that it dissociated into actin and myosin ATP. Then the ATP was cleaved on the myosin but the hydrolysis products ADP and Pi remained bound to the myosin, and dissociated only very slowly until combination with actin took place again. When combination did take place, the products were released and the cycle was completed. It was possible to measure the rate constants for the various steps in the cycle, and the general principle of the model has been shown to be correct by a very large number of experiments over the long period of time since it was first proposed. Of course, the details of the cycle have become increasingly sophisticated over the years, the main advance lying in the recognition of the reversibility of the various steps in the process so that, for instance, dissociation became a transition from a tight binding state to a loose binding state, with an appropriate equilibrium between bound and unbound states in each case. The number of identifiable steps in the process has grown too, and there is still some controversy over the minimum number needed to explain the data, as there is over the question of which steps are rate limiting [8]. However, there is universal agreement that what is being studied during ATP splitting is a cyclic process involving states of association and dissociation of the myosin S_1 head subunits with actin. In the relaxed state (i.e. in the presence of the regulatory proteins, but absence of calcium) actin and myosin are predominantly dissociated under physiological conditions.

Now these are all very well known facts and there is no controversy over the basic phenomena so far as I am aware, certainly not among the numerous very eminent people working in the enzyme kinetic field. It would therefore seem to be essential to take them into account when trying to arrive at a model of the contractile process in muscle. Given that actin and myosin are located in separate filaments, and that the crossbridges have been identified as the S_1 head subunits of myosin, attached into the myosin filament backbone via the S_2 linkage, it is inescapable that the crossbridges are involved in a cyclical structural interaction with actin to split ATP and provide energy for contraction. Since the energy required to lift near maximal loads would call for the splitting of an ATP molecule by more than half the myosin heads present in a muscle for every 12 nm of sliding of actin past myosin filaments (or approximately 1% of muscle length change), a high proportion of all the crossbridges must be acting in parallel all the time to generate tension.

I think these are very compelling arguments, and we should be absolutely clear about them. There is no other energy source in muscle except the one that works this way, and so the problem is not *whether* the crossbridges are responsible for energy transduction in muscle by some type of cyclical and parallel process, but *how* they transduce the energy from that process into force and movement.

4

Constancy of filament length

There is an abundance of good evidence published that no significant change in filament length or in axial repeat takes place in the actin or myosin filaments in vertebrate skeletal muscle down to a sarcomere length of $2.0\,\mu$m. (For a recent summary see [9]). The contrary reports that are sometimes quoted derive in considerable part from early Russian work describing large changes in A-band length and carried out before certain technical pitfalls were generally appreciated, and from other studies that have similar limitations. This was an argument that was settled to most people's satisfaction about 20 years ago [10, 11], and I do not think there is any good cause to rehearse it again now. However, as an example of recent independent work I will quote the conclusion of Dr. Dreizen who was invited by Dr. Pollack to attend the Seattle Symposium [12] in order to describe his work on A-band lengths. Dreizen et al. [12] state 'In sarcomeres above $2.0\,\mu$m in length, A-band length is constant (... In fibres treated with ATP), as in the absence of ATP'. It is also worth recording the following opinion 'The results of electron- and optical micrographic studies in vertebrate muscles are consistent. Above rest length, variations of sarcomere length are brought about by variations in thick/thin filament interdigitation; thick filament lengths remain constant. The several reported instances of thick filament shortening above rest length must be viewed skeptically in light of the substantial body of evidence to the contrary [13]. I think it would be entirely reasonable to accept these conclusions.

The possibility that myosin filaments in vertebrate striated muscle start to shorten when sarcomere lengths fall below $2.0\,\mu$m is less easy to disprove, but I have looked into all the reports of such shortening very carefully and can find no evidence to suggest that any significant overall shortening process occurs. It is conceivable that some disruption of the very tips of the tapered myosin filaments may take place when the I-bands become very short, leading to length changes of a few percent, but the changes by 10–15% (i.e. by up to 200 nm in A-band length) sometimes reported [12] at apparently shorter sarcomere lengths can be very well accounted for by lack of perpendicularity between the fibre axis and the viewing direction in the electron microscope (i.e. plane of section not parallel to filaments), reducing sarcomere lengths and all apparent filament lengths and internal periodicities by the same factor. Observations of a reduced 14.3 nm axial period are diagnostic of this type of artefact. Below sarcomere lengths of about $1.6\,\mu$m, of course, A-band lengths must necessarily be reduced by mechanical compression.

Evidence that muscle length change takes place by filament sliding is, on the other hand, very abundant, and I have already referred briefly to reconstituted systems in which it can be seen. It is also very nicely demonstrated in Yanagida's recent work [14], using fluorescently labelled I-filaments in a crab muscle long sarcomeres.

Basic mechanism of cross bridge action

The significant questions that we need to address are concerned with the detailed structural mechanism by which the crossbridge-actin interaction develops the sliding force. In principle, there are many ways in which this could happen, and it would be as well to mention some of these before describing the actual evidence, so that one can see that there is plenty of scope for further discoveries even if one restricts oneself to a relatively constrained model. Thus the motive force could be generated by a local change in actin structure, sliding of the myosin S_1 head along the actin filament, a change of structure in the myosin head, a change in length of S_2, or a local change of structure in the myosin backbone, or some combination of these. It is not possible at present to positively eliminate any one of these conceivable sites of force generation, but some seem much less plausible than others.

Thus, there is very good evidence that the overall extent of the relative movement of actin filaments past myosin in the course of the attachment cycle of one myosin head is about 12 nm [15] although force development by the attached bridge does not have to take place throughout this distance. Nevertheless, the extent of movement seems too large to be plausibly accommodated for by a local structural change in the actin filament alone, for it is a compact and apparently axially very stable structure without very large protuberances which could be capable of such large shifts.

The myosin head itself is the prime candidate for the local structural change, because it functions as the major part of the enzyme complex which splits ATP, and because it is suitably placed in the structure to bring about relative sliding between actin and myosin filaments.

The S_2 portion of myosin is a less promising candidate although its interesting physical properties are likely to play a very important role in the passive mechanical properties of the overall crossbridge structure. But its spatial separation from the ATPase site would make it necessary to invoke additional mechanisms to transmit both the signal and the energy over long distances. Changes in myosin backbone structure face a similar difficulty because of their distance from the site of energy release, plus an even greater difficulty in explaining what the driving force could be and producing any experimental evidence for such a change taking place.

All in all therefore, most people think that the immediate behaviour of the myosin head itself is the most likely source of contractile force. Obviously, if it were a straightforward mechanism based on such changes, it would have been elucidated a long time ago. The likelihood is that it is indeed a mechanism of this general type but one which has certain features that make it peculiarly difficult to unravel. However, before dealing with the more subtle aspects of the problem, there are a number of further basic facts about the mechanism which need to be kept in mind.

6

I refer to recent structural studies which seek to determine what the myosin crossbridges actually do in a contracting muscle (and by 'crossbridge' I should say that I include both the S heads, and the S_2 chain alpha-helical linear structure that connects them into the thick filament backbone made up of the LMM tails of myosin).

X-ray studies of activation

The first change in structure that we can detect in a muscle after it has been stimulated is in the actin filaments. It consists of the appearance of a new reflection in the X-ray diffraction pattern on the actin second layer line at a spacing of about 18 nm (half the actin repeat and readily distinguishable from the myosin periodicities at orders of 43 nm). (Fig. 1-1 and 1-2.) This happens with a half-time of about 17 msec. at 6° C and 3 msec. at 20° C, and is probably caused by tropomyosin movement brought about by calcium binding to troponin, switching on the thin filaments. This occurs before significant amounts of tension are developed, and is still seen in muscles stretched to non-overlap, i.e. it is an autonomous structural change in the thin filaments [18].

This is followed, with a delay of about 10–15 msec. by a large change in the equatorial X-ray pattern, which we believe is brought about by the net movement of large numbers of myosin crossbridges to the vicinity of the actin filaments, and there is very strong evidence, which I can't go into now, that they are actually attached to actin in some way. I think the myosin heads are already spending part of their time near actin in a relaxed muscle, and then become trapped there by attachment when muscle is switched on. At the same time, there are large changes in the myosin layer line reflections, showing that the myosin crossbridges have been disordered from their original regular helical arrangement around the myosin backbone, which is what one might expect when they become attached to actin [17, 18]. However, this initial attached state seems to be one which does not produce tension (or not much tension anyway) since tension development is delayed by another 10–15 msec. following the equatorial and layer line changes. This is still the case where most of the internal shortening in the muscle has been prevented by stretch, i.e. when there is no reason to think that the tension rise is being delayed by force-velocity effects. The process of tension development, which we would assume corresponds to some further transition in the attached crossbridge, does not lead to any new changes in these parts of the X-ray pattern. The patterns show that in a fully developed isometric contraction, a large proportion of the crossbridges is attached to actin [19, 20].

When a single twitch and a tetanus are compared at 6° C, it is apparent that thin filament activation is already maximal in the single twitch, (Fig. 1-3) and cross-bridge attachment is found to be virtually maximal too as judged from the equatorial pattern. Presumably it is the rate of transition of bridges from the

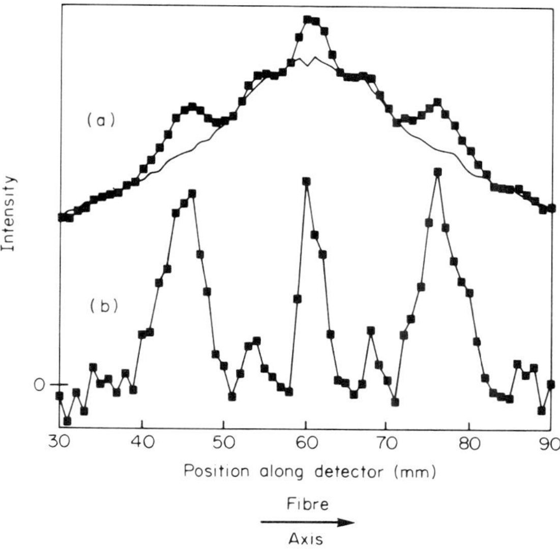

Figure 1-1. (a) The X-ray diffraction pattern from resting and contracting muscle recorded by a position sensitive detector crossing the second actin layer-line at a radial spacing of 0.023 Å^{-1}. No second layer-line is apparent in resting muscle, but a strong reflection appears during contraction. (b) Subtracting the resting from the contracting pattern makes the second layer-line more obvious. Intensity and position can be easily determined and the reflection corresponds to an axial spacing of about 179 Å, i.e. one half of the actin helical repeat. The patterns shown here were collected in the time frames beginning 50 ms after the first stimulus and ending 50 ms before the last stimulus and were averaged for the contracting pattern.

attached stage – to the tension generating state which is the limiting factor in the shorter time available during the single twitch which leads to somewhat lower tension development. At higher temperatures, (14°C for example), it appears that activation is not maximal in a single twitch, (Fig. 1-3b) and crossbridge attachment is also found to be incomplete.

During relaxation, the thin filaments begin to revert back toward their resting state as soon as stimulation ceases, whereas crossbridge detachment and tension decay are significantly delayed (i.e. by 100–150 msec. at 6°C to the halfway point). The rate of return of the thin filament structure is faster in muscles stretched beyond overlap, so it may be that the tropomyosin movement is impeded by attached crossbridges.

Now, what evidence is there for an attachment-detachment cycle during muscle shortening? In a sense, this is selfevident from what we know of the dimensions of crossbridges and of actin molecules (i.e. in the range 5–20 nm) and of the extent of the relative movement of the actin and myosin filaments during shortening (i.e. several hundred nanometers). It is also of interest to enquire whether there is any evidence that the crossbridges do actually come off the actin filament in the course of their movement from one actin monomer to other ones along the

8

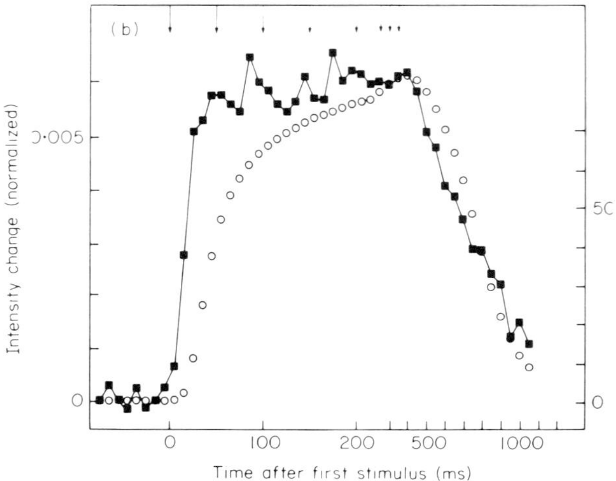

Figure 1-2. Time course of second layer line intensity during tetani at 6° C (average of 6 experiments). (■ Intensity; ○ Tension.) The arrows indicate the 350 ms long train of 20 Hz electrical pulses used for the tetanic stimulation. Note that the time frame duration is 10 msec. for the 5th to the 29th time frame, and 50 msec. otherwise. This gives the apparent kink in the tension time course.

actin filament. We (Huxley, Faruqi & Simmons, unpublished) have looked at the behaviour of the equatorial pattern during rapid shortening, and we see that it does indeed change part of the way back to a relaxed pattern, though it does so more slowly after the shortening starts than one would expect on the basis of free diffusion of crossbridges. (Perhaps this is also the reason why initial attachment is relatively slow.) At the same time, at higher temperatures at least, one can, during rapid shortening, also see a partial recovery of the myosin layer-line pattern and of the meridional 21.4 nm reflection which is characteristic of relaxed muscle. So it is clear that there is indeed a detached crossbridge population at higher shortening velocities, though more work is needed to quantitate it. When the contraction becomes isometric again, the normal active pattern is restored, with a delay.

There is also X-ray evidence for the transfer of crossbridges from one site on actin to a neighbouring one during shortening [21]. If we apply a quick release or a quick stretch to a muscle, we produce an axial disordering of the crossbridges. This disordering is delayed by about half a millisecond on the length change and tension fall, indicating that the release of the undamped elastic component in the crossbridge takes place ahead of any change in crossbridge configuration, as would be the case, for instance, if we were releasing an elastic stretch of the S_2 element of the crossbridge, and the rest of the crossbridge just moved along with the actin filaments. A possible explanation for the observed disordering of the 14.3 nm-crossbridge axial repeat is that the rapid sliding between actin and myosin filaments brings about a compression of S_2 by variable amounts depend-

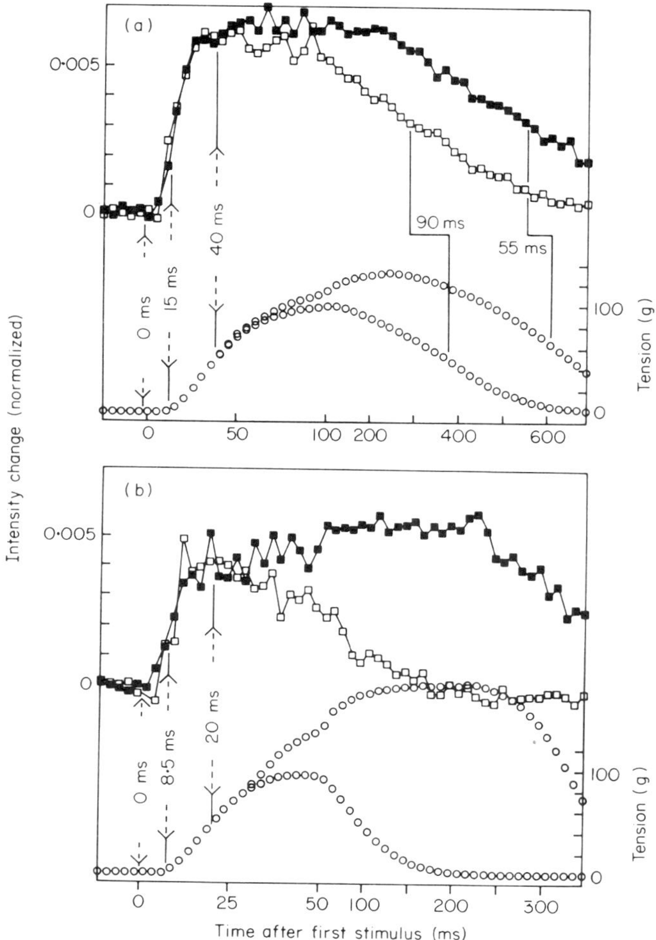

Figure 1-3. (a) Time course of the second layer line intensity in twitches and tetani at 6°C. The measurements on several muscles were added before the analysis. The upper part of the panel shows the intensity traces, the lower part shows tension (O) The 20 time frames immediately after the stimulus were of 5 ms duration, the rest 20 ms. (b) Same experiment at 14°C. Time frames of 2.5 and 10 ms were used. The half-times for the rise and fall of tension and intensity are indicated on the diagrams.

ing on how far through the attached phase of the cycle the individual bridges have progressed. So, the observed drop in the 14.3 nm intensity does give an indication of a relative axial movement, taking place during the working stroke, between the attachment site of the crossbridge on actin and the end of the crossbridge where it is anchored to S_2. However, the argument is rather an intricate one and I would not expect it to carry complete conviction.

The more straightforward characteristic of the intensity fall is that it can be reversed during the first one or two milliseconds after the length change by restretching the muscle to the original length. This indicates that cross- bridges initially are still attached and can be pulled back to their original state. After 5 or 6 milliseconds, however, the change cannot be reversed and the muscle now behaves like one which started at the new length, as though many of the cross-bridges had now transferred themselves to new positions on actin.

Another feature of the X-ray diagram from contracting musce is an intensification of the 5.9 nm and 5.1 nm actin reflections. Part of the 5.9 nm change may be associated with activation, but another part (and probably all of the 5.1 nm change) seems to be associated with myosin attachment and tension development. This would imply a specific steric relationship between at least part of the structure of the attached myosin heads and the actin monomer repeat. Interestingly, the strength of these reflections appears to be unchanged during shortening at moderate speed. This indicates that the myosin heads attach to actin at sites which always have the same steric relationship to the actin subunit repeat. The heads do not just slide smoothly along the actin filaments.

In summary, the X-ray studies give very satisfactory evidence supporting the attaching, cycling crossbridge model for contraction. However, these studies have not been so productive as far as giving information about what the attached crossbridges actually do to produce force and movement, other than that they undergo some internal structural change. And so let me indicate the lines along which I think the different determinations of crossbridge behaviour might fit together.

The X-ray results show (by virtue of the absence of a strong labelled actin pattern in the layer line pattern from contracting muscle) that a considerable proportion of the attached myosin heads, although they are likely to be attached to a specific site on actin, are not attached in a specific conformation relative to the actin structure. It could therefore be argued that this variable configuration represents the range of configurations through which the myosin head goes in the course of its working stroke. As an example, just for illustration, one could think of a rigid myosin head going through a large range of angles of tilt about its attachment site to actin. A more realistic model on the same basic principle would be to have a fixed attachment of a domain of myosin to actin and a substantial range of different shapes of the myosin head. However, I have always felt somewhat uneasy with the concept of the myosin head undergoing a very large and progressive shape change, and much prefer the picture of two well defined structural states with a very rapid transition between them. One apparent difficulty with such a model is that the rapid tension recovery following small quick-releases of an isometrically contracting muscle [15] seems to indicate the presence of a substantial number of crossbridges which are still near the beginning of their power stroke. Yet the EPR measurements [22] seem only to show a rigor type attachment, which is more likely to represent the end of the power stroke. Another apparent difficulty is that if all the attached crossbridges are in one or other of these two states, then they should give rise to some kind of labelled actin

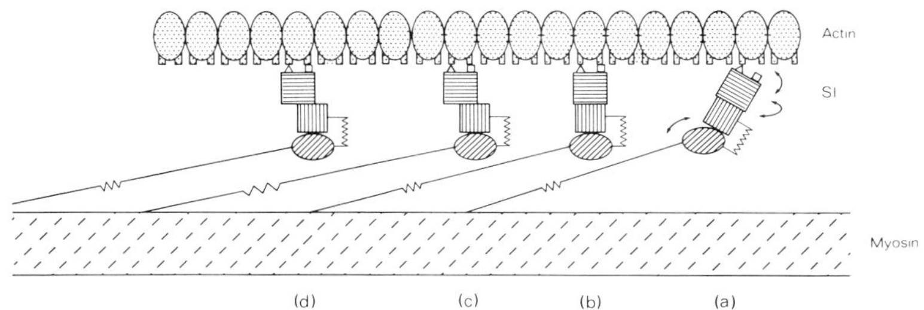

Figure 1-4. Schematic diagram illustrating different configurations of myosin crossbridges during the part of the crossbridge cycle when they are attached to actin. (a) represents the initial weakly attached state (possibly one-site binding) in which it is supposed that the S_1 head can adapt a variety of orientations relative to the actin filament and may also have considerable internal flexibility. (b) represents a short-lived configuration in which the transition to strong attachment (possibly two-site binding) can first take place. This quickly triggers a structural change in the S_1 head which extends the elastic element (possibly but not necessarily in S_2) by about 40 Å so that the crossbridge goes over into configuration (c). (c) represents the configuration of the tension-generating crossbridges, in which the form of attachment of the S_1 head is close to, but not identical to, that in the rigor state. The elastic part of the crossbridge (shown here diagrammatically as an extensible element in S_2) has been stretched and is generating tension and shortening as the actin and myosin filaments slide past each other. (d) represents the configuration at the end of the working stroke. The elastic element has shortened back to its equilibrium length and is no longer generating tension. The S_1 head can now adopt the normal rigor-like attachment (perhaps by dissociation of ADP) and can be detached from actin following the binding of the next molecule of ATP. (For simplicity, only single myosin heads are shown.)

pattern. It was such a pattern that we had originally, of course, hoped to see in a contracting muscle. However, we have to remember that the intensity of such a pattern will be proportional to the *square* of the number of crossbridges which contribute, so that if 20% of all crossbridges are attached in some specific structural state, the intensity will be only 20% of 20% of that given by all the crossbridges acting together, i.e. 4%, and any such pattern would be extremely difficult to see.

This provides a clue as to how the paradox mentioned above might be resolved. If this 20% of crossbridges are the ones that are producing all the contractile force, then taking reasonable values for the free energy available from ATP splitting, one can calculate a working stroke of about 4.0 nm. This happens to be about the same value as the extension accommodated in the undamped elastic element in the crossbridges [23], so one could visualize a very rapid transition to the final structural state of the myosin head, with the energy being stored elastically and released as the muscle shortened. The initial state representing the beginning of the working stroke could be a very short lived structural intermediate that was too transient to be detected readily.

The rest of the attached bridges would be in a much more flexibly attached state in respect of their orientation on actin, and would possibly have a considerable

12

internal flexibility as well. These would correspond to be initially attached crossbridges and though there might be a large number of myosin heads in this state, which would show up on the equatorial X-ray pattern as being near actin, their variable axial and azimuthal position would cause them not to contribute to the layer line pattern, and, if they were undergoing Brownian movement about their attachment sites, would make them difficult to distinguish from randomly arranged unattached heads by optical or spin-label techniques.

I describe this particular model (Fig. 1-4), not because I'm convinced it must necessarily be right, but simply to show that one should keep a rather open mind about how crossbridges are behaving, and that negative evidence – for example, absence of probe or X-ray evidence for more than one attached state – should be interpreted quite carefully. One should always bear in mind that it is not only the structural evidence which indicates a crossbridge cycle, but all the transient mechanical kinetic experiments and all the biochemical kinetics. I think there can be no doubt that the sliding force for contraction is generated by a step-wise interaction of crossbridges and actin. What we have to determine is what part of the crossbridge undergoes the active structural change, and where that energy is stored until the quantum of shortening has taken place. In practical terms, what one needs to do, I believe, is to find better ways of getting structural information about mobile but attached myosin heads, and to discover whether these too can be involved in tension generation.

References

1. Sheetz M.P., Chasan R. and Spudich J.A.: ATP-dependent movement of myosin in-vitro: Characterisation of a quantitative assay. J. Cell Biol. 99: 1867–1871, 1984.
2. Spudich J.A.: Movement of myosin coated beads on oriented filaments reconstituted from purified actin. Nature 315: 584–586, 1985.
3. Goldman Y.E., Hibberd M.G. and Trentham D.R.: Relaxation of rabbit psoas muscle fibers from rigor by photochemical generation of adenosine-5'-triphosphate. J. Physiol. 354: 577–604, 605–624, 1984.
4. Hibberd M.G. and Trentham D.R.: Relationships between chemical and mechanical events during muscular contraction. Ann. Rev. of Biophysics & Biophys. Chem. 15: 119–161, 1986.
5. Eisenberg E. and Hill T.L.: Muscle Contraction and free energy transduction in biological systems. Science, 227: 999–1006, 1985.
6. Taylor E.W.: mechanism of actomyosin ATPase and the problem of muscle contraction. CRC Crit. Rev. Biochem. 6: 103–164, 1979.
7. Lymn R.W. and Taylor E.W.: Mechanism of adenosine triphosphate hydrolysis by actomyosin. Biochemistry 10: 4617–4624, 1971.
8. Stein L.A., Chock P.B. and Eisenberg E.: The rate limiting step in the actomyosin adenosinetriphosphate cycle. Biochemistry 23: 1555–1563, 1984.
9. Huxley H.E.: The crossbridge mechanism of muscle contraction and its implications. J. Exp. Biol. 115: 17–30, 1985.
10. Huxley H.E. Structural arrangements and the contraction mechanism in striated muscle. Proc. Roy. Soc. B160: 442–448, 1964.

11. Huxley H.E.: Structural evidence concerning the mechanism of contraction in striated muscle; in *Muscle* (Eds. Paul, Daniel, Kay and Monckton) pp 3–28. Pergamon, New York, 1965.

12. Dreizen P., Herman L. and Berger J.E.: Contractile Mechanisms in Muscle (Eds. Pollack & Sugi) pp 135–149. Plenum Press, New York, 1984.

13. Pollack G.E.: The crossbridge theory. Physiol. Rev. 63: 1049–1113, 1983.

14. Yanagida T., Nakase M, Nishiyama K. and Oosawa F.: Direct observation of motion of single F-actin filaments in the presence of myosin. Nature 307: 58–60, 1984.

15. Huxley A.F. and Simmons R.M.: Proposed mechanism of force generation in striated muscle. Nature 233: 533–538, 1971.

16. Harrington W.F.: On the origin of the contractile force in skeletal muscle. Proc. Nat. Acad. Sci. USA 76: 5066–5070, 1979.

17. Huxley H.E. and Brown W.: The low angle X-ray diagram of vertebrate striated muscle and its behaviour during contraction and rigor. J. Mol. Biol. 30: 383–434, 1967.

18. Huxley H.E., Faruqi A.R., Kress M., Bordas J. and Koch M.H.J.: Time resolved x-ray diffraction studies of the myosin layer-line reflections during muscle contraction. J. Mol. Biol. 158: 737–684, 1982.

19. Haselgrove J.C. and Huxley H.E.: X-ray evidence for radial cross bridge movement and for the sliding filament model in actively contracting skeletal muscle. J. Mol. Biol. 77: 549–568, 1973.

20. Yagi N., Ito M.H., Nakajima H., Izumi T. and Matsubara I.: Return of the myosin heads to thick filaments after muscle contraction. Science 197: 685–687, 1977.

21. Huxley H.E., Simmons R.M., Faruqi A.R., Kress M., Bordas J. and Koch M.H.J.: Changes in the X-ray reflections from contracting muscle during rapid mechanical transients and their structural implication. J. Mol. Biol. 169: 469–506, 1983.

22. Cooke R. et al.: Muscle crossbridges: Do they rotate? Adv. Exp. Med. Biol. 170: 413–477, 1984.

23. Ford L.E., Huxley A.F. and Simmons R.M.: Tension responses to sudden length change in stimulated frog muscle fibers near slack length. J. Physiol. 269: 441–515, 1977.

2. Stepwise shortening and the mechanism of contraction

GERALD H. POLLACK, HENK L.M. GRANZIER, ALICIA MATTIAZZI,
CHARLES TROMBITAS, AMMASAI PERIASAMY,
PETER H.W.W. BAATSEN, and DAVID H. BURNS

Introduction

As Sir Andrew Huxley [1] concluded in his response to a review article on
stepwise shortening, [2] 'before the presence of steps can be claimed to imply a
fundamental rethinking of the mechanism of contraction, three questions need to
be answered:
- (i) Are the steps genuine?
- (ii) If they are genuine, are they necessarily related to the contractile mechanism itself?
- (iii) If in some cases the steps do arise in the contractile mechanism, does this
  imply that current theories are incorrect?'

All three questions will be considered here. Although this chapter is not the place
for a detailed discussion of the technical aspects of the measurements, we will
consider recent approaches that bear directly on the validity of the phenomenon.
We will then speak to the mechanism: why the present theory appears incompati-
ble with the existence of steps; and what alternative kinds of theories might
account for their presence.

Are steps real?

More than a decade ago, we stumbled upon an unexpected result, which led to an
even more unexpected result. Struggling with the question of basic principles of
cardiac mechanics, we [3] noted a serious problem with commonly used preparations of cardiac muscle. Microscopic observation revealed that the clamped
ends of papillary muscle specimens were seriously damaged; that the striations
were disrupted not only at the sites immediately adjacent to the clamps, but often
well into the specimen. It soon became clear that if the principles of cardiac
mechanics were to be inferred from such preparations, studies would need to
focus on the central, viable region.

The advent of lasers and high-resolution optical sensors made it possible to track the time course of sarcomere shortening in this viable region with high precision. Because of the regularity of the muscle's striation pattern, the muscle can be treated, to a first approximation, as a diffraction grating. This has been known for years [4], controversy about interpretational details notwithstanding [5, 6, 7].

Armed with a high-resolution optical diffractometer, we set out to measure the characteristics of sarcomere shortening in cardiac muscle. To our surprise, we found that sarcomere shortening was punctuated by periods of pause, during which there was little or no length change, conferring a staircase-like character on the shortening waveform [8]. Examples are shown in Fig. 2-1.

The pauses intrigued us. The diffraction pattern reflects the collective behaviour of a sizeable fraction of sarcomeres ranging over the field illuminated by the laser. This ensemble could pause two ways. In the more complicated way, some sarcomeres could shorten while others lengthened such that the mean velocity remained zero for a period; if this recurred fortuitously time and again as contraction progressed, the train of pauses could be explained.

The simpler explanation is that the entire ensemble pauses and shortens synchronously. Because the intensity profile of the diffraction pattern remained steady during the pause this simpler explanation seemed more probable. At the same time [9], we checked for several potential artifacts, and could find no reason to suspect the steps were not genuine.

This simpler explanation poses a difficulty [8, 9]. It implies that molecular elements must somehow act in concert; otherwise pauses would not be detectable in an ensemble so large. A typical region sampled by the laser beam may contain 100 million filaments. Could an ensemble of this magnitude (or even a fraction of it) act synchronously?

This question lies at the root of the present controversy. According to the accepted theory of contraction, there is no provision to synchronize the action of bridges [10, 11]. Active shortening ought to occur smoothly. Unless the steps are peripheral to the contractile mechanism, either the theory must be inadequate or the steps must be artifacts.

In order to test whether the steps were artifacts, we have devised methods alternative to diffraction to measure shortening – three published and a fourth in progress. All four methods have shown steps similar to those measured by diffraction [12, 13, 14]. All but the newest are considered in the review article mentioned above, and the criticisms presented in the response by A.F. Huxley. The interested reader is encouraged to read the original papers as well as the criticisms, in order to render judgment as to the adequacy of controls.

Meanwhile, since the criticisms had been directed primarily toward earlier, striation-based methods, we redirected our efforts toward methods that were independent of the optical properties of the muscle striations. Following the pioneering work of Gordon, Huxley and Julian [15], and more recent work by

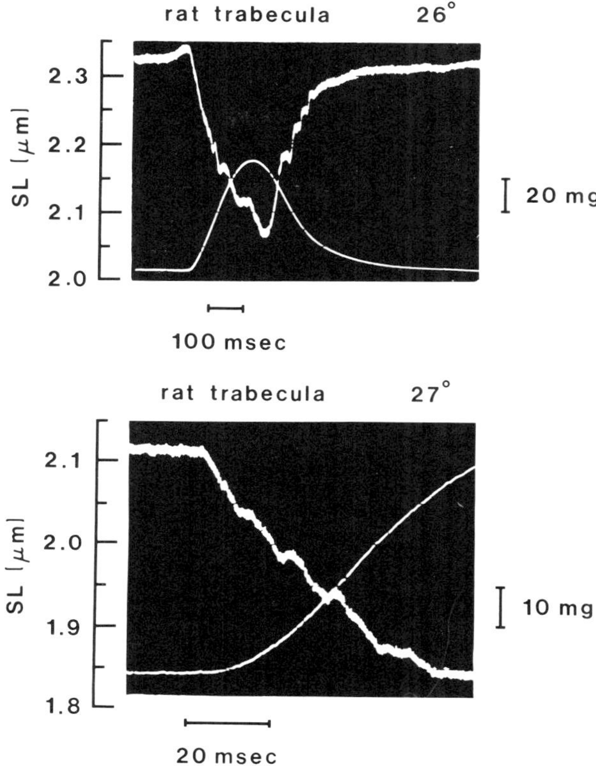

Figure 2-1. Stepwise sarcomere shortening in cardiac muscle, as measured by the optical diffraction technique. Specimens were mounted between fixed clamps, and stimulated. The central, viable region shortened at the expense of end compliance. Sarcomere length changes are interspersed with pauses during shortening and relengthening. Tension trace shown below on each panel.

Edman and Hoglund [16], we devised a method to track the length of a fiber segment. The segment was demarcated by a pair of thin hairs from the ear of a black cat. Segment length was tracked optically [14].

The results confirmed all of the optical methods. Stepwise shortening was seen regularly during both active shortening and unstimulated releases. Shortening patterns bore close resemblance to those obtained with the microscopic methods. In fact, when segment length and diffraction methods were employed on the same fiber during the same contraction, records were generally superimposable [17].

The above-mentioned study contained systematic controls for possible artifact: To check for translation-induced artifact, we translated the fiber bodily along each of three orthogonal axes. Induced fluctuations were just above the noise floor, and could not have given rise to artifactual steps. Possible distortions of the hair image waveform were considered quantitatively, and were ruled out as an alternative source of steps. Thus, segment length steps appear genuine.

18

Segment steps have been confirmed in two other laboratories. Housmans [8] plunged microelectrode tips into the belly of a papillary muscle, and used an optical scanner to follow intermarker spacing. Although some records showed smooth shortening, many showed shortening with 'hesitations' interposed between steps. Stepwise behavior was particularly evident when the load was kept modest. The stepping pattern was repeatable from contraction to contraction.

In a more detailed study, Tameyasu [19] used a high-speed video system to follow shortening in single isolated frog heart cells. Segments were demarcated by natural markers such as glycogen granules. Stepwise shortening was found regularly. The number of detectable steps was limited, as the records became progressively less distinct with shortening. Nevertheless, the step pattern was repeatable from contraction to contraction, as well as from preparation to preparation. Pause durations were found to be decreased by catecholamines, possibly explaining their positive inotropic action.

In summary, though each of the three independent optical methods used to measure stepwise shortening has been the target of criticism, a fourth method, not based on the optical properties of the striations, gives the same result. This segment-length method has also been used in several other laboratories, and the presence of steps has been confirmed in each.

Muscle length steps

Recently, a fifth approach has been initiated. When a single fiber under tetanic isometric stimulation is suddenly clamped to a load slightly less than isometric, the muscle shortens, but not smoothly. Several groups have shown that the velocity undergoes one or more 'isotonic velocity transients' [20, 21, 22]. Examples of such transients are shown in Figs. 2-2 and 2-3. In Figure 2-3, multiple transients can be seen.

A.F. Huxley has suggested more than once [21, 1] that these isotonic transients might be related to stepwise shortening. In our preliminary investigations of this questions, we compared the global shortening pattern measured by a standard servomotor position sensor with the local shortening pattern measured by optical diffraction. The question was whether the transient reductions of muscle shortening velocity might correspond to sarcomere length pauses.

Preliminary results are shown in Fig. 2-4. The initial muscle shortening transient clearly shows up in the sarcomere shortening trace. Provided the muscle length transient was distinct, in no case was it absent from the sarcomere length record. All regions along the fiber showed this pause.

Less frequently, additional muscle length transients followed the first; generally they damped out after several oscillations, When additional transients were found in the muscle length signal, they inevitably appeared in the sarcomere length signal as well (Fig. 2–5). On the other hand, the sarcomere length signal

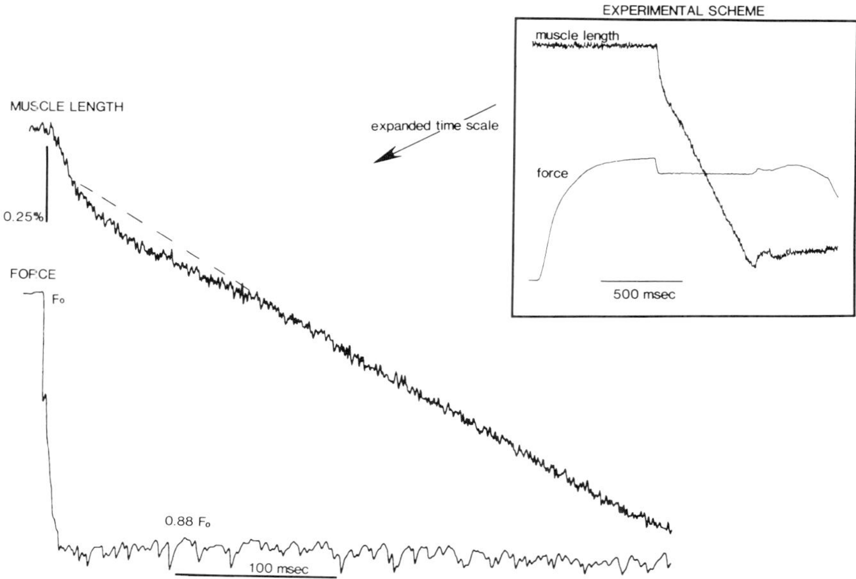

Figure 2-2. Isotonic velocity transient. Inset shows the experimental scheme. Tetanically stimulated single fiber is clamped to a new load. Muscle shortening velocity does not settle immediately to its final value. It first undergoes a transient, shown more clearly on the expanded scale, below. Experiment 1/7/86; semitendinosus fiber; resting sarcomere length – 2.65 μm; temperature 0.8° C.

sometimes showed additional pauses and steps that were not reflected in the muscle length signal.

We tentatively conclude that the 'isotonic velocity transients' are indeed manifestations of stepwise shortening; that the quick release perturbation is sufficiently strong to synchronize stepping along much of the length of the fiber, though synchrony may fade progressively with time – or on occasion it may not (Figs. 2-3 and 2-5). Considering the known inhomogeneities along the length of a fiber [23], progressive loss of synchrony over so long a span is to be expected. Indeed, it is impressive that the steps in muscle length remain as clear as they do.

The finding that sarcomere length steps are manifested in the muscle length signal confirms the prediction of A.F. Huxley. Further it provides yet another method – a fifth – by which the presence of stepwise shortening has been confirmed.

While the presence of unsuspected artifact can never be fully dismissed in any method, the consistency among methods (and among laboratories) implies that if some common artifact is lurking, it must be an insidiously subtle one. Though the criticisms have been substantial, ten years of consistent results with diverse methods convinces us that the answer to question (i) is likely to be – yes.

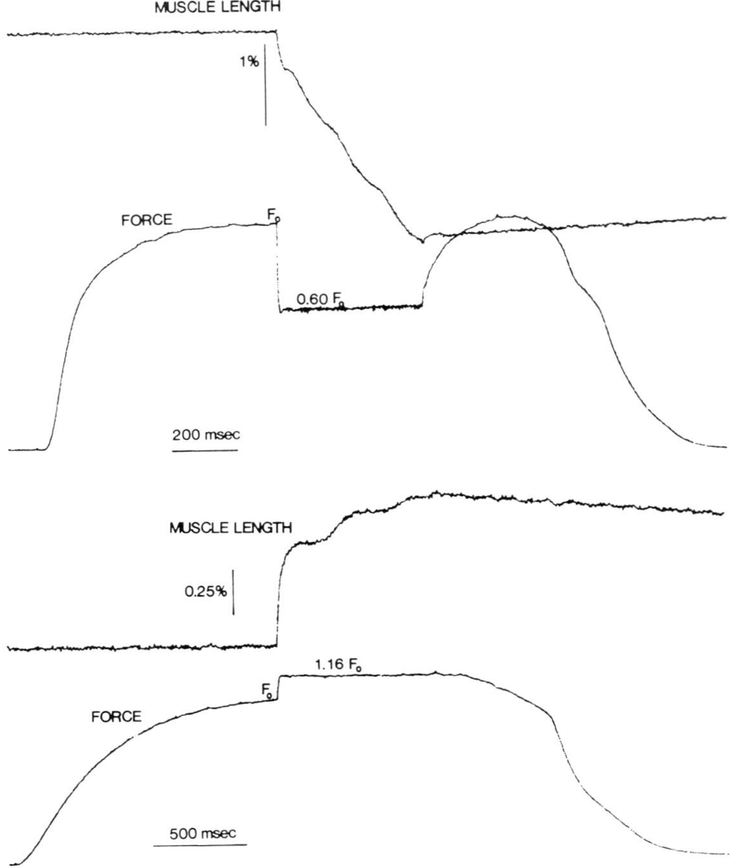

Figure 2-3. Load-clamp experiments in which more than one transient was observed. Top: Experiment 1/3/86; semitendinosus single fiber; resting sarcomere length – 2.35 μm; temperature 1.5° C. Bottom: Load clamp above isometric. Experiment 1/7/86; semitendinosus fiber; resting sarcomere length – 2.5 μm; temperature 2.3° C.

Are steps related to contraction?

To answer Huxley's question (ii), it is necessary to know both the source of the steps and the nature of the contractile mechanism. Thus, we need to consider each of these issues before we can conclude whether or not the steps are extraneous to contraction.

As for the contractile mechanism, the sliding filament/cross-bridge theory has been around for more than three decades. Although literally hundreds of alternative mechanisms have been proposed in the modern era, most investigators consider the essentials of the theory to be adequate. Thus, one may begin by

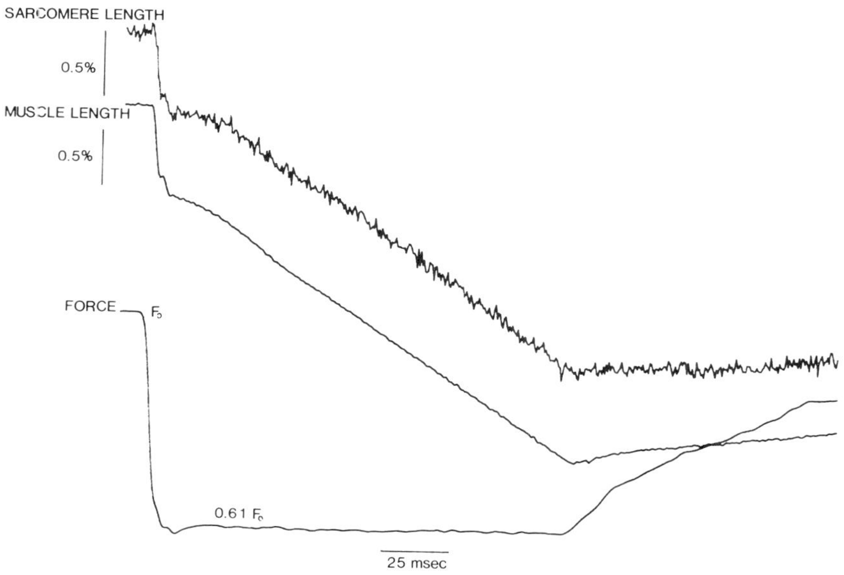

Figure 2-4. Load-clamp experiment with simultaneous muscle length and sarcomere length measurements. The low velocity phase of the muscle length transient shows up as a pause in sarcomere length. Experiment 12/30/85; semitendinosus fiber; sarcomere length just before clamp 2.71 μm; temperature 3.9° C.

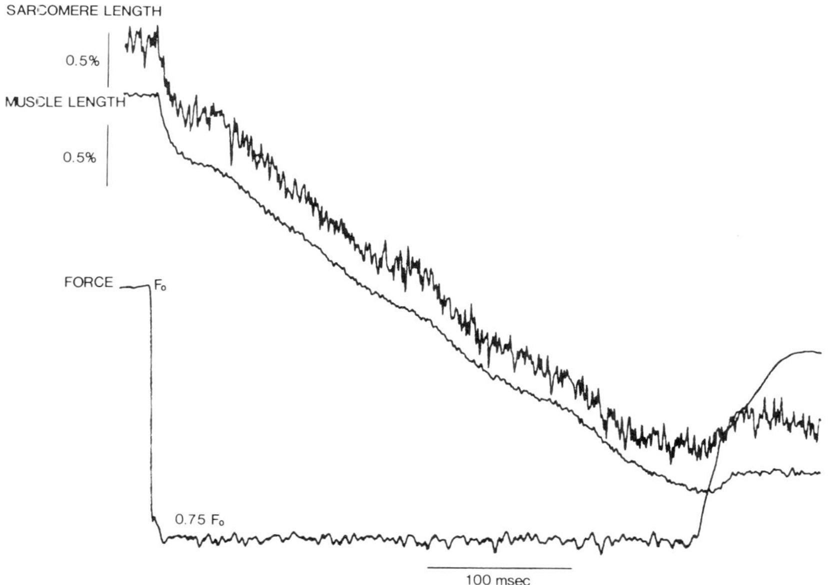

Figure 2-5. Load-clamp experiment with simultaneous muscle length and sarcomere length measurement. Three muscle length transients can be seen. The low velocity phases of muscle shortening show up as pauses or periods of reduced velocity on the sarcomere length trace. Experiment 1/7/86; tibialis anterior single fiber; sarcomere length just before clamp 2.15 μm; temperature 1.8° C.

22

assuming the theory to be correct, and work toward uncovering the stepping mechanism on that basis. Alternatively, one may ignore the theory and begin afresh. In this latter approach, the steps themselves are potentially useful in devising the theory; whether primary or secondary, their presence needs to be explained.

We choose this latter course. The reasons why the presently accepted theory may be inadequate are detailed in a comprehensive review [24]; the arguments cannot be done justice in the space allotted here. Briefly, the concerns include: whether thick filaments shorten; how the history-dependence of contraction can be accounted for; why the shape of the length-tension relation often differs from the 'classical' result; how to reconcile the absence of bridge rotation implied by recent probe results; and some half dozen other basic issues.

We therefore approach question (ii) backwards. We begin by considering the source of the steps. We then use the constraints imposed by the presence of steps to help deduce a more satisfactory contraction model. At that stage we may consider whether or not the steps are intimately tied to the contractile mechanism or are only peripherally related. By preview, both may be accurate.

Source of steps

Two clues help narrow the potential mechanisms [14]:
(1) Activation is not required. Relaxed fibers that are stretched or released by a servomotor show stepwise shortening. This implies that actomyosin interaction is probably not required to generate the steps.
(2) Steps remain in presence when fibers extended beyond thick-thin overlap are stretched or released. This confirms that actomyosin interaction is not required.

These two clues could be taken as immediate evidence that steps are unrelated to contraction (A.F. Huxley's point (ii), above). However, this conclusion is premature. The fact that steps can be observed in the absence of actomyosin interaction does not necessarily imply that actomyosin interaction, when it occurs during active contraction, does not also occur in steps. Judgment needs to be reserved.

The above-mentioned clues, on the other hand, lead directly to a proposal for step generation in unstimulated fibers. When to fiber is stretched beyond overlap, continuity between Z-lines is not lost. It is retained through a set of filaments that interconnect each end of the thick filament with the nearest Z-line. When the fiber is stretched, these 'connecting filaments' are likewise stretched. Probably these filaments support much of the resting tension [25].

Connecting filaments are not well-known, though they are now well-studied and apparently uncontroversial. Initially, they were identified in insect flight muscle [26], with direct evidence for their existence coming later from [27]. In vertebrate muscle, connecting filaments were identified by Huxley and Peachey

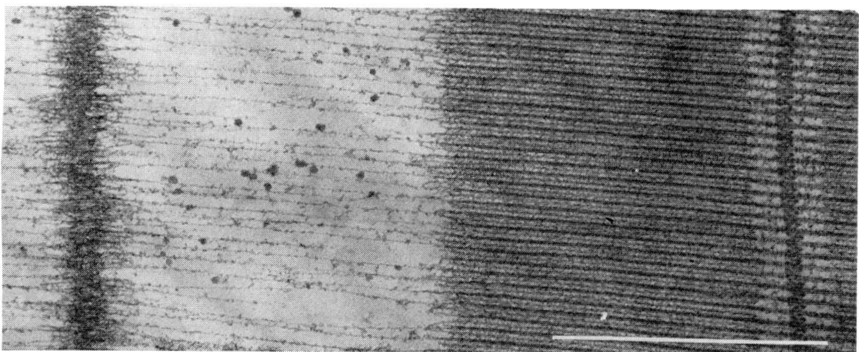

Figure 2-6. Honeybee flight muscle stretched in rigor. Stretch tore thin filaments from their anchor points on the Z-line; the length change was therefore conferred only on the connecting filaments. The latter are clearly seen on the left side of the micrograph, interconnecting the thick filaments (right) with the Z-line (far left). Scale bar – 1 μm.

[23], confirmed by Sjostrand [28] and by Carlsen et al. [29], examined for structural detail by Locker and Leet [30], and characterized biochemically in a series of experiments from the laboratories of K. Maruyama and K. Wang [31].

An example in which connecting filaments can be seen particularly well is shown in Fig. 2-6. This was prepared from insect flight muscle. The specimen was placed in rigor, then stretched. As shown previously [32, 33], this procedure tears the thin filaments from their anchor points at the Z-line; thin filaments remain bound to the bridges. Connecting filaments are extended by the stretch.

Since thick and thin filament lengths remain constant in unactivated fibers, imposed length changes must be fully conferred on the connecting filament; this is an inescapable feature of the structural arrangement. If sarcomere length changes occur stepwise, the connecting filament must change length in steps. In unactivated fibers, then, the source of the steps likely resides in the connecting filaments.

An entirely different possibility is that the source of the steps lies somewhere outside the myofibril – e.g. in the membrane, sarcoplasmic reticulum, T-tubules, etc. However, we have been able to detect step-like shortening patterns in small myofibrillar preparations [34], where such structures are presumably disrupted. Thus, the responsible element probably lies within the myofibril. This is not surprising, for nowhere else can one find the structural regularity that must be necessary to synchronize the steps over vast regions of space.

The inference that connecting filaments change length stepwise is consistent with their structure. Isolated connecting filament proteins are thread-like, but often contain isolated nodules distributed along their length, where the filament appears to have gathered up [35, 36]. These knot-like nodules may represent discrete, localized regions of shortening.

Occam's razor would have it that connecting filaments were the unique source of steps; but the data, alas, do not support this pleasingly simple explanation. Stepwise shortening can be detected at sarcomere length well below those at which resting tension is present [37], where connecting filaments are presumably slack. Under these conditions, another element is probably responsible for the steps.

Thick filament shortening

Logically, the second source of steps ought to be mechanistically similar to the first. Or, it might not. For example, one may propose connecting-filament shortening for the unactivated fiber and, say, cross-bridge cycling for the activated. But this would posit mechanisms that are fundamentally different, and one may question whether steps of similar character might reasonably arise out of mechanisms so fundamentally different.

A more likely possibility for the activated fiber is stepwise shortening of another of the sarcomere's filaments; this would preserve the same class of mechanism in both situations. The thin filament is unlikely, for may studies have confirmed the constancy of thin-filament length under a broad spectrum of conditions. This leaves the thick filament. Could a thick-filament shortening mechanism be responsible?

Figure 2-7 shows the sarcome structure obtained by freezefracture. Structures revealed by this method are based on their physical presence, not on a pattern of chemical staining. Thus, the thick filament does not terminate; it interconnects with a (connecting) filament of slightly smaller diameter, which, together with the thin filaments, forms a crowded I-band. The main point of this Figure (and Fig. 2-6) is that apart from thin filaments, the sarcomere may be thought of as having

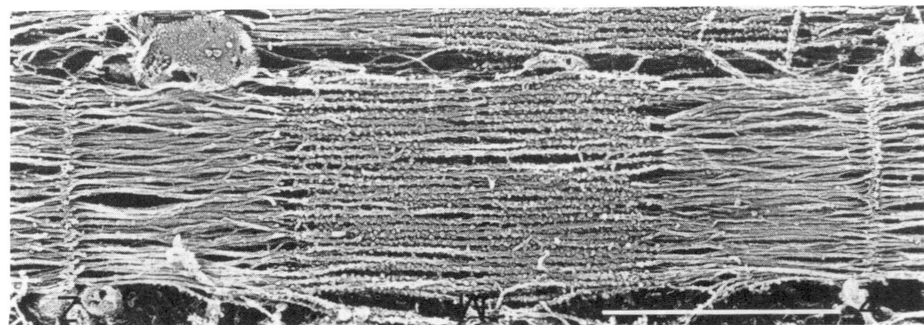

Figure 2-7. Freeze-fracture image of relaxed frog semitendinosus muscle, stretched beyond thick/thin filament overlap (from Suzuki and Pollack, 1986). The gap between the tips of thin filaments and ends of thick filaments is spanned by connecting filaments, which run from thick filaments to Z-lines. Scale bar – 1 μm.

one continuous filament running from Z-line to Z-line. The central region of this continuous filament is thicker and more robust than flanking elements. But the essential point is that it is continuous.

From such a perspective, the proposition that stepwise shortening of activated fibers arises from thick filament shortening is not at all preposterous – provided the data support such a contention. The division of labor would then be simple: connecting filaments in the absence of activation; thick filaments during activation. The mechanism derives from two regions of a single filament. Occam's razor is not seriously blunted.

Do thick filaments really shorten?

The suggestion that thick filaments shorten in steps, or for that matter shorten at all, is obviously at odds with accepted views. However, the classical observations of Huxley and Hanson [38] and Huxley and Niedergerke [39] that showed constancy of A-band width have not been broadly confirmed. On the contrary, a surprisingly large number of papers published since the midfifties have reported A-band shortening or thick-filament shortening of substantial magnitude [24]. These include cardiac as well as skeletal muscle.

In this laboratory, a number of studies have been launched to pursue this question. Preliminary results are shown below. We have approached the question using both optical microscopy and electron microscopy.

In the first study, single fibers of frog tibialis anterior muscle were stimulated to contract tetanically. During tetanus, the fibers were allowed to shorten slowly. Typically, fibers shortened from $3\,\mu$m sarcomere length to $2\,\mu$m in two to three seconds. Because of this low velocity, active tension remained high during shortening, so the muscle performed substantial work.

Figure 2-8a shows a representative result. Since polarization microscopy was used, A-bands are light, I-bands dark. We found that A-bands and I-bands both shortened during active contraction. We have detected A-band shortening to well below $1.0\,\mu$m. As a control, we measured the changes of band pattern occurring during shortening of the unstimulated fiber. Figure 2-8b shows that length changes were restricted largely to the I-band, as expected. Thus, A and I bands could not have been confused.

Although these studies have not yet been completed, several novel features which improve the reliability of the result should be mentioned. First, lenses with highest available numerical aperture have been used, thereby optimizing the resolution. Second, a flash-lamp with pulse duration on the order of 25 microseconds virtually eliminates any blurring arising out of fiber translation. Finally, image processing algorithms are being applied; these can enhance image quality and allow more systematic and objective identification of A/I boundaries.

A-band shortening has also been noted electron microscopically, though a

26

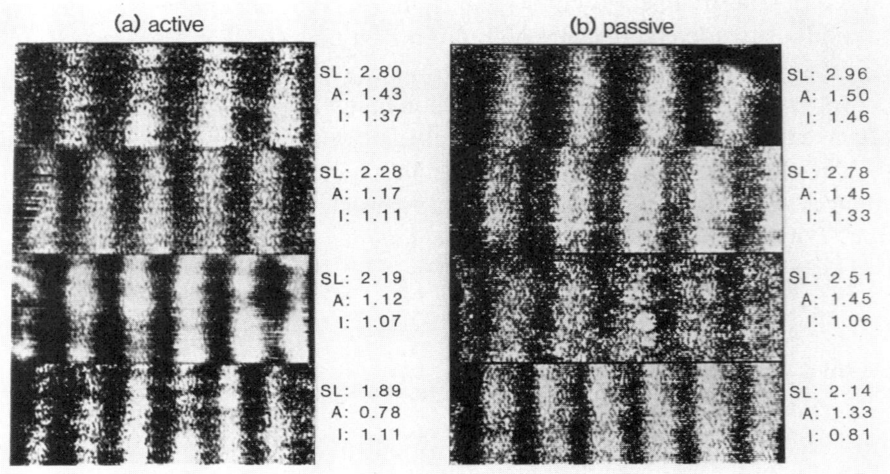

Figure 2-8. Polarization microscopic images of frog tibialis anterior muscle. A-bands light; I-bands dark. Fibers were pre-stretched, then shortened with a servomotor. (a) In stimulated fibers, sarcomere shortening was associated with both A- and I-band shortening. (b) In unstimulated fibers, most shortening was confined to the I-band. Panels show representative images, each taken from a different fiber.

systematic series of experiments has not yet been undertaken. Figure 2-9, for example, shows a specimen of dog cardiac muscle fixed during an hypoxic episode. A region just outside this field has shortened extremely and irreversibly. Sarcomeres in the field are on the borderline between damaged and surviving regions. Note that these sarcomeres are of variable length, some near normal, others short. The shortened sarcomeres contain short thick filaments. Although the sarcomeres under observation cannot by any stretch of the imagination be considered 'physiological', the micrograph clearly demonstrates that the thick filament possesses the capacity to shorten.

Another example is shown in Fig. 2-10. This insect flight muscle specimen was fixed during the induction of rigor. In sarcomeres that retained their normal length, thick filament length also remained normal; shorter sarcomes contained shorter thick filaments. The images shown were taken from the same section, eliminating many potential artifacts. Apparently, during the induction of rigor, as ATP is withdrawn and tension is built up, sarcomeres can shorten. This shortening seems to be associated with thick filament shortening. Note that the crossbridges are spaced more closely in the shortened thick filaments than in the unshortened ones. This implies that a molecular rearrangement may drive thick filament shortening.

Figure 2-11 shows an example of thick filament shortening in frog skeletal muscle. Fibers were activated by brief glycerination at low temperature, which

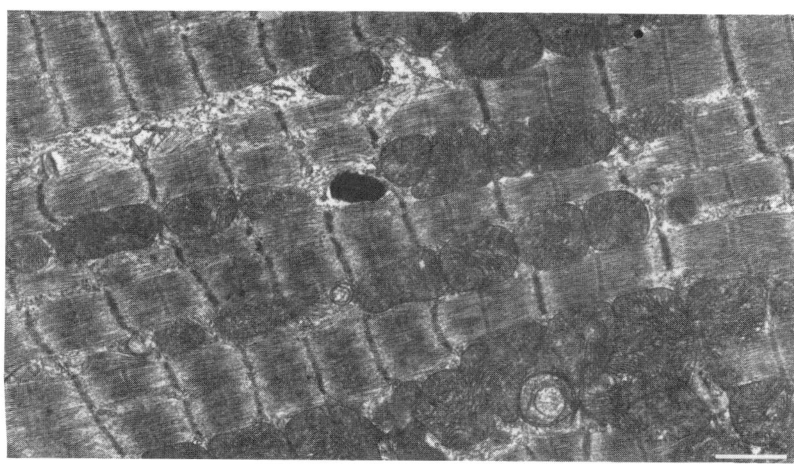

Figure 2-9. Dog cardiac muscle subjected to acute hypoxia. (K. Trombitas, E. Roth and B. Torok, unpublished). Both normal and shortened sarcomeres are observed in the field. In shortened sarcomeres, thick filaments are correspondingly shorter. Scale bar – 1 μm.

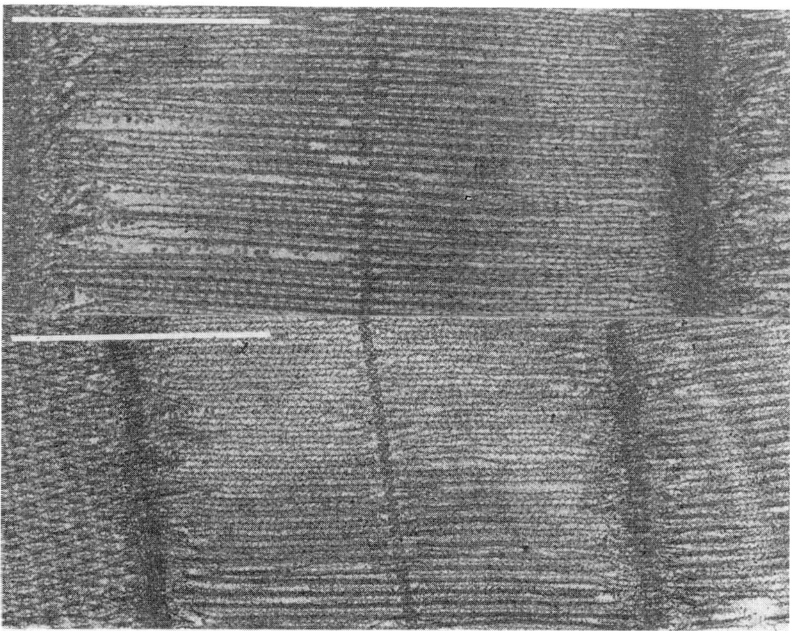

Figure 2-10. Honeybee flight muscle in rigor. Section is extremely thin, grazing thick filaments in some areas. This specimen tore during the induction of rigor, allowing shortening in some regions. Representative regions are shown. Sarcomeres that shortened during the induction of rigor had shorter thick filaments, as is apparent. Scale bar – 1 μm.

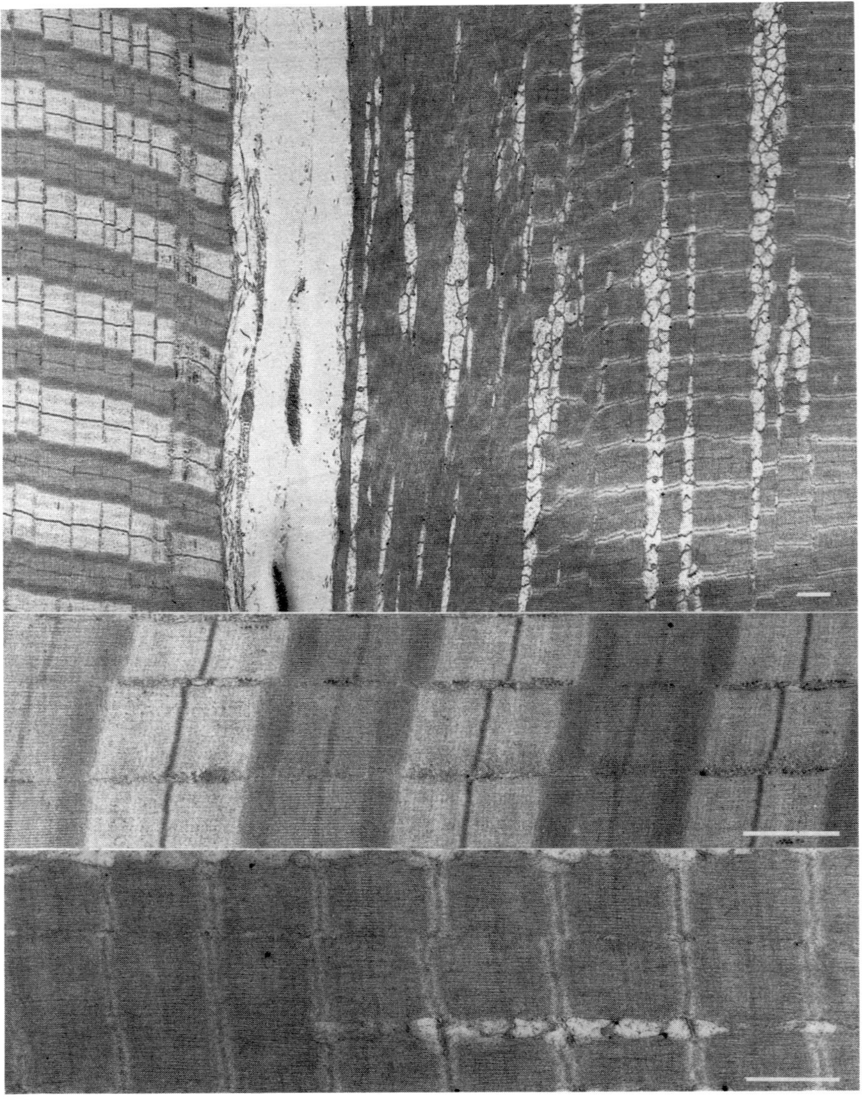

Figure 2-11. Unloaded frog sartorius muscle activated by brief immersion in cold glycerol solution, then stretched. Top panel shows unshortened and shortened sarcomeres in neighboring fibers, implying that activation was localized. Higher magnification of unshortened and shortened regions (below) shows substantial thick filament shortening in the shortened sarcomeres. Magnification of two lower panels is identical. Scale bars 1 μm.

caused immediate local activation and shortening. Sarcomeres of normal length contained thick filaments of normal length, while shortened sarcomeres contained shortened thick filaments. In the example shown, thick filaments shortened to 1.1 μm, and where A-band periodicity could be detected, it, too, had diminished by some 30–40%.

Like others, we too have found examples of sarcomere shortening with little or no thick filament shortening, in contrast to the examples shown above. We are entertaining the possibility that regions of suprathreshold activation shorten primarily by A-band shortening, while those of subthreshold activation shorten by I-band (connecting filament) shortening.

A possibility to consider is that shortening of the thick filament occurs in steps; that in activated muscle, stepwise shortening of the thick filament mediates stepwise shortening of the sarcomere. This mechanism would be parallel to that in connecting filaments – the one we surmised might apply in unstimulated muscle.

Since X-ray diffraction patterns preclude uniform shrinkage of the filament, the remaining possibility is that the thick filament shortens molecule by molecule; in steps. A detailed description of such a mechanism will be described in a forthcoming book (Pollack, in preparation). Meanwhile, it is relevant to ask whether the thick filament structure lends itself to such a possibility.

Figure 2-12 shows a molecular model of the vertebrate thick filament. This model does not follow along accepted lines; however, many features of the model appear consistent with electron micrographic images. The most obvious feature is that the filament comprises three sub-filaments [40]. In the figure, the sub-filaments are drawn splayed to emphasize the three-stranded underlying structure.

Within each sub-filament, molecules can pack at intervals of 14.3 nm or 43 nm [41]. The first produces a filament with far too many projected bridges. The second produces two possible filament structures: In one, heads of each molecule subtend an angle of 60 degrees; in the other, 180 degrees. The latter one is shown, as it appears more consistent with published micrographs. Note that the S-2 arm is buried within the filament. Except for the fact that each pair of projected heads stems from one myosin rod, not two, this model is basically similar to the one originally described by Huxley and Brown [42].

In this model, rods are packed more or less parallel to the filament axis; the helical twist is most gentle, even though the helical track followed by head origins is steeper (pitch 2 × 43 nm). Thus, shortening of a single rod – e.g. by a helix-coil transition – would cause neighboring rods to slide by the shortening molecule, diminishing the filament length by a step [43]. This could not happen if the rods twisted steeply around one another.

The implication of this model is that active shortening is mediated by thick filament shortening – segment by segment. As the number of shortened segments increases, the degree of sarcomere shortening increases. In the case of unstimul-

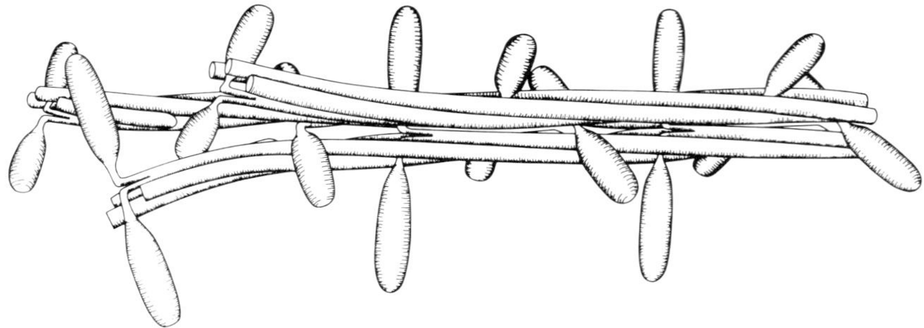

Figure 2-12. Proposed model of vertebrate thick filament structure. For clarity, filament is shown splayed. Essence of model is that the filament is built of three sub-filaments; that heads of each molecule project at 180° C from one another; and that rods twist gently.

ated fibers, or insufficiently activated myofibrils in stimulated fibers, shortening would occur in the connecting filament instead of the thick filament. Thus, the dual mechanism. A more detailed discussion of this preliminary model will appear in the forthcoming book mentioned above.

One final aspect of stepwise shortening that has not been touched on so far is the issue of synchrony. How may one account for the vast synchrony implied by this phenomenon?

Synchronization of steps and pauses

The chief element underlying synchrony may be the cross-bridge – though not as generally conceived. The textbook view of cross-bridge structure has it that the bridge consists of a long (S-2) arm angled slightly from the filament axis, connected to two globular (S-1) heads. 'Hinges' at either end of the arm allow the bridge to swing as necessary to complete its stroke. Some micrographs of negatively stained, isolated thick filaments give credence to the two-hinged structure.

On the other hand, electron micrographs of the intact lattice do not support so complicated a structure. In early micrographs, bridges were identified as simple, rod-like structure projecting approximately normally from the filament axis [44]. More recent electron micrographs of living (non-rigor) specimens have consistently supported this simple structure; a casual flip through one's file of reprints on muscle structure will confirm it.

Several years ago we noted that in the non-overlap zone, these simple, rod-like bridges appeared to project all the way from one thick filament to the next, forming rung-like interconnections [24]. These thick-thick interconnections resembled those in the M-region, except that they were localized within the cross-bridge zone.

If thick filaments were really interconnected along their length, this would

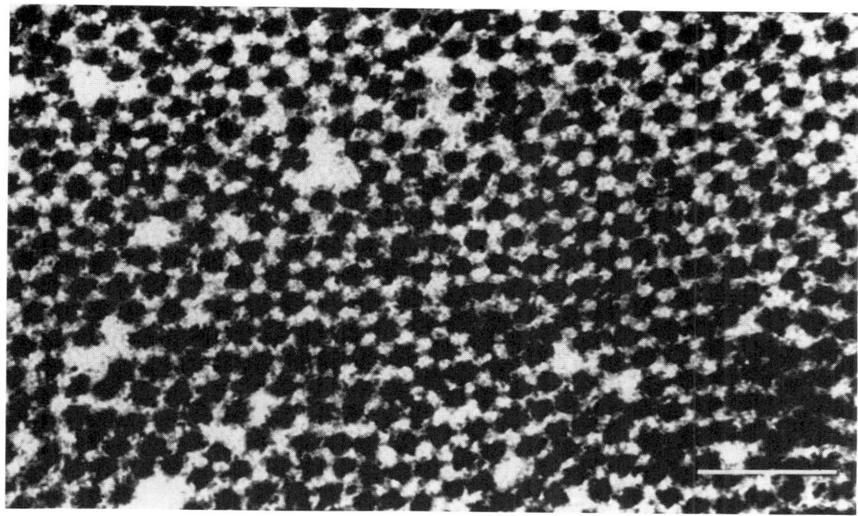

Figure 2-13. Cross-section of relaxed, stretched frog semitendinosus muscle in the non-overlap zone. Abundant interconnections between thick filaments can be seen. Scale bar – $0.1\,\mu$m.

constitute a starting point for synchrony: one segment of a thick filament could not shorten unless corresponding segments in parallel filaments shortened simultaneously. Segment shortening would be an all-or-none event throughout the cross-section of the myofibril. And given the known lateral interconnections between myofibrils, all-or-none behavior would extend throughout the width of the fiber. Thus, the basis for synchrony.

For this reason, we launched a detailed study of cross-bridge structure. We first considered the possibility that the interconnections were artifacts of chemical fixation. To test this, we employed the freeze-fracture method, where no chemical fixatives are required. The results [45] showed clear evidence of interconnections in relaxed, contracting, and rigor states. It appeared that the interconnections were formed by two cross-bridge heads binding at their tips.

Additional studies are now being carried out with diverse methods. Representative results are shown below:

Figure 2-13 shows a cross-section from the non-overlap zone of relaxed frog semitendinosus muscle (one of a serial set). Interconnections between thick filaments can be seen. These interconnections are less robust and somewhat less regular than those in the M-region. Nevertheless, they are abundant and clear. Figure 2-14 shows a freeze-fracture image prepared from honeybee flight muscle in rigor. Interconnections in the non-overlap zone can be clearly seen. No fixatives were used during preparation. Interconnections cannot be a fixation or staining artifact.

Figure 2-15 shows another freeze-fracture image, this one prepared from frog

32

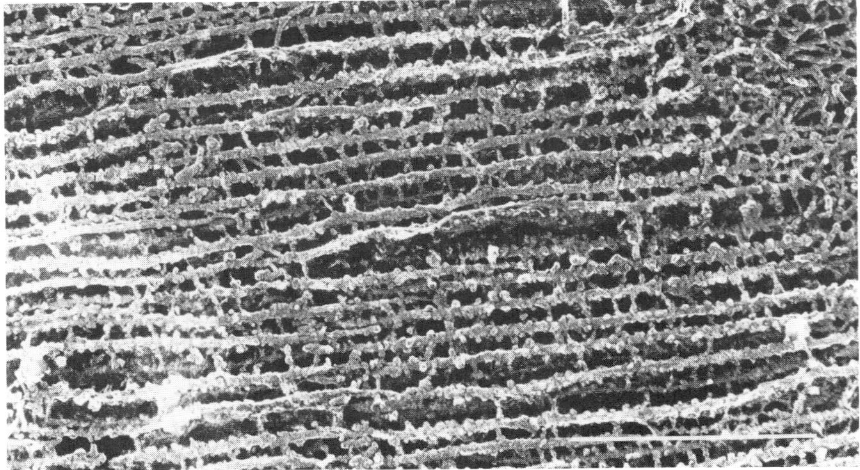

Figure 2-14. Honeybee flight muscle, prestretched to withdraw thin filaments from the A-band. The specimen was placed in rigor, released, and prepared by the freeze-fracture method. The A-band lattice is shown. Note that adjacent thick filaments are interconnected by bridge-like structures.

cardiac muscle. Again, interconnections can be seen, though not quite so clearly as in the insect preparation.

The micrographs shown in Figs. 2-13–2-15 are not unique; they are representative of images published earlier. Interconnections can be seen even in early micrographs [29]. With painstaking care and modern methodology, we have managed to preserve these structures somewhat better than has been possible in

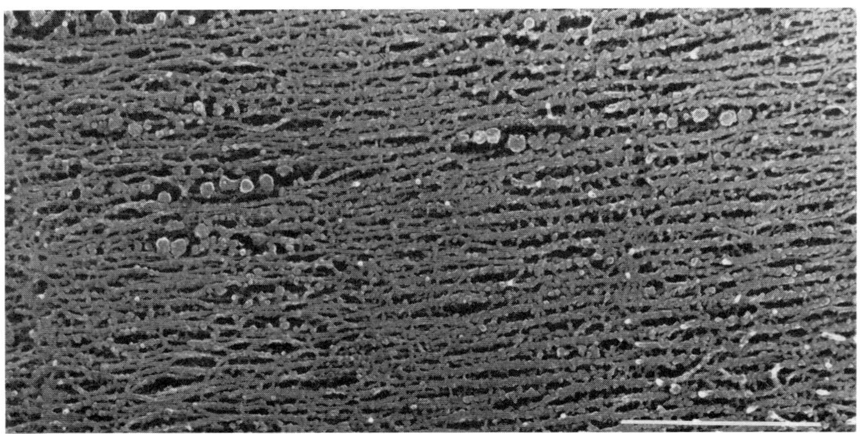

Figure 2-15. Freeze-fracture replica of relaxed, moderately stretched frog heart. Interconnections between thick filaments are discernible, but less clear than in other Figures. Scale bar – 0.5 μm.

the past. The fact that the interconnections are now clearly visible with diverse methods implies that they are not likely to be preparation artifacts, but genuine structures. As mentioned, these interconnections may constitute the basis for synchrony.

On the other hand, the existence of interconnections raises the question of whether activated bridges have the capacity to rotate: If bridges remain interconnected to apposing bridges, particularly in the overlap zone, they could experience difficulty rotating; the negative results of the probe studies might then be explained. This issue evidently bears directly on the validity of the cross-bridge theory.

Conclusion

It appears, then, that the answer to question (ii) is both yes and no. If the steps arise as proposed, they stem from both thick filament shortening and connecting filament shortening. The first is directly associated with active contraction, the second not.

Meanwhile, we have implicitly approached question (iii) – implications for the validity of the cross-bridge theory. We found that the most plausible hypothesis for active stepwise shortening was thick filament shortening. It is of course possible that thick filament shortening could occur above and beyond cross-bridge cycling, but such a mechanism would seem unnecessarily complex. Why not thick filament shortening alone? Especially in light of the large number of observations in conflict with the swinging cross-bridge theory [24].

Although the cross-bridge theory is nominally accepted, many in the field quietly (some not so quietly!) question its validity. It is certainly the dissatisfaction with this theory that has prompted the emergence of the very many alternative theories that have appeared. The late Graham Hoyle, in his recent book, describes 'Why muscle scientists lose knowledge'. In the context of the work presented here, his views are probably worth pondering [46].

References

1. Huxley A.F.: Comments on Quantal mechanisms in cardiac contraction. Circ. Res. 59: 9–14, 1986.
2. Pollack G.H.: Quantal mechanisms in cardiac contraction. Circ. Res. 59: 1–8, 1986.
3. Krueger J.W., Pollack G.H.: Myocardial sarcomere dynamics during isometric contraction. J. Physiol. (London) 251: 627–643, 1975.
4. Ranvier L.: Du spectre produit par les muscles stries. Arch. Physiol: 274–281, 1874.
5. Rudel R., Zite-Ferenczy R.: Interpretation of light diffraction by cross-striated muscle as Bragg reflexion of light by the lattice of contractile proteins. J. Physiol. (London) 29: 509–522, 1979.
6. Goldman Y.E., Simmons R.M.: Control of sarcomere length in skinned muscle fibres of Rana Temporaria during mechanical transients. J. Physiol. 350: 496–518, 1984.

34

7. Sundell C.L., Goldman Y.E., Peachey L.D.: Fine structure in near-field and far-field laser diffraction pattern from skeletal muscle fibers. Biophys. J. 49: 521–530, 1986.

8. Pollack G.H., Iwazumi T., ter Keurs H.E.D.J., Shibata E.F.: Sarcomere shortening in striated muscle occurs in stepwise fashion. Nature 268: 757–759, 1977.

9. Pollack G.H., Vassallo D.V., Jacobson R.C., Iwazumi T., Delay M.J.: Discrete nature of sarcomere shortening in striated muscle. In: Cross-bridge Mechanism in Muscle Contraction, eds., H. Sugi and G.H. Pollack. University of Tokyo Press, Tokyo, 1979, pp. 23–40.

10. Huxley H.E.: The double array of filaments in cross-striated muscle. J. Biophys. Biochem. Cytol.: 631–646, 1957.

11. Huxley H.E.: The mechanism of muscular contraction. Science 164: 1356–1366, 1969.

12. Delay M.J., Ishide N., Jacobson R.C., Pollack G.H., Tirosh R.: Stepwise sarcomere shortening: Analysis by high-speed cinemicrography. Science 213: 1523–1525, 1981.

13. Jacobson R.C., Tirosh R., Delay M.J., Pollack G.H.: Quantitized nature of sarcomere shortening steps. J. Muscle Res. and Cell Motility 4: 529–542, 1983.

14. Granzier H.L.M., Pollack G.H.: Stepwise shortening in unstimulated skeletal muscle fibers. J. Physiol. 362: 173–188, 1985.

15. Gordon A.M., Huxley A.F., Julian F.J.: Tension development in highly stretched vertebrate muscle fibers. J. Physiol. (London) 184: 143–169, 1966.

16. Edman K.A.P., Hoglund O.: A technique for measuring length changes of individual segments of an isolated muscle fiber. J. Physiol. 317: 8–9 p, 1981.

17. Granzier H.L.M., Myers J.A., Pollack G.H.: Stepwise shortening of muscle fiber segments. Submitted for publication.

18. Housmans P.: Discussion, in: Contractile Mechanisms in Muscle. Ed., G.H. Pollack and H. Sugi. Plenum Press, N.Y., pp. 782–784, 1984.

19. Tameyasu T., Toyoki T., Sugi H.: Nonsteady motion in unloaded contractions of single frog cardiac cells. Biophys. J. 48: 461–465, 1985.

20. Civan M.M., Podolsky R.J.: Contraction kinetics of striated muscle fibers following quick changes in load. J. Physiol. 184: 511–534, 1966.

21. Armstrong C.M., Huxley A.F., Julian F.J.: Oscillatory responses in frog skeletal muscle fibres. J. Physiol. (London) 186: 26–27P, 1966.

22. Sugi H., Tuschiya T.: Isotonic velocity transients in frog muscle fibres following quick changes in load. J. Physiol. 319: 219–238, 1981.

23. Huxley A.F., Peachey L.D.: The maximum length for contraction in vertebrate striated muscle. J. Physiol. 156: 150–165, 1961.

24. Pollack G.H.: The sliding filament/cross-bridge theory: a critical review. Physiol. Reviews 63: 1049–1113, 1983.

25. Magid A., Ting-Beall H.P., Carvell M., Kontis T., Lucaveche C.: Connecting filaments, core filaments, and side-struts: a proposal to add three new load-bearing structures to the sliding filament model. In: Contractile Mechanisms in Muscle. Ed., G.H. Pollack and H. Sugi. Plenum Press. N.Y., 1984, pp. 307–328.

26. Auber J., Couteaux R.: L'attache des myofilaments secondaires au niveau de la strie Z dans les muscles des Dipteres. C.R. Acad. Sci. 254: 3425–3443, 1962.

27. Trombitas K., Tigyi-Sebes A.: Direct evidence for connecting filaments in flight muscle of honeybee. Acta Biochim. Biophys. Hung. 9: 243–253, 1974.

28. Sjostrand F.S.: The connections between A- and I-band filaments in striated frog muscle. J. Ultrast. Res. 7: 225–246, 1962.

29. Carlsen F., Fuchs F., Knappeis G.G.: Contractility and ultrastructure in glycerol-extracted muscle fibers. J. Cell Biol. 7: 225–246, 1965.

30. Locker R.H., Leet N.G.: Histology of highly stretched beef muscle. 11. Further evidence on the location and nature of gap filaments. J. Ultrast. Res. 55: 157–172, 1976.

31. Locker R.H.: The role of gap filaments in muscle and meat. Food Microstructure 3: 17–32, 1984.

32. Trombitas K., Tigyi-Sebes A.: Fine structure and mechanical properties of insect muscle. In:

Insect Flight Muscle, ed. R.T. Tregear, Elsevier/North Holland, Amsterdam, 1977, pp. 79–90.

33. White D.C.S.: Structural and mechanical properties of insect fibrillar flight muscle in the relaxed and rigor states. D.Phil. thesis, Oxford University, 1967.

34. Pollack G.H., Tirosh R., Brozovich F.V., Lacktis J.W., Jacobson R.C., Tameyasu T.: Stepwise shortening: evidence and implications. In: Contractile Mechanisms in Muscle. eds., G.H. Pollack and H. Sugi. Plenum Press. N.Y., pp. 765–786, 1984.

35. Trinick J., Knight P., Whiting A.: Purification and properties of native titin. J. Mol. Biol. 180: 331–356, 1984.

36. Wang K., Ramirez-Mitchell R., Palter D.: Titin is an extraordinarily long, flexible, and slender myofibrillar protein. Proc. Natl. Acad. Sci. (USA) 81: 3685–3689, 1984.

37. Vassallo D.V., Pollack G.H.: The force-velocity relation and stepwise sarcomere shortening in cardiac muscle. Circulation Research 51 (1): 37–42, 1982.

38. Huxley H.E., Hanson J.: Changes in the cross-striations of muscle during contraction and stretch and their structural interpretation. Nature 173: 973–976, 1954.

39. Huxley A.F., Niedergerke R.: Structural changes in muscle during contraction. Interference microscopy of living muscle fibres. Nature 173: 971–973, 1954.

40. Maw M.C., Rowe A.J.: Fraying of A-Filaments into three subfilaments. Nature 286: 412–414, 1980.

41. McLachlan A.D., Karn J.: Periodic charge distributions in the myosin rod amino acid sequence match cross-bridge spacings in muscle. Nature 299: 226–231, 1982.

42. Huxley H.E., Brown W.: The low-angle x-ray diagram of vertebrate striated muscle and its behavior during contraction and rigor. J. Mol. Biol. 30: 383–434, 1967.

43. Pollack G.H.: A proposed mechanism of contraction in which stepwise shortening is a basic feature. In: Contractile Mechanisms in Muscle. Plenum Press N.Y., 1984, pp. 787–792.

44. Huxley A.F.: Muscle structure and theories of contraction. Prog. Biophys. Chem. 7: 255–318, 1957.

45. Hoyle G.: Muscles and Their Neural Control. Wiley, N.Y., 1983.

3. Mechanics of the myofibril

TATSUO IWAZUMI

Introduction

In nearly every field of science deeper understanding of nature led to investigations into ever smaller features of the object, from macroscopic to microscopic to molecular to atomic to nuclear. At each step change of size we have made a quantum jump in our knowledge about the object. In the field of muscle mechanics, investigations started from whole muscle tissue but soon moved into single fiber level then to single cell level. Single cell mechanics have not been well developed yet at this moment because of many technical difficulties involved, but I decided a few years ago to leap-frog the single cell level and directly move to single myofibril level where only 10 sarcomeres or so would be dealt with. It is my aim in this chapter to give a preliminary account of observations that have not been made in macroscopic studies of muscle mechanics and to discuss their consequences for our concepts of muscle contraction.

Methods: instrumentation

Two essential requirements for the study of single myofibril mechanics are to measure forces in nanograms (10 pN) and to control the myofibrillar length in nanometers, both on a time scale of microseconds. To satisfy these requirements special tranducers were developed. The details were described elsewhere [1] and only the principle of operation is briefly explained below.

Figure 3-1 shows a perspective view of the force transducer and length control activator. They are functionally different but the shapes and working priciples are identical and their roles are interchangeable. Each transducer is made of a very fine insulated copper wire (12 μm dia) formed into U-shape (1 mm wide and 1.5 mm high) and welded to platinum posts. A myofibril is attached at the bottom with silicone glue at right angles with respect to both wires. The assembly is immersed in a solution filled chamber and magnetic field (B) is applied in vertical

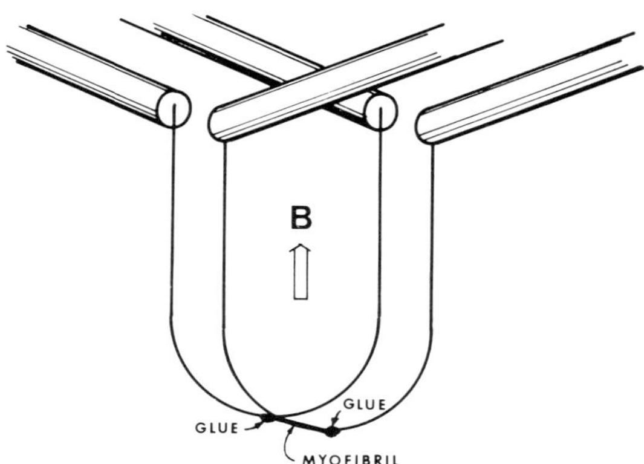

Figure 3-1. Perspective view of force and length control transducers. Very fine copper wire (12 μm) is formed into U-shape using a special jig and spot welded to two supporting posts. A myofibril is microdissected in a very small chamber through which relaxing solution that contains muscle extract continuously flows. A dissected single or double myofibril lying on a glass bottom of the chamber is oriented horizontally and placed in the center of the microscope field ($\times$400). A wire transducer with a very small bead of silicone glue at the bottom is introduced into the chamber and lowered on the one end of the myofibril then lightly rubbed against it so that the myofibril is completely incorporated into the body of the glue which polymerizes in water in a minute.

direction as indicated by an arrow. A halogen lamp light source is situated above the assembly and a microscope objective lens is located directly below the myofibril. The lens projects images of the two wires and the myofibril onto three separate sensors; a photo position detector for each wire and a 1024 element photodiode array for the myofibril. The position detector consists of a dual photodiode with a very narrow gap, and the dark image of the wire falls onto the gap and a portion of each photodiode. When the wire image deviates from the center (at the gap), one photodiode is exposed to more light and another less light; therefore, the difference of two photo-currents is proportional to the wire position deviation. Actually, the difference is divided by the sum of two photo-currents for normalization which eliminates the effect of light intensity variations. Servo control of the wire position is exerted by passing a current through the wire while the position signal is fed back to an error amplifier which compares the signal with the position command and drives a current amplifier. When similar servo control loop is formed for the force transducer, the current that flows through and keeps this wire in a stationary position is proportional to the force applied to the wire. The wire transducers can also be used without servo controls. In this case, the length control is performed by sending a current through the wire, and the force is measured from the deviation of the wire position from the stationary position upon application of a force. The following is a summary of the system performance.

Length Controller
Resolution	:	$0.2\,\text{Å}\sqrt{\text{Hz}}$ over 0–5 KHz bandwidth
		$20\,\text{Å}$ rms over 0–50 KHz bandwidth
Step response	:	$10\,\mu s$
Frequency response	:	50 KHz, 2 KHz without servo

Force Transducer
Resolution	:	$0.5\,\text{ng}/\sqrt{\text{Hz}}$ over 0–5 KHz bandwidth
Frequency response	:	50 KHz, 2 KHz without servo
Maximum force	:	1 mg

Preparations

Most experiments reported here were performed on the myofibrils from bullfrog atrium. This is because the bullfrog atrial cells contain only two myofibrils at their tapered ends. Other cardiac myofibrils from Rana Pipiens, toads, turtles and skeletal myofibrils from rabbits and rats have been used, but they were much harder to dissect out of large bundles.

Microdissections

Every step of the single myofibril experiment is critical and nerve racking, but the micro-dissection procedure is by far the most difficult and frustrating. Myofibrils were mechanically dissected by using super fine needles and four specially built remotely controlled micromanipulators. Homogenization is a very simple method to produce myofibrils in large number, but they all suffered damages, even if they appeared intact in optical microscopy, and showed much less tension and slow tension development compared with manually dissected good quality myofibrils. It is likely that the cause of damages is excessive stretch of sarcomeres during homogenization since the manually dissected myofibrils also behaved similarly if their sarcomeres were stretched more than 50% of the slack length. When sarcomeres were over-stretched, the optical contrast of the A-band diminished even if they were promptly returned to the normal length, suggesting misregistration of the thick filaments.

Solutions

The compositions were determined according to the procedures by Fabiato & Fabiato [2] using stability constants suggested by him [3]. The key parameters were: pMg = 2.5, pMgATP = 2.5, pH = 7.10, Imidazole = 30 mM, Creatine-phosphate (CP) = 12 mM, Creatinephosphokinase (CPK) = 15 U/ml, Total

EGTA = 10 mM, and $\mu = 0.16$. The pCA values were 9.0, 6.5, 6.0, 5.5, and 5.0. 50 M Leupeptin was added to pCA 9.0 solution. CP and CPK were most likely unnecessary because the myofibrils were so small (1–2 μm) that ATP diffusion would be unimpeded, but they were nevertheless added to allow direct comparison of the myofibril data with other skinned fiber data.

Muscle extract

Muscle extract is required to keep myofibrils viable during microdissection. Without it the myofibril gradually lost Ca^{2+} sensitivity and also developed high resting tension over a period of one hour. This phenomenon appeared to be due to soluble protein washout from the myofibril, and the relaxing solution containing the extract was essential since microdissection often took more than an hour. The extract was made as follows: I. 0.1–0.5 g muscle tissue from which a small piece has been set aside for myofibril dissection is minced by a small pair of scissors; II. Suspend the minced tissue in pCa 9.0 solution at 1 g/0.1 ml proportion; III. Homogenize gently (5000 rpm) for 30 min. at room temperature; IV. Centrifuge at 10,000 g for 10 min. at room temperature; V. Collect supernatant. Dilute it with pCa 9.0 solution 2 to 3 times. Too concentrated extract will cause slight contraction of myofibrils; VI. Filtrate with a 0.2 μm nylon filter before use.

Results

Time course of tension development

Figure 3-2 shows a time course of tension produced by a good quality double myofibril from bullfrog atrium activated by pCa 5.5 solution. Identification of single or double myofibril is easy because single myofibrils produced a maximum tension of about 50 μg. The tension rise time is a reliable indicator of the quality of the myofibril; it should be 2 seconds or less at $\mu = 0.16$. As the myofibril quality deteriorated after many contractions, the rise time became longer with a concomitant diminution of active tension, and the optical contrast of the A-band diminished. When the myofibril was damaged either during microdissection or excessive activations with high Ca^{2+} solutions, the rise time became longer than 10 seconds, sometimes more than one minute. In such damaged myofibrils, tension levels were lower than normal and deteriorated rapidly with time, and the resting tension increased after each contraction.

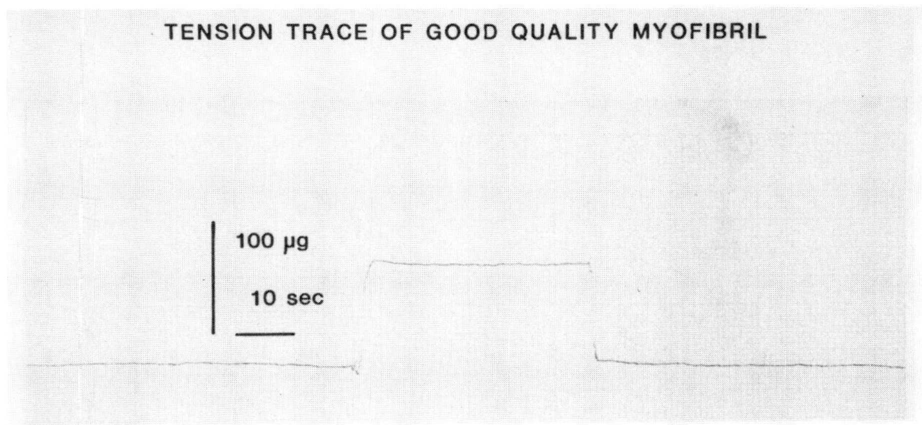

Figure 3-2. Time course of isometric tension from a good quality myofibril. Small ripples of the trace are building vibrations. The rise and fall times of active tension are not limited by Ca^{2+} diffusion time but a function of ionic strength.

Sarcomere length-tension relations

SL-tension curves were constructed for pCa values of 6.0, 5.5, and 5.0 at sarcomere lengths 2.2 (slack length), 2.55, 2.9, 3.25, and 3.6 µm Activation-relaxation cycles always began at 2.2 µm, went up to sarcomere length SL of 3.6 µm, while stretches were imposed only during the relaxed state, then came down to 2.2 µm again. This protocol was repeated or each pCa value. The tension value at each SL was taken from the average of two measurements (except at the longest SL values) to account for tension reduction due to myofibril deterioration. The result is summarized in Fig. 3. It is emphasized that increasing active tension with stretch was observed without exception in all types of good quality myofibrils tested and that the myofibrils were never stretched during contraction. The active tension dropped steeply beyond 3.6 µm, but after such activation signs of damage to the myofibril were found, such as slower tension development a skewed appearance of the sarcomeres and the A-band optical contrast diminished substantially. As mentioned in the dissection procedure above, even passive stretches beyond overlap were harmful for sarcomeres.

Activations at pCa less than 5.0 caused sarcomere skewing and distortions which became more severe at longer sarcomere lengths, and active tension deteriorated rapidly with time thus making it impossible to obtain reliable tension values at longer sarcomere lengths. Increasing active tension as a function of increasing sarcomere length is not a peculiar phenomenon only associated with myofibrils. Skinned skeletal fibers, when activated with utmost care to maintain good sarcomere uniformity, showed the same property [4] and also skinned cardiac trabeculae [5], although only up to 2.3 µm beyond which trabeculae could not be stretched.

42

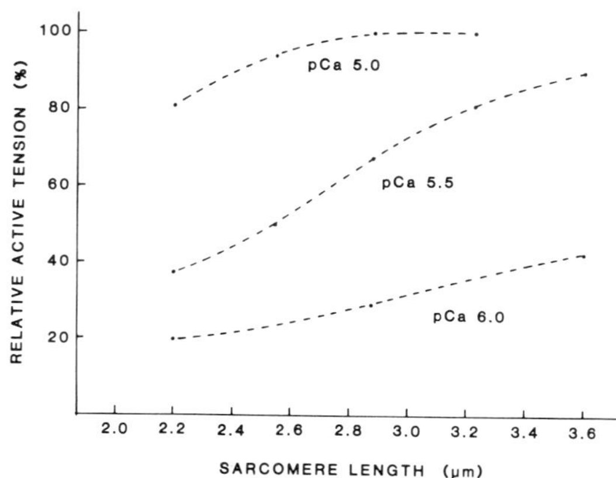

Figure 3-3. Sarcomere length vs. tension curves of a bullfrog atrium myofibril. See text for protocol explanation. No exception has been found to the increasing active tension with sarcomere length so long as the sarcomeres were regular and tension rise times were short.

Spontaneous resting tension fluctuations

When fresh muscle extract was added at too high a concentration to the pCa 9.0 solution, slight shortening of myofibrils was observed. If the frequency spectrum of the resting tension is analyzed one can clearly demonstrate that the myofibril is producing spontaneous random vibrations. The spectrum of the force fluctuations has a second order slope with roll-off frequencies which continuously shift with time from about 20 Hz in the beginning then to lower values until the vibrations die out about an hour later. The maximum noise power in the beginning is about $0.1\,\mu g$ rms. That this disappearance of the fluctuations of resting tension is not due to loss of contractile ability of the myofibril, can be shown by demonstrating normal tension development with Ca^{2+}. Apparently, there is a substance in the extract that induces random vibrations in the myofibril, but identification of the substance and the elucidation of the mechanism of the vibration have not been made yet. It is possible that the substance actually consists of very small vesicles containing Ca^{2+} which, as the solution reaches the myofibril, release a small amount of Ca^{2+} upon contact with myofilaments.

Oscillation in damaged myofibrils

An entirely different kind of vibrations from the one just described above were observed in damaged myofibrils. When bullfrog atrium myofibrils were dissected out, most of them suffered minor damages which were not apparent on visual inspection. Upon activation by pCa 6.0 solution, tension slowly developed, as common to all damaged myofibrils, then violent oscillations set in as the tension approached plateau as shown in Fig. 3-4.

Microscopic observation revealed that a tug-of-war between healthy and damaged sarcomeres was taking place; at the start healthy ones shorten while stretching damaged ones, then this pattern reversed at a rate of few times a second. If this war was allowed to continue for a minute or two, the oscillations diminished and finally the damaged sarcomeres were completely stretched out and healthy ones went into supercontracture. If activation was aborted much before such a terminal situation, sarcomeres partially recovered to their original lengths with obvious sarcomere length inhomogeneity. The tension fluctuation spectrum is shown in Fig. 3-5 which shows second order kinetics with a roll-off frequency of about 10 Hz. This spectrum shape is very similar to one that appears during resting tension fluctuations in the presence of the muscle extract except for much greater intensity.

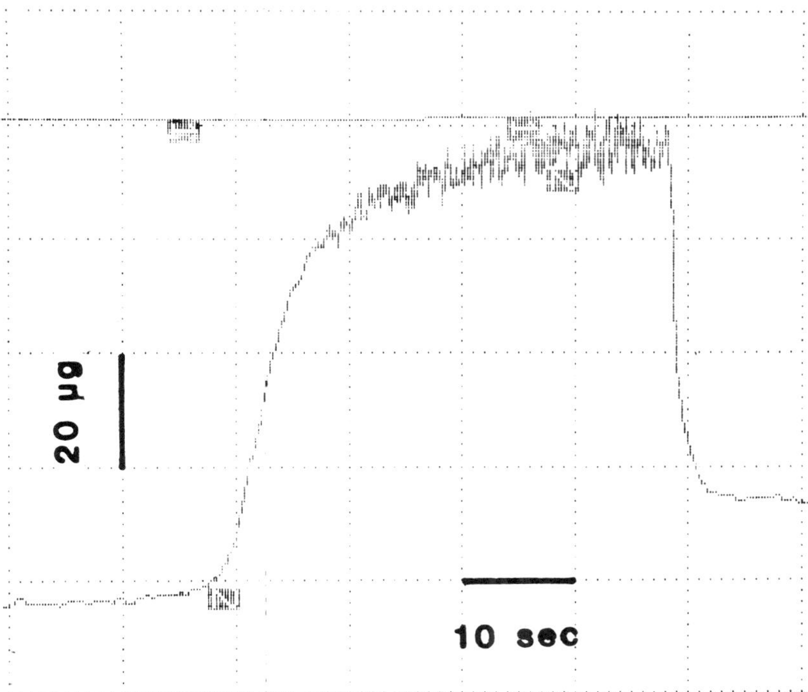

Figure 3-4. Violent oscillations of damaged myofibrils. Bullfrog atrium myofibrils, when some of the sarcomeres suffer minor damages, tend to fall into a tug-of-war between healthy and damaged sarcomeres. Not slow tension rise and substantially raised resting tension after relaxation.

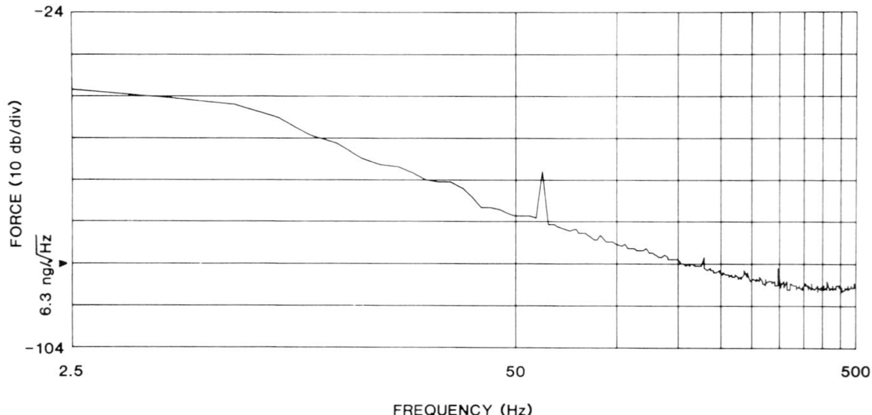

Figure 3-5. Tension fluctuation spectrum during the tug-of-war. The total power of the fluctuations is about $2\,\mu g$ rms which is about 20 times greater than the resting tension fluctuations described in Section 3, although the spectral shapes of the fluctuations are very similar.

The mechanism of the tug-of-war is likely due to the difference of tension rise times, stretch activations and shortening deactivations between healthy and damaged sarcomeres. As described before, damaged sarcomeres produce active tension much more slowly than good ones. Therefore, when all sarcomeres in the myofibril are activated by Ca^{2+} at the same time healthy ones produce tension faster than damaged sarcomeres thus healthy ones shorten while stretching damaged sarcomeres. However, the capability of the damaged sarcomeres to produce tension increases due to the combination of action of a slow rise time and delayed stretch activation, above that of the healthy sarcomeres. As damaged sarcomeres shorten the tension generating capacity of the healthy sarcomeres increases by stretch activation and so on, the process repeats many times until the slow rise of tension of damaged sarcomeres (which can last many minutes) ends, upon which the tug-of-war ceases and damaged ones are continuously stretched until healthy ones go into super-contracture.

It is of interest to note that the tug-of-war did not seem to occur in skeletal myofibrils. Obviously, a set of conditions must exist between tension rise times, stretch activation, and shortening deactivations in order to produce the tug-of-war. Computer simulations will be necessary to find the conditions since these factors are of highly non-linear and complex characteristics.

Elastic transfer function of myofibrils

Outstanding advantages of the new transducers are their extraordinary sensitivities and frequency bandwidths both of which are essential to investigating the elastic properties of myofibrils. The force transducer is capable of detecting $0.5\,ng/\sqrt{Hz}$; therefore, vibrations of only a few tenth of nanometer amplitude produced at the length controller are detectable at the other end of the myofibril. White noise perturbations combined with cross-correlation technique are a more convenient and faster way to measure the elastic transfer function but a much greater amplitude is required. Even so, only a few nanometer rms perturbation is sufficient. Since surrounding water medium can also conduct vibrations, it is necessary to subtract its effect. Fortunately, the transfer function of water is negligible below 500 Hz.

The elastic transfer functions of cardiac myofibrils under various conditions (rest, contraction, rigor, etc.) were similar to those of skeletal myofibrils. Therefore, the characteristic high resting stiffness in intact cardiac muscle must be associated with extra-myofibrillar structures.

Another important consideration of the elastic transfer function is the spectral analysis of spontaneous vibrations of the myofibril. As evident in Fig. 3-5, the spectrum has a curved slope. This is due to the fact that the elastic transfer function has a magnitude which increases with frequency as shown in Fig. 3-6. Therefore, fluctuations of force are transmitted through a structure which has greater stiffness at high frequencies.

The effect of slow stretch or release on tension fluctuations during contraction

Probably the most interesting experiments of the myofibril mechanics will be to investigate whether or not the random vibrations produced by cross-bridge attachment and detachment to the thin filament during contraction could be detected. A prevailing hypothesis for the molecular mechanism of striated muscle contraction is based upon a notion that active tension is brought about by the cyclic attachments between cross-bridges and thin filaments in conjunction with the enzymatic hydrolysis of ATP, and each cross-bridge acts independently of others. Consequently, the force imparted to the thin filament is necessarily intermittent and the total force will vary randomly with time about the average force, i.e., the tension will fluctuate about a mean value.

Mathematical theory of random vibrations is a well established field of physics, and derivation of theoretical predictions is straightforward if a concrete model is given. There are several models of cross-bridge kinetics proposed [6–11], and each will produce somewhat different results. For example, those models that produce negative forces during cross-bridge cycles necessarily yield greater fluctuation figures than those without negative forces. Regardless of a particular model chosen, however, the rms value of force fluctuations increases with N, where N is the number of cross-bridges, while the mean tension increases in direct proportion to N. In a half-sarcomere N is about 50,000 at full overlap length, and the

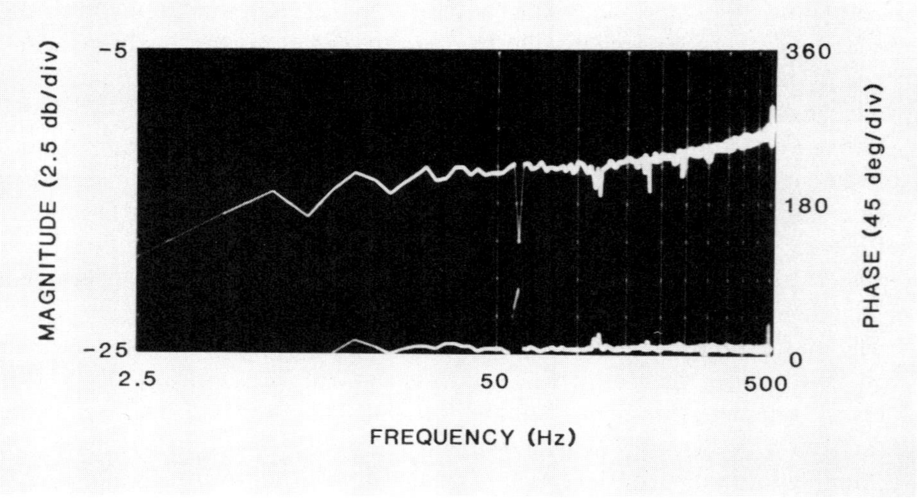

Figure 3-6. Elastic transfer function of myofibril during contraction. The solid curve is magnitude and the broken curve is phase. Stiffness magnitude 0 db = 100 ng/nm.

estimates of the ratio of fluctuation over the mean tension range between 0.001 and 0.01. Since actually measured maximum mean tension per sarcomere is about 50 μg, the expected fluctuation rms values should fall between 50 and 500 ng. For instance, Boredjo [12] estimated it to be 190 ng by adopting Hill's model. N can be reduced by stretching the sarcomere thereby increasing the ratio of fluctuation over the mean; for example, by stretching the sarcomere to 3.46 μm the ratio can be increased by a factor of 3.16.

The fluctuation rms values given above are total power, i.e., integration of power spectrum density. The shape of the spectrum density depends upon the kinetics involved, but when the cycling processes are dominated by the fastest step, the spectrum exhibits approximately the first order characteristics with a roll-off frequency corresponding to the fastest step and a slope of 20 db/decade. Figure 3-7 shows expected fluctuation spectra assuming the lowest rms value above (50 ng rms) with 1, 10, 100 Hz roll-off frequencies.

In actual experiments resting tension fluctuation intensity (= a) spectrum and active tension fluctuation intensity (= b) spectrum were measured separately and the difference between them ($\sqrt{a^2 - b^2}$) is the spectrum of interest. Because of this differential measurement the resolution of the spectrum is at least 10 db better than the system resolution. In Fig. 3-8 the broken curve is the spectrum during rest and the solid curve is one during isometric contraction. Each spectrum was averaged over 16 continuous measurements. Evidently, there is no significant difference between the rest and contraction spectra at the differential resolution level of 0.1 ng/$\sqrt{\text{Hz}}$ which is more than 100 times (40 db) below the level that was predicted to observe the fluctuations. It could be argued, however, that the

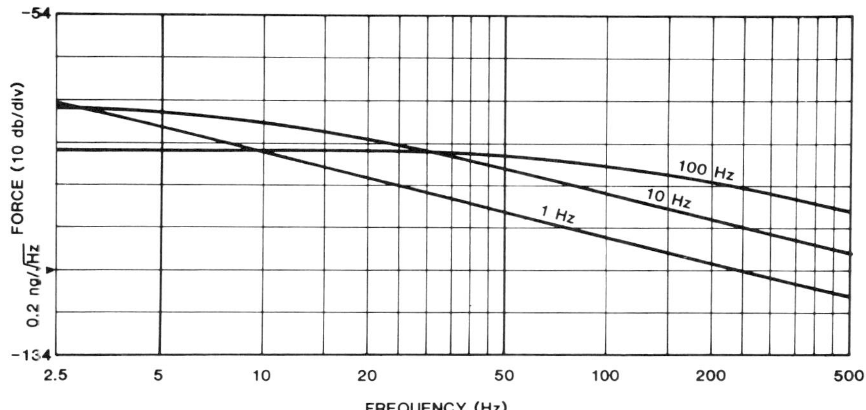

Figure 3-7. Expected tension fluctuation spectra arising from cross-bridge cycling. Assumptions: Total fluctuation power = 50 ng rms; Kinetics = First order; Roll-off frequencies = 1, 10, 100 Hz.

isometric contraction might result in all cross-bridges at strained positions thus locked-up and unable to cycle. To eliminate this possibility the myofibril was slowly stretched and released 16 times by up to 5% of the slack length (about 5 nm per half-sarcomere) during contraction. Each stretch or release lasted one second, and the spectrum measurement was made in the later 0.5 seconds so as to make sure that transients after each direction change had died out.

The results were identical to Fig. 3-8, i.e., there were no significant differences between rest and contraction spectra. In other words, no tension fluctuations

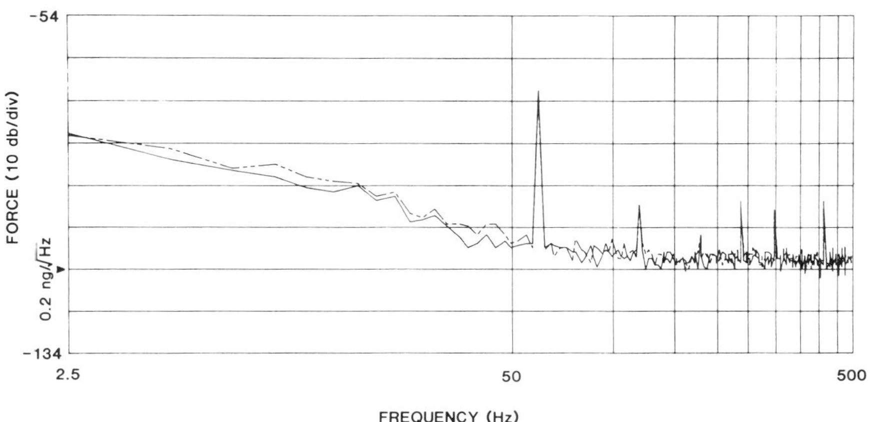

Figure 3-8. Measured tension fluctuation spectra during rest and contraction. Broken curve is of during rest and solid curve during isometric contraction. Indistinguishable results were obtained also during slow stretch and release contractions. The difference of these two spectra is: fluctuations generated by the cross-bridges, but there is no significant difference between them. The first order slope at the low frequencies was due to refractive index fluctuations of heated air in the light housing.

48

were detectable down to the level of 2 nanograms rms over 500 Hz bandwidth during isometric or slow stretch and release contractions. An argument that the cross-bridge vibrations were attenuated while propagating in the sarcomeres is implausible since elastic transfer functions measured during rest and contraction clearly demonstrated dramatic increase if stiffness during contraction, which has been interpreted as the evidence of cross-bridge attachment. Thus, we are faced with incontrovertible evidence that challenges the fundamental concept of the cross-bridge action in muscle contraction.

Conclusions

The myofibril mechanics required a great deal of effort in the development of instrumentation and methodology. I believe that the effort was worthwhile since the results, although still preliminary, have revealed vast and fertile world of unknowns. Just as was the case in physics, when it moved from classical mechanics to quantum mechanics people discovered things did not just scale down in proportion, the same is true in muscle mechanics. Typical preparations contain only 10 sarcomeres or so allowing us to observe the behavior of each sarcomere. Detailed observation of individual sarcomeres in action will lead to elucidation of not only the fundamental contractile processes but also more pragmatic aspects of sarcomere pathology such as failure mode analyses.

References

1. Iwazumi, T.: High speed and ultra sensitive instrumentation for myofibril mechanics measurements. Am. J. Physiol., 1986.
2. Fabiato, A. and Fabiato, F.: Calculator programs for computing the composition of the solutions containing multiple metal and ligands used for experiments in skinned muscle cells. J. de Physiol. (Paris) 75: 463–505, 1979.
3. Fabiato. A.: Myoplasmic free calcium concentrations reached during the twitch of an intact isolated cardiac cell and during calcium-induced release of calcium from the sarcoplasmic reticulum of a skinned cardiac cell from the adult rat or rabbit ventricle. J. gen. Physiol. 78: 457–497, 1981.
4. Iwazumi, T. and Pollack, G.H.: The effect of sarcomere non-uniformity on the sarcomere length-tension relationship of skinned fibers. J. Cell. Physiol. 106: 321–337.
5. Kentish, J.C., Ter Keurs, H.E.D.J., Noble, M.I.M., Ricciardi, L., Schouten, V.J.A.: The relationships between force, Ca^{2+} and sarcomere length in skinned trabeculae from rat ventricle. J. Physiol. 345: 24P, 1983.
6. Huxley, A.F.: Muscle structure and theories of contraction. Prog. Biophys. Biophys. Chem. 7: 255–318, 1957.
7. Lymn, R.W. and Taylor, E.W.: Mechanism of adenosine triphosphate hydrolysis by actomyosin. Biochem. 10: 4617–4624, 1971.
8. Hill, T.L.: Theoretical formalism for the sliding filament model of contraction of striated muscle. Pt. I. Prog. Biophys. Molec. Biol. 28: 267–340, 1974.

9. Hill, T.L.: ibid. Pt. II. Prog. Biophys. Molec. Biol. 29: 105–159, 1975.
10. Eisenberg, A. and Greene, L.E.: The relation of muscle biochemistry to muscle physiology. Ann. Rev. Physiol. 42: 293–309, 1980.
11. Eisenberg, E. and Hill, T.L.: Muscle contraction and free energy transduction in biological systems. Science 227: 999–1006, 1985.
12. Borejdo, J.: Tension fluctuations in contracting myofibrils and their interpretation. Biophys. J. 29 49–64, 1980.

General discussion of the contractile properties of the sarcomere

A possible role of calcium during stepwise length changes was considered unlikely as the steps can be seen in unactivated fibres, upon stretch of a fibre, in skinned fibres and beyond overlap. Dr. Pollack proposed that the synchrony that exists during the steps can be explained by a gradual development of tension such that most elements will make a length transition at about the same time. Dr. Huxley pointed out that that cross bridges, even though they hydrolyse ATP independently, are coupled to each other by rigid filaments. This must impose synchrony on the crossbridges as is shown by the response of muscle to a quick release and the behaviour of insect flight muscle. As to the source of the steps which occur beyond overlap other structures than connecting filaments, e.g. the cell membrane, should be investigated. The resolution of the sarcomere length measurement in the study of single myofibrils does not allow the detection of steps as reported by Dr. Pollack. However, the absence of steps in force development in single myofibrils was interpreted as evidence that the structures responsible for steps must reside outside the sarcomere.

Dr. Iwazumi related his observation that the force-sarcomere length relation is flat to the greater uniformity of the myofibril compared to larger preparations, and emphasized that a high concentration of activating calcium always causes non uniformity of the A-band specially in long sarcomeres.

It was agreed that a model, simulating the power spectrum or force fluctuations should incorporate both the force generators in parallel and in series as well as the transfer function of the elements in series. The low noise level of the force during contraction does not necessarily rule out a mechanism of independent pulsatile force generators but constrains the degree of cooperativity strongly. The observation however, still seems paradoxical in the face of the fact that the energy source of contraction, ATP, is provided in quantal form.

The slow rise of force in the single myofibril, whether obtained from slow or fast muscle fibres despite the rapid flow of activating solution over the myofibril and a short diffusion distance is unexplained, but may have been related to the ionic strength (.16) of the solutions used.

4. Excitation-contraction coupling in myocardium: implications of calcium release and Na/Ca exchange

HENK E.D.J. TER KEURS, VINCENT J.A. SCHOUTEN, JEROEN J. BUCX, BARBARA M. MULDER and PETER P. DE TOMBE

Introduction

It is well accepted that during excitation-contraction coupling calcium entry into cardiac cell, following the upstroke of the action potential, triggers calcium release from the sarcoplasmic reticulum [1, 2, 3]. The released calcium activates the contractile apparatus and is subsequently together with calcium that entered the cell during the action potential partially sequestered in the sarcoplasmic reticulum. The remainder of the calcium leaves the cell through the membrane, partly [4] in exchange for Na^+ partly transported by the Ca^{2+} pump. Ca^{2+} efflux through the membrane must in the steady state balance the influx during the action potential, while the calcium that is sequestered by the sarcoplasmic reticulum returns with some delay to the release sites [5]. The Ca^{2+} transport processes are reflected in: i) the electrical properties of the cell and ii) the relation between twitch force and the preceeding interval.

This chapter is concerned with the interrelationships between the cardiac action potential, calcium turnover by the sarcoplasmic reticulum and the cell membrane and mechanics of the muscle. We will, in the following, first present evidence that Ca^{++} extrusion from the cell delays the repolarization phase of the action potential in rat heart as a result of the electrogenic properties of the Na/Ca exchange mechanism. Subsequently, we will describe spontaneous contractions which arise in areas of damage in rat cardiac trabeculae. These contractions travel along the muscle and induce synchronous twitches and triggered arrhythmias. Propagation of spontaneous contractions and the observation that they precede each twitch of a triggered arrhythmia can be explained by i) Ca^{++} overload induced spontaneous Ca^{++} release in the area of damage followed by ii) propagation of Ca^{++} induced Ca^{++} release as a result of Ca^{++} diffusion in longitudinal direction in the cells. Ca^{++} extrusion by the Na/Ca exchanger, then, provides the depolarization to elicit the twitches of a triggered arrhythmia [6, 7].

Method

Dissection and mounting of the preparation

Trabeculae were dissected from the heart of Wistar rats. The hearts were excised from animals under ether anaesthesia. Dissection was performed under a binocular microscope, while the heart was perfused with a modified Krebs-Henseleit solution. Thin trabeculae, running between the free wall of the right ventricle and the atrioventricular ring were selected. Preparations were mounted in a glass covered chamber; the volume of the chamber was .5 ml. The preparation was superfused at a flow rate of 2 ml/min. The solutions used during dissection and experiments contained (in mM): Na^+, 147.4; K^+, 5.0; Cl^-, 98.5; Mg^{2+}, 1.2; PO_4^{2-}; 2.0; SO_4^{2-}; 1.2; $H_2CO_3^-$ 28.0; glucose, 11.0; $CaCl_2$ as specified in the results section. The temperature of the fluid in the experimental chamber, was kept at 25.0° C. In the study of spontaneous contractions the temperature was kept at 21° C. The solutions were in equilibrium with 95% O_2 and 5% CO_2 pH was 7.4.

Experimental apparatus

Stimulus pulses of 3 ms duration and of a strength 50% above threshold were derived from a programmable timing unit via a stimulus isolator, and two platinum wire electrodes.

A region of the muscle that was illuminated by a laser beam (cross section 400 μm) was observed using an inverted microscope and television system [8]. Sarcomere length in the illuminated area was measured from diffraction patterns generated by the muscle in HeNe laser light [8]. Sarcomere behavior of different areas of the trabecula could be recorded and compared by translating the microscope stage that supported the preparation in a direction parallel to the longitudinal axis of the specimen. The displacement of the microscope stage was measured from a linear potentiometer by means of a bridge amplifier. The muscle was connected to a quartz strain gauge force transducer via a stainless steel hook. The opposite end of the preparation was connected to a servomotor via a stainless steel hook.

The membrane potential was measured by means of glass microelectrodes with a 3 mm long highly flexible shaft [9]. The resistance of the microelectrodes (filled with 3 M KCl) was 60–140 MΩ. Frequently single cell impalements lasted up to 8 hours even if the preparation contracted vigorously and the site of impalement moved more than 100 μm. The measured membrane potential was amplified and was fed into an action potential analyser; its output of resting membrane potential (V_{rest}), sampled 20 ms prior to the stimulus and the duration of the action potential at 20% (APD20) or at 50% (APD50) of the amplitude were recorded on a chart recorder. Action potentials were photographed from the screen of an oscilloscope.

Results

Action potential properties and twitch force

Characteristic for the action potential of rat myocardium is a short plateau and a slow final repolarization phase (Fig. 4-1a). As a result of variations in stimulus frequency (protocol used Fig. 4-1b) the duration of the plateau phase and of slow repolarization phase varied characteristically with peak force of the concomittant twitches (Fig. 4-1c). The duration phase of the plateau phase decreased in proportion to twitch force, whereas the duration of the slow repolarization phase increased in proportion to twitch force (Fig. 4-1c). An increase of Ca^{2+} at constant force level caused the duration of the slow phase of repolarization to shorten. Lowering of the Na_o^+ caused an increase in twitch force while the duration of the slow phase decreased markedly. Upon return to normal Na_o^+, when Na_i^+ is known to be depleted [10], the duration of the slow phase increased transiently up to 5 times the control value (not shown; cf. Schouten, ter Keurs (1985) [11]), while force was reduced.

Spontaneous contractions and arrhythmias

Reduction of Na_{o2}^+ caused spontaneous contractions particularly at elevated Ca_o^{2+}. Similar spontaneous contractile activity was observed at high Ca_o^{2+} alone (i.e. ≥ 2.5 mM) and in regions of the muscle close to a damaged area e.g. close to a dissected branch or close to the original insertions of the muscle into the free wall of the right ventricle or atrio ventricular ring.

During the first hour after excision spontaneous activity in the terminal ends of a preparations developed into a strikingly reproducible chain of events specially if the muscle was kept at 20–22° C and stimulated with stimulus trains of 2 Hz interspersed by 12 sec rest periods. Following the last electrically stimulated contraction of the train a spontaneous contraction started in an area of approximately 250μm length close to the damaged end of unbranched muscles and travelled as a localized contraction along the length of the otherwise 'silent' muscle. We observed propagation of spontaneous contractions by direct microscopy and by recording local sarcomere shortening (AC)in different regions of the trabecular (Fig. 4-2).

Force development during the spontaneous contractions was small and lasted as long as the contraction wave travelled. Propagation velocity of spontaneous contractions ranged between 0.05 and 15 mm/sec and increased with the external Ca^{2+} concentration and with the number of stimuli in the train (as did the number of spontaneous contractions and their coupling interval to the last stimulated twitch [12]. At high Ca_o^{2+} or following a large number of stimuli nearly all preparations showed spontaneous twitches. The time-course of force develop-

54

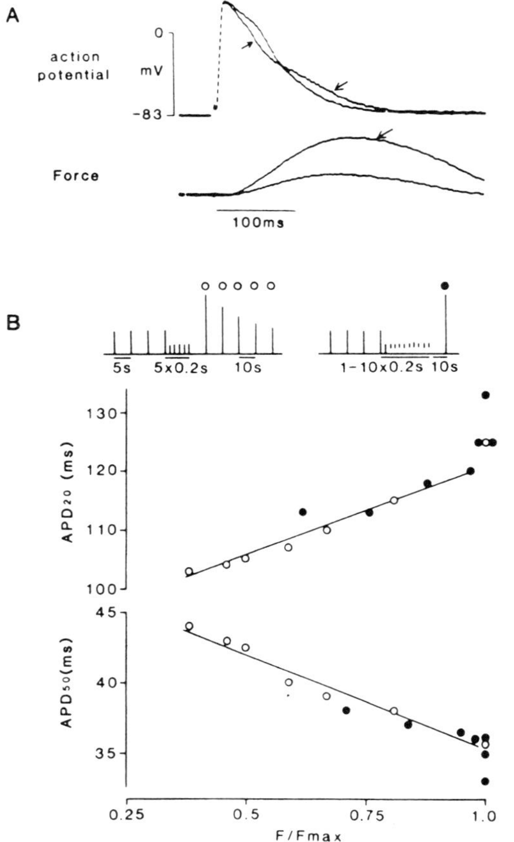

Figure 4-1. A.p.d.–F relationships during post-extrasystolic potentiation. A, traces show action potentials and contractions of the first (arrows) and the tenth beat during the negative force staircase following ten extrasystoles. B, the negative a.p.d.$_{50}$–F relationship and the positive a.p.d.$_{20}$–F relationship measured from potentiated beats. O, data obtained from the negative staircase following five extrasystoles (see left part of the inset). ● O, data of the first potentiated beat only following different numbers of extrasystoles (see right part of the inset). Results in A and B were from different trabeculae. [Ca^{2+}]$_o$ was 0.8 mM. (Reproduced with permission from, Schouten V.J.A. and ter Keurs H.E.D.J. ter Keurs; The slow repolarization phase of the action potential in rat heart; J. Physiol. 360: 13–25, 1985.)

ment and of sarcomere shortening of the spontaneous twitches was comparable to the time-course of an electrically elicited twitch. Spontaneous twitches started during the rising phase of the propagated contraction. The rapid increase of the rate of rise of force of such a spontaneous twitch is clearly noticeable in Fig. 4-3.

The occurrence of a spontaneous twitch was frequently followed by a series of spontaneous twitches, i.e. a triggered arrhythmia (Fig. 4-4). It is noteworthy that the intervals between the spontaneous twitches were initially short, but then increased progressively. Stable spontaneous tachycardias could persist for many

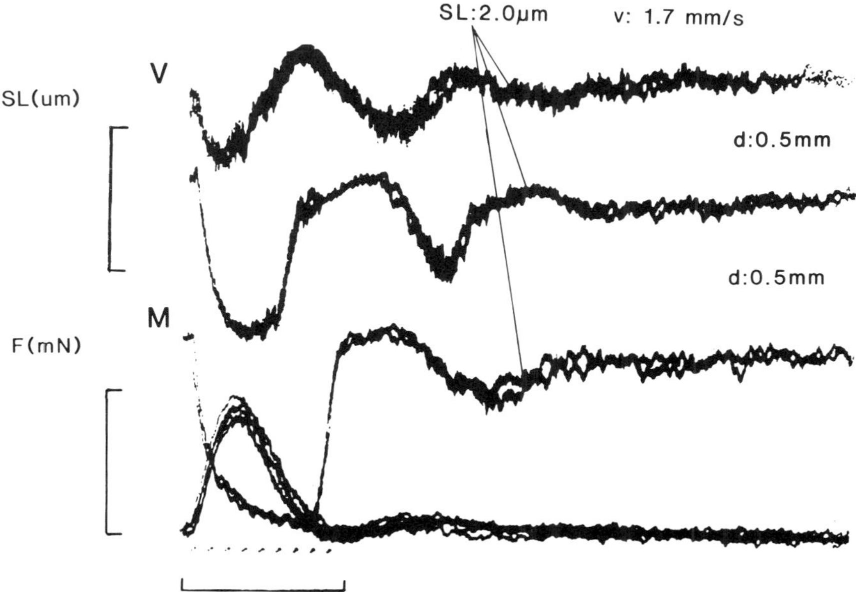

Figure 4-2. Sarcomere length (SL) and force (F) recorded during a focal AC, following the 1st of a train of ten electrically stimulated twitches, at three positions spaced (d) 0.5 mm apart. The AC started at the valvular end (V) and travelled to the myocardial end (M). $[Ca^{2+}]_o$, 2.5 mM; T, 21° C. Reproduced with permission from ter Keurs H.E.D.J., and Mulder B.M.; Propagation of after contractions in cardiac muscle of rat, J. Physiol. 353: 59 p., 1984.

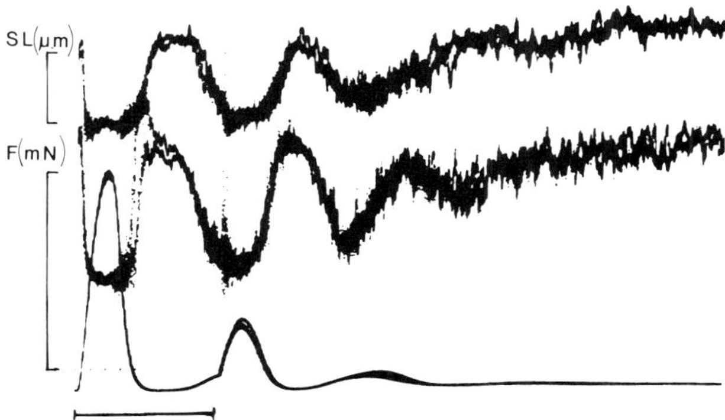

Figure 4-3 shows an example of the development of a spontaneous twitch that is triggered by an aftercontraction. Note the acute increase of the rate of rise of force development during the first aftercontraction, and the similarity of the time-course of subsequent twitch and that of the electrically elicited twitch. For further explanation see text.

56

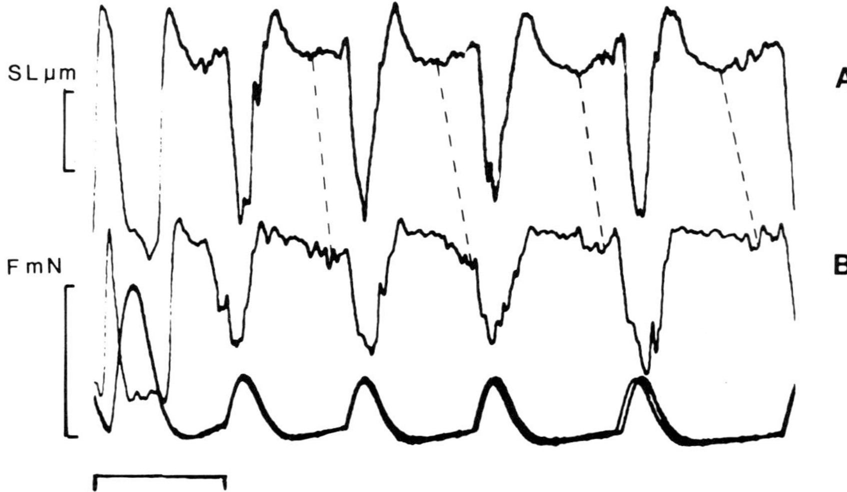

Figure 4-4. shows an example of a short lasting triggered arrhythmia. Note the gradual increase of the interval between the spontaneous twitches. The aftercontraction started at the valvular end (A) of the preparation and travelled toward the myocardial end (B). Note that synchronized contractions were triggered at the moment that the propagated aftercontractions arrived at B. Note furthermore that the propagation velocity decreased while the interval between the synchronized twitches increased.

minutes before the intervals between the spontaneous twitches increased and the arrhythmia stopped while only an aftercontraction was observed as the final event of the sequence. It was observed that the spontaneous twitches were usually initiated at the moment of arrival of the propagating contraction at a fixed site along the trabecula (Fig. 4-4) irrespective of the propagation velocity of the regional contraction. The increase of the interval time between the spontaneous twitches corresponded to the decrease of the velocity of propagation of the sarcomere shortening wave.

Discussion

Na/Ca exchange and the slow phase of repolarization

The slow phase of repolarization of the action potential may result from current generated by: 1) membranes of the sarcoplasmic reticulum during Ca^{2+} release [13], 2) a Ca^{2+} activated cation channel [14] and 3) electrogenic Na/Ca exchange [4, 15]. The latter hypothesis provides an explanation [11] for the effects of modification of the Na^+ and Ca^{2+} gradients over the cell membrane on the action potential. Ca^{2+} extrusion by the Na/Ca exchanger occurs against the electro-chemical gradient of Ca^{2+} driven by the electrochemical gradient of Na^+ (see for review ref 10). Our results suggested [11] that the slow phase of repolarization is prolonged by an increase of Na^+ (cf. results) and lowered Na_i^+ (cf. results) while the converse changes occurred if the Na^+ concentrations were modified in the opposite way. On the other hand the duration of the slow phase of the action potential increased with an increase of Ca_i^{2+} as reflected by an increase in developed force (cf. results) and shortened with an increase of Ca_o^{2+}. This hypothesis was recently corroborated by the studies of Hilgemann [16] who showed that in rabbit atrium which exhibits a similar slow phase of repolarization of the action potential as the rat ventricle, that this phase is accompanied by extrusion of calcium from the cell into the extracellular fluid. Model simulations also predict an influence of electrogenic Na^+/Ca^{2+} exchange on the action potential [17].

Spontaneous contractions and arrhythmias

The observations reported here suggest that spontaneous contractions arise in areas in which damage has caused considerable influx of calcium into the cells. Calcium overloading of the sarcoplasmic reticulum in these cells [18, 19] may cause spontaneous Ca^{2+} release by the sarcoplasmic reticulum by a mechanism that is not precisely understood [20] but which occurs at a moment that is coupled to the last electrically stimulated contraction (see Fig. 4-2). The contraction encompasses the whole muscle over 1-3 cell-lengths and travels over several millimeters at a constant velocity away from the damaged area along otherwise quiescent myocardial cells. The velocity of conduction is too low and too variable to be explained by electrotonic conduction, suggesting that an electrical event generated and conducted by the cell membrane cannot be the causal mechanism. However, the phenomena of propagated spontaneous contractions and the concomitant arrhythmias can be explained on the basis of the model shown in Fig. 4-5.

Calcium release in the area of damage induces a local elevation of the cytosolic Ca^{2+} concentration which causes Ca^{2+} induced Ca^{2+} release of the adjacent sarcomeres [3]. Repetition of this process gives rise to propagation of the release of calcium and the resulting contraction. It is to be expected that when the Ca^{2+} concentration in the cytosol and in the release compartment of the sarcoplasmic reticulum rise, either as a result of an increase of the extracellular Ca^{2+} concentration or as a consequence of an increase in the number of stimuli, the threshold for Ca^{2+} release will be reached more rapidly. Model simulations of the process of Ca^{2+} induced Ca^{2+} release based on the kinetics of the release process [19] and of Ca^{2+} binding [21] and sequestration in the cell predict that propagation velocity may vary between 0.1 and 25 mm/s (Backx et al. in preparation) as was observed experimentally.

The observation that a small force was generated as long as the wave of sarcomere shortening travelled along the muscles is consistent with the fact that

58

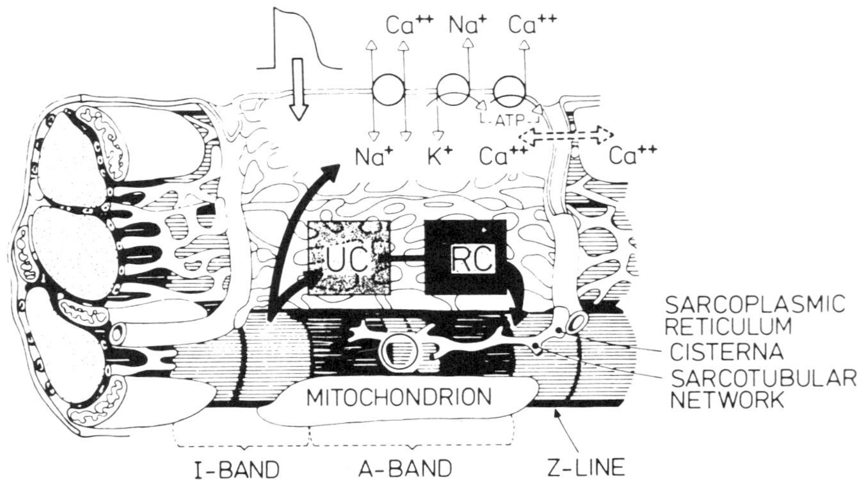

Figure 4-5. Depicts a model of the cardiac cell after Katz [19] and the events that take place during excitation-contraction coupling. The dashed squares above the sarcoplasmic reticulum depict the uptake compartment and the release compartment of calcium in the sarcoplasmic reticulum. Diffusion of calcium ions from one sarcomere to another is indicated by the dashed arrows. For further explanation see text.

the contraction occurred in a small region that was in series with the otherwise resting, i.e. compliant muscle. This contrasted the time-course of the spontaneous twitches that were observed under conditions of a high calcium load (Fig. 4-3). The occurrence of twitches that were preceded by propagating contractions is consistent with the assumption that a spontaneous twitch was elicited by a transient depolarization that resulted from electrogenic Na/Ca exchange mediated extrusion of the calcium that was released by the sarcoplasmic reticulum during the spontaneous contraction. This depolarization triggered action potential generation as has been observed in other studies [22, 6, 7]. We frequently found that spontaneous arrhythmias occurred in the presence of spontaneous contractions in combination with transient depolarizations.

The termination of these tachycardias is in this respect of particular interest (Fig. 4-4). The interval between the twitches increased exponentially from 750 msec, initially, to 2500 msec just before termination of the tachycardia. The observed decrease of the velocity of propagation of the spontaneous contractions preceding the twitches is consistent with the hypothesis that (Fig. 4-5) the propagated contraction which travels through the preparation, elicits an action potential as a result of the concomittant transient depolarization when it reaches a region with a low threshold for action potential generation. The interval between spontaneous twitches should depend on both the distance between the damaged area, where the propagated contractions start, and the area where the threshold for action potential generation is lowest and on the propagation velocity of the spontaneous contraction, which in turn depends on the intracellular calcium concentration.

We conclude that the observed propagation of spontaneous contractions is consistent with a model in which calcium induced calcium release occurs, as has been proposed by Fabiato, whilst propagation of release at the observed velocities can be accounted for by: i) diffusion of calcium ii) calcium binding to cytosolic binding sites and iii) the properties of the release and sequestration process.

Moreover, our observations suggest that spontaneous contractions occur, and trigger arrhythmias, in recently damaged cardiac muscle as in a heart with a recent myocardial infarction. These observations are compatible with the hypothesis that propagated contractions lead to triggered arrhythmias as a result of the electrogenic character of the Na/Ca exchanger.

Conclusions

In this chapter, we presented evidence in support of the hypothesis that electrogenic Na/Ca exchange is responsible in rat cardiac muscle for: 1) the slow repolarization phase of the action potential and; 2) the development of triggered arrhythmias.

It was shown that the duration of the slow phase of repolarization of the action potential varies in proportion to the Na^+ concentration gradient and inversely with the Ca^+ concentration gradient over the cell membrane. This suggested that Na/Ca exchange can generate a current of sufficient magnitude to maintain the membrane depolarized at $-60\,mV$.

In damaged trabeculae we observed triggered arrhythmias which were always preceded by propagating spontaneous contractions. Propagation of spontaneous contractions was consistent with spontaneous calcium release in the region of damage of the trabeculae as a result of a calcium overload of the sarcoplasmic reticulum. Calcium release in the damaged area causes calcium induced calcium release in adjacent sites as a result of diffusion of calcium. Propagation velocity of the spontaneous contraction was consistent with this model. The occurrence of arrythmias was consistent with the hypothesis that the release of calcium during this process leads to a depolarization as a result of electrogenic Na/Ca exchange. The triggered action potential adds to the calcium load of the cells and thereby causes another spontaneous calcium release to repeat the cycle.

Acknowledgements

Supported by Grants from the: Alberta Heritage Foundation for Medical Research of which Dr. ter Keurs is a Medical Scientist; Alberta Heart & Stroke Foundation; Netherlands Heart Foundation; Netherlands Association for the Advancement of Pure Science.

References

1. Wood, E.H., Heppner, R.L. and Weidmann, S.: Inotropic effects of electric currents. Circulation Research 24: 409–445, 1969.
2. Morad, M. and Goldman, Y.: Excitation-contraction coupling in heart muscle: membrane control of development of tension. Progress in Biophysical and Molecular Biology 27: 257–31, 1973.
3. Fabiato, A.: Calcium-induced release of calcium from the cardiac sarcoplasmic reticulum. American Journal of Physiology 245: C1–C14, 1983.
4. Mullins, L.J.: The generation of electric currents in cardiac fibers by Na/Ca exchange. American Journal of Physiology 236: C103–C110, 1979.
5. Koch-Weser, J. and Blinks, J.R.: The influence of the interval between beats on the myocardial contractility. Pharmacological Reviews 15: 601–652, 1963.
6. Kass, R.S., Lederer, W.J., Tsien, R.W. and Weingart, R.: Role of calcium ions in TI currents and aftercontractions induced by strophantidin in cardiac Purkinje fibers. Journal of Physiology 281: 187–208, 1978a.
7. Kass, R.S.and Tsien, R.W.: Fluctuations in membrane current driven by intracellular calcium in cardiac Purkinje fibers. Biophysical Journal 38: 259–269, 1982.
8. Daniels, M., Noble, M.I.M., ter Keurs, H.E.D.J. and Wohlfart, B.: Velocity of sarcomere shortening in rat cardiac muscle: relationship to force, sarcomere length, calcium and time. Journal of Physiology 355: 367–382, 1984.
9. Schouten, V.J.A.S. Thesis: Excitation-contraction coupling in heart muscle. Leiden, 1985.
10. Chapman, R.A.: Control of cardiac contractility at the cellular level. American Journal of Physiology 245 (Heart Circulation Physiology 14): H535–H552, 1983.
11. Schouten, V.J.A. and ter Keurs, H.E.D.J.: The slow repolarization phase of the action potential in rat heart. Journal of Physiology 360: 13–25, 1985.
12. Ter Keurs, H.E.D.J. and Mulder, B.M.: Propagation of aftercontractions in cardiac muscle of the rat. J. Physiol. 353: 59P, 1984.
13. Simurda, J., Simurdova, M., Braveny, P. and Sumbera, J.: Activity-dependent changes of slow inward current in ventricular heart muscle. Pflugers Archiv. ges. Physiologie 391: 277–283, 1981.
14. Colquhoun, D., Neher, E., Reuter, H. and Stevens, C.F.: Inward current channels activated by intracellular calcium in cultured cardiac cells. Nature 294: 752–754, 1981.
15. Noble, D.: Ionic mechanisms controlling the action potential duration and the timing of repolarization. Japanese Heart Journal 27: 3–19, 1986.
16. Hilgemann, D.W.: Extracellular calcium transients and action potential configuration changes related to poststimulatory potentiation in rabbit myocardium. J Gen. Physiol., 87: 675–706, 1986.
17. DiFrancesco, D., Hart, G. and Noble, D.: Ionic current transients attribute to the Na-Ca exchange process in the heart: computer model. Journal of Physiology 328: 15–16P, 1982.
18. Kort, A.A. and Lakatta, E.G.: Calcium-dependent mechanical oscillations occur spontaneously in unstimulated mammalian cardiac tissues. Circulation Research 54: 396–404, 1984.
19. Allen, D.F., Eisner, D.A., Priolo, J.S. and Smith, G.L.: The relationship between intracellular calcium and contraction in calcium-overloaded ferret papillary muscles. Journal of Physiology 364: 169–182, 1985.
20. Fabiato, A.: Calcium-induced release of calcium from the sarcoplasmic reticulum. Journal of General Physiology 85: 189–320, 1985.
21. Cannel, M.B., Allen, D.: Model of calcium movements during activation in the sarcomere of frog skeletal muscle. Biophysical Journal 45: 913–925, 1984.
22. Cranefield, P: Action potentials, afterpotentials and arrhythmias. Circulation Research 41: 415–423, 1977.

5. Calcium influx and sarcoplasmic reticulum calcium release in cardiac excitation-contraction coupling

DONALD M. BERS

Introduction

It has now been over 100 years since Ringer [1] demonstrated that extracellular Ca plays a critical role in cardiac muscle contraction. It is now clear that Ca influx is an important factor in cardiac excitation-contraction coupling (ECC). However, whether this Ca influx does in fact contribute directly to the activation of the myofilaments remains controversial. Part of this controversy is quantitative. That is, does enough Ca enter the cell to directly activate the myofilaments during a single cardiac muscle beat? The answer to this, until quite recently would have been, simply, no. Recently, single cell voltage and patch clamp studies [2, 3, 4], radiotracer flux measurements [5], and extracellular Ca-selective microelectrodes and dyes [6, 7] have increased estimates of the Ca influx during a beat (to about $10–183\,\mu$mol/kg wet tissue) into the range required for half-maximum activation of the myofilaments ($[15–42]\,\mu$mol/kg wet tissue) [8, 9]. These ranges are large and at this time neither of these values is known with sufficient precision to provide unequivocal evidence for or against a direct role for Ca influx in myofilament activation.

Several cellular sites have been suggested to be the immediate source of Ca which activates the myofilaments, but the most widely accepted possibilities today are probably transsarcolemmal Ca influx (e.g. as described by Langer and coworkers [10–14]), and Ca release from the sarcoplasmic reticulum (SR) (e.g. as described by Fabiato, [15, 16]). Fabiato has proposed a model where Ca influx is insufficient to activate the myofilaments directly, but serves primarily to induce release of additional Ca from the SR which would then activate the myofilaments. This Ca induced release of Ca from the SR in Fabiato's mechanically skinned fibers is graded such that a larger or faster Ca influx may be expected to induce greater SR Ca release. This facet of Fabiato's model means that tension development will vary with Ca influx, whether this Ca influx activates the myofilaments directly or simply serves to induce release of Ca from the SR. One way to examine whether Ca influx can activate tension development is to inhibit SR Ca release and examine tension development under various conditions. Caffeine and ryano-dine are two agents which inhibit SR Ca release although they may do so by different mechanisms. Caffeine simply renders the SR permeable to Ca so that it can neither accumulate nor release Ca [17, 18]. Ryanodine also inhibits SR Ca release, but does not prevent Ca uptake by the SR [19]. While the action of ryanodine appears to be specifically on the SR, caffeine produces several other effects (e.g. increased Ca influx and myofilament Ca sensitivity, [20, 23]) which would tend to increase tension development.

Table 5-1 shows the effects of these two agents on steady state tension develop-ment (at $30°$ C and 0.5 Hz in a HEPES buffered physiological superfusate). It can be seen that in frog ventricle, ryanodine had almost no effect on tension develop-ment, while caffeine produced a positive inotropic effects which may be at-tributed to the non-SR affects of caffeine. These results are consistent with Fabiato's finding that frog ventricle does not display Ca-induced SR Ca release [24, 25] and the widely held conclusion that frog ventricle depends primarily on Ca influx for myofilament activation (e.g. see [26]). Tension development was only modestly depressed by these agents in rabbit ventricle but strongly depressed in rat ventricle, with rabbit atrium having an intermediate sensitivity. These results suggest that Ca influx can activate nearly normal tension development in rabbit ventricle, but that Ca influx is inadequate in rat ventricle (with rabbit atrium intermediate). Fabiato [24, 25] has also found this sequence in terms of Ca-induced release of SR Ca in cardiac tissue. That is, this phenomenon is most strongly displayed in rat ventricle and least in rabbit ventricle, with rabbit atrium being intermediate. Bers et al. [27] demonstrated an identical sequence for these four tissues in terms of sensitivity to $[Ca]_o$ with rat being most sensitive. Neonatal rat ventricle also behaves very much like adult rabbit ventricle with respect to all the above indices. Thus there appear to be substantial species (rat vs. rabbit), regional (atrium vs. ventricle) and developmental (neonate vs. adult rat) differ-ences in the relative contributions of Ca influx and SR Ca release to the activation of the myofilaments.

The relative contributions may also change in different experimental condi-tions. Ca influx associated with individual twitches has been measured using

Table 1. Effects of caffeine and ryanodine on steady state twitch tension in several cardiac tissues.

	Developed tension (% of control)	
	5 mM Caffeine (n)	100 nM Ryanodine (n)
Frog ventricle	$120 \pm 8\%$ (3)	$96 \pm 1\%$ (4)
Rabbit ventricle	89 ± 9 (8)	78 ± 3 (9)
Rabbit atrium	63 ± 10 (4)	49 ± 7 (4)
Rat ventricle	33 ± 2 (4)	13 ± 3 (8)

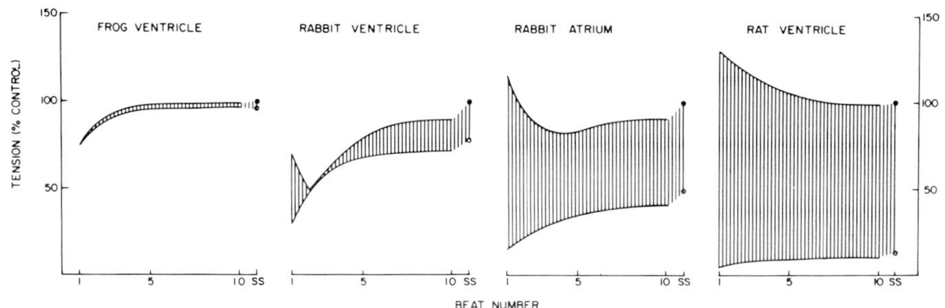

Figure 5-1. A summary of tension recovery from 30-s rest intervals in frog, rabbit, and rat ventricle, and rabbit atrium in absence (upper curves and o) and presence of ryanodine and o). Final points (SS) are steady-state values. Relative SR contribution to activation of any beat in any tissue is indicated by shaded area and relative influx by area below shading. (From 3, with permission from the American Physiological Society.)

extracellular Ca-selective microelectrodes. After a rest period, the Ca influx that accompanies the contraction is initially small and then increases monotonically to a steady state level with each subsequent contraction [6, 20]. Twitch tension recovers in a similar fashion to this in the presence of caffeine or ryanodine in all of the above tissues (see lower curves in Fig. 5-1).

The upper curves in Fig. 5-1 illustrate the manner in which twitches return to steady state in the absence of these agents. Thus, one may conclude that the shaded area between the curves is a rough index of the relative contribution of SR Ca release to tension development. For example, in rabbit ventricle, the first post-rest contraction is relatively strongly dependent on SR Ca release, for the next few beats (Ca influx may dominate and finally as the SR is 'reloaded' by increasing Ca influx it reaches a new steady relative contribution. Figure 5-2 is a simple working model of cellular Ca movements associated with cardiac ECC which indicates that both Ca influx and SR Ca release may contribute to myofilament activation and the relative contributions will vary in different tissues and under different conditions.

If there are really two sources of Ca which can activate cardiac myofilaments, then one may be able to find some conditions that can partially separate these two components during a single contraction. Indeed, such biphasic contractions have been reported under a variety of conditions [28–34]. We observed biphasic contractions during some experiments with milrinone in ferret ventricular muscle (which is highly SR dependent by the above criteria) and these are shown in Figs. 5-3 and 5-4 [35].

Milrinone increases the slow inward Ca current under these conditions and also exerts a mild caffeine-like action on the SR [35–37]. When milrinone is added there is a transient positive inotropic effect and substantial shortening of the twitch. This, we think, is due to rapid enhancement of Ca current, which would accelerate and increase the magnitude of the SR Ca release. Over the next few

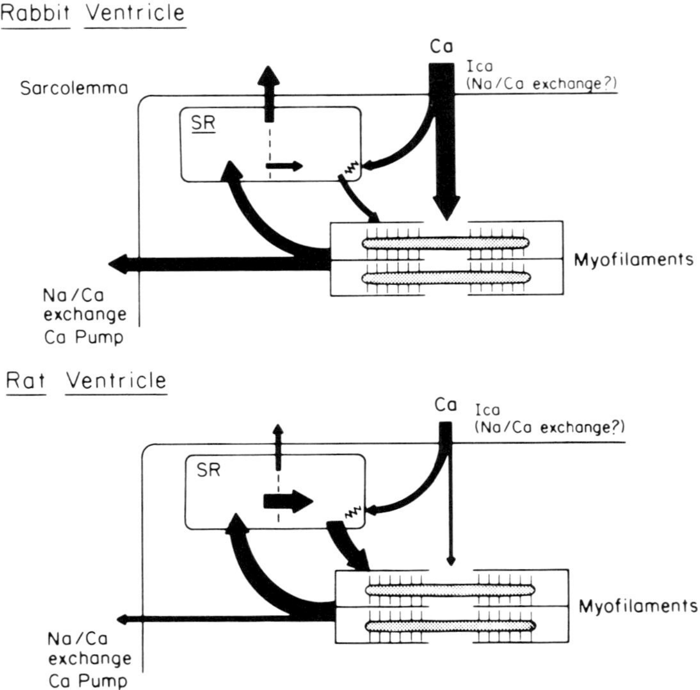

Figure 5-2. A simple working model for Ca cycling that is involved in excitation-contraction coupling in cardiac muscle. Thickness of arrows is meant to imply relative magnitudes of Ca movements. The division of sarcoplasmic reticulum (SR) is a kinetically defined construct. (From 3, with permission from the American Physiological Society.)

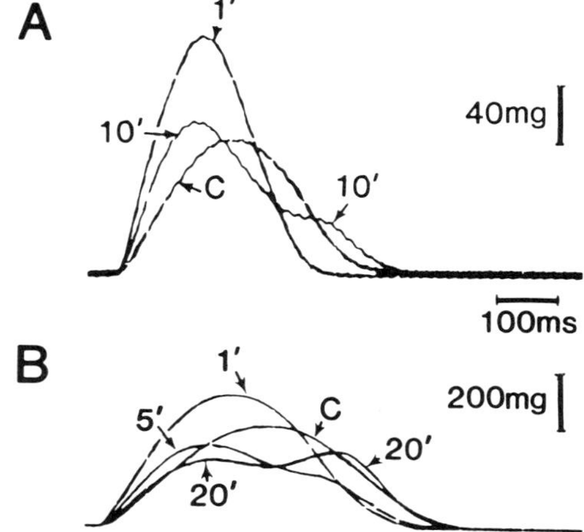

Figure 5-3. Effect of 50 μg/ml milrinone on action potential-elicited twitch tension in two different papillary muscles at 28° C. Control twitches (C) and twitches at the various times indicated after addition of milrinone are shown. The tracing corresponding to 5 minutes after drug application in panel B indicates that both components of the biphasic twitch can be seen without prolongation of the total twitch duration. (From 32, with permission of the American Heart Association.)

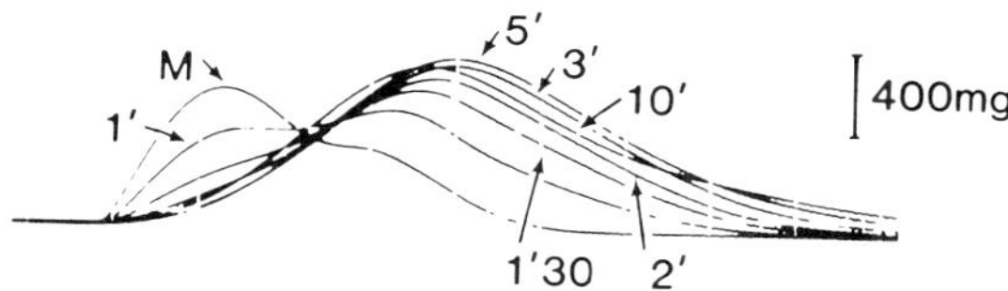

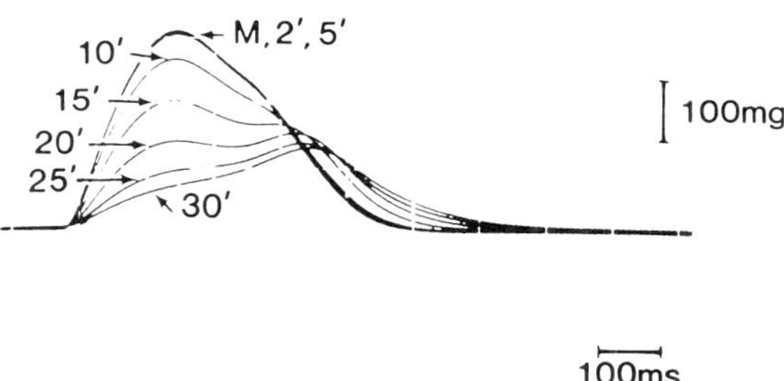

Figure 5-4. Effects of caffeine and ryanodine on the biphasic twitches induced by 50 µg/ml milrinone at 28° C and 0.5 Hz. Top panel: time course of action of 10 mM caffeine. Bottom panel: time course of action of 100 nM ryanodine. The trace labelled M corresponds to a steady-state twitch in the presence of milrinone prior to the addition of caffeine or ryanodine. The numbers refer to the time (minutes) after addition of caffeine or ryanodine to the perfusate. (From 32, with permission of the American Heart Association.)

minutes, this fast peak decreases in magnitude and a second component of contraction becomes increasingly apparent. This, we think, is due to the depressant effect of milrinone on SR Ca uptake and release. That is, now the increased influx can activate a slower component of contraction.

Figure 5-4 demonstrates the effects of caffeine and ryanodine on biphasic contractions observed during steady state exposure to milrinone. Caffeine eliminates the first component, while enhancing the second component and ryanodine simply eliminates the first component. These results are consistent with the first component of the biphasic twitches being due to SR Ca release and the second component being due to Ca influx. Thus it appears clear that both transsarcolemmal Ca influx and SR Ca release can contribute to activation of mammalian myofilaments during contractions and the relative contributions can vary.

References

1. Ringer, S.: A further contribution regarding the influence of the different constituents of the blood on the contraction of the heart. J. Physiol. London 4: 29, 1983.
2. Hume, J.R. and Giles, W.: Ionic currents in single isolated bullfrog atrial cells. J. Gen. Physiol. 81: 153–194, 1983.
3. Isenberg, G.: Ca entry and contraction as studied in isolated bovine ventricular myocytes. Z. Naturforch. 37: 502–512, 1982.
4. Lee, K.S. and Tsien, R.W.: Reversal of current through calcium channels in dialysed single heart cells. Nature 297: 498–501, 1982.
5. Lewartowski, B., Pytkowski, B., Prokopczuk, A., Wasilewska-Dziubinska, E. and Otwinowski, W.: Amount and turnover of calcium entering the cells of ventricular myocardium of guinea pig heart in a single excitation. In: Advances in Myocardiology, edited by E. Chazov, V. Smirnov and N.S. Dhalla, New York, Plenum Press, Vol. 3, pp. 345–357, 1982.
6. Bers, D.M.: Early transient depletion of extracellular [Ca] during individual cardiac muscle contractions. Amer. J. Physiol. 244: H462–H468, 1983.
7. Hilgemann, D.W., Delay, M.J. and Langer, G.A.: Activation-dependent cumulative depletions of extracellular free calcium in guinea pig atrium measured with antipyrylazo III and tetra-methylmurexine. Circ. Res. 53: 779–793, 1983.
8. Fabiato, A.: Calcium-induced release of calcium from the cardiac sarcoplasmic reticulum. Am. J. Physiol. 245: C1–C14, 1983.
9. Solaro, R.J., Wise, W.M., Shiner, J.S. and Briggs, F.N.: Calcium requirements for cardiac myofibrillar activation. Circ. Res. 34: 525–530, 1974.
10. Bers, D.M. and Langer, G.A.: Uncoupling cation effects on cardiac contractility and sarcolemmal Ca2+ binding. Amer. J. Physiol. 237: H332–H341, 1979.
11. Langer, G.A.: Heart: Excitation-contraction coupling. Ann. Rev. Physiol. 35: 55–86, 1973.
12. Langer, G.A.: Editorial: The role of calcium in the control of myocardial contractility: an update. J. Mol. Cell. Cardiol. 12: 231–239, 1980.
13. Langer, G.A., Frank, J.S. and Brady, A.J.: The myocardium. In: Cardiovascular Physiology II, edited ty A.F. Guyton and A.W. Cowley. Baltimore, MD: University Park, 1976, vol. 9, p. 191–237. (Int. Rev. Physiol. Ser.)
14. Philipson, K.D. and Langer, G.A.: Sarcolemmal-bound calcium and contractility in the mammalian myocardium. J. Mol. Cell. Cardiol. 11: 857–875, 1979.
15. Fabiato, A.: Effects of cyclic AMP and phosphodiesterase inhibitors on the contractile activation and the CA2+ transient detected with aequorin in skinned cardiac cells from rat and rabbit ventricles (abstr.). J. Gen. Physiol. 78: 15a–16a, 1981.
16. Fabiato, A. and Fabiato, F.: Calcium and cardiac excitation-contraction coupling. Ann. Rev. Physiol. 41: 473–484, 1979.
17. Fabiato, A.: Simulated calcium current can both cause calcium loading in and trigger calcium release from the sarcoplasmic reticulum of a skinned canine cardiac Purkinje cell. J. Gen. Physiol. 85: 291–320, 1985.
18. Sutko, J.L., Thompson, L.J., Kort, A.A. and Lakatta, E.G.: Comparison of effects of ryanodine and caffeine on ventricular myocardium. Am. J. Physiol. 250: H786–H795, 1986.
19. Sutko, J.L., Ito, K. and Kenyon, J.L.: Ryanodine: a modifier of sarcoplasmic reticulum calcium release in striated muscle. Fed. Proc. 44: 2984–2988, 1985.
20. Bers, D.M.: Ca influx and sarcoplasmic reticulum Ca release in cardiac muscle activation during post-rest recovery. Am. J. Physiol. 248: H366–H381, 1985.
21. Blinks, J.R., Olson, C.B., Jewell, B.R. and Braveny, P.: Influence of caffeine and other methylxanthines on mechanical properties of isolated mammalian heart muscle. Evidence for a dual mechanism of action. Circ. Res. 30: 367–392, 1972.
22. Fabiato, A.: Myoplasmic free calcium concentration reached during the twitch of an intact

isolated cardiac cell and during calcium-induced release of calcium from the sarcoplasmic reticulum of a skinned cardiac cell from the adult rat or rabbit ventricle. J. Gen. Physiol. 78: 457–497, 1981.
23. Wendt, I.R. and Stephenson, D.G.: Effects of caffeine on Ca-activated force production in skinned cardiac and skeletal muscle fibres of the rat. Pflugers Arch. 398: 210–216, 1983.
24. Fabiato, A.: Calcium release in skinned cardiac cells: variations with species, tissues and development. Fed. Proc. 41: 2238–2244, 1982.
25. Fabiato, A. and Fabiato, F.: Calcium-induced release of calcium from the sarcoplasmic reticulum of skinned cells from adult human, dog, cat, rabbit, rat, and frog hearts and from fetal and newborn rat ventricles. Ann. N.Y. Acad. Sci. 307: 491–522, 1978.
26. Morad, M., Goldman, Y.E. and Trentham, D.R.: Rapid photochemical inactivation of Ca2+-antagonists shows that CA2+ entry directly activates contraction in frog heart. Nature 304: 635–638, 1983.
27. Bers, D.M., Philipson, K.D. and Langer, G.A.: Cardiac contractility and sarcolemmal calcium binding in several cardiac preparations. Am. J. Physiol. 240: H576–H583, 1981.
28. Bogdanov, K.Y., Zakharov, S.I. and Rosenshtraukh, L.V.: The origin of two components in contraction of guinea pig papillary muscle in the presence of noradrenaline. Can. J. Physiol. Pharmacol. 57: 866–872, 1979.
29. Braveny, P. and Sumbera, J.: Electromechanical correlations in the mammalian heart muscle. Pfluegers Arch. 319: 36–48, 1970.
30. Coraboeuf, E.: Membrane electrical activity and double component contraction in cardiac tissue. J. Mol. Cell. Cardiol. 6: 215–255, 1974.
31. Endoh, M., Tijima, T. and Motomura, S.: Inhibition by theophylline of the early component of canine ventricular contraction. Am. J. Physiol. 242: H349–HY358, 1982.
32. King, B.W. and Bose, D.: Mechanism of biphasic contractions in strontium-treated ventricular muscle. Circ. Res. 52: 65–75, 1983.
33. Reiter, M., Vierling, W. and Seibel, K.: Excitation-contraction coupling in rested-state contractions of guinea pig ventricular myocardium. Naunyn-Schmiedeberg's Arch. Pharmacol. 325: 159–169, 1984.
34. Seibel, K., Karema, E., Takeya, K. and Reiter, M.: Effect of noradrenaline on an early and late component of the myocardial contraction. Naunyn-Schmiedeberg's Arch. Pharmacol. 305: 65–74, 1978.
35. Malecot, C.O., Bers, D.M. and Katzung, B.G.: Biphasic contractions induced by milrinone at low temperature in ferret cardiac muscle: Role of the sarcoplasmic reticulum and transmembrane calcium influx. Circ. Res. (In press), 1986.
36. Rapundalo, S.T., Grupp, I., Grupp, G., Matlib, M.A., Solaro, R.J. and Schwartz, A.: Myocardial actions of milrinone: Characterization of its mechanism of action. Circulation 73: III–134–III–144, 1986.
37. Su, J.Y., Mechanism of milrinone-induced positive inotropic action (Abstract). Biophys. J. 47: 283a, 1985.

General discussion of excitation-contraction coupling

The after-contractions described here were observed in muscles in which only one site of damage was manifest. In case of preparations with multiple loci of injury one observes multiple waves of contractions travelling in different directions and frequently colliding. The latter phenomenon has been observed in many laboratories.

The most important determinants of velocity of propagation in the model was an increased cytosolic calcium concentration with occupation of the calcium binding sites, enhanced SR loading, a lowered threshold for release of the SR.

The suggestion that after-contractions might be related to incomplete relaxation of the working heart was raised. This possibility is supported by the observation (Bucx & ter Keurs, unpublished) that during anoxia secondary shortening of sarcomeres may be seen in relation to delayed relaxation.

Species differences in excitation-contraction coupling are important; the question whether the sarcoplasmic reticulum in human myocardium contributes to activation has not been settled. Neither is there complete agreement on the stoichiometry of the Na/Ca exchanger, although its electrogenic character is generally accepted.

6. Cardiac energetics

C.L. GIBBS

Introduction

In this chapter I wish to consider the energy balance sheet for cardiac muscle and to discuss some of the uncertainties that exist in current measurements. Many of the problems I will highlight are not specific to cardiac muscle and certainly exist to varying degrees in skeletal and smooth muscle studies. I will be mainly concerned with results coming from my own laboratory and for that reason would like to acknowledge the debt that I owe to my colleagues and in particular to Dr. Brian Chapman, Dr. Denis Loiselle, Dr. Igor Wendt and Mr. George Kotsanas. I will be reporting energetic data obtained in myothermic and polarographic studies on papillary muscles together with some whole heart oxygen consumption data and will compare our results with those of other investigators.

The immediate energy source in cardiac muscle is ATP and in terms of the contractile event we can identify three major enzyme systems that are primarily responsible for the measured energy flux. They are (i) the Na^+-K^+-ATPase of the sarcolemmal Na^+ pump (ii) the sarcoreticular and sarcolemmal Ca^{++}-ATPases and (iii) the actomyosin ATPase of the myofibrillar contractile unit. The background to this statement has been provided several times [1, 2, 3]. The free energy supply made available when ATP is hydrolysed is buffered by supplies of creatine phosphate and it seems as if the enzyme involved (creatine phosphokinase) has an important function as part of an energy shuttle system within the cardiac cell [4]. Although we believe that the three enzymes systems listed above will satisfactorily account for the initial energy flux the reader need to be warned that in amphibian skeletal muscle the observed initial energy output is usually not in balance with the underlying high energy phosphate breakdown until well after the contractile event [5, 6].

In the classical amphibian skeletal muscle studies (see Hill [7], for the most thorough discussion) it was possible to show that the rapid initial metabolism (I) was followed by the slow evolution of a second phase of heat production. This heat was called the recovery heat (R) and in skeletal muscle takes 20 to 30 min to be released at $0°C$ [8]. Its rate of evolution increases with temperature, the Q_{10} lying between 2 and 3. Now in amphibian skeletal muscle it is clear that providing we are examining twitch or brief tetanic responses the inital and recovery processes are temporally separated even at temperatures as high as $20°C$. The situation is more controversial in cardiac muscle.

Brian Chapman and I maintain that even with glucose as the sole exogenous substrate there is some overlap of the inital and recovery metabolisms in the rabbit myocardium at $20°C$ [9] but Alpert and Mulieri [10] believe that there is virtually complete temporal separation. At normal body temperature and heart rate there can be little doubt that there is substantial overlap. We have calculated on theoretical grounds, and on the basis of our own results, that the recovery heat/initial energy ratio should be close to 0.72. A value very close to this (0.65) has been found experimentally by Alpert's group [11] for rat myocardium but somewhat suprisingly Alpert and Mulieri [10] report a value of 1.46 for the rabbit. The two protocols were quite different (i.e. rat versus rabbit) but the reason for the discrepancy with our rabbit data remains to be resolved. There is general agreement amongst muscle physiologists, however, that the recovery heat can be attributed to the oxidation of carbohydrates, fatty acids and lactate (Krebs cycle) supplemented to a minor extent by substrate level phosphorylations occurring in the cytoplasmic glycolytic and mitochondrial citric acid cycle.

In nearly all the experiments that I will describe the *total* heat (initial & recovery) in a train of contractions has been recorded. My colleagues and I believe that the heat production so measured, including any degraded internal or external work, is a direct measure of the total enthalpy of all the chemical reactions underwriting the mechanical event, see Chapman [3]. Nearly all our experiments over the last 12 years have been run at $27°C$. This represents the highest temperature that we feel is safe for the adequate oxygenation of our preparations with our experimental techniques and protocols [1].

Basal metabolism

Before we can attempt to quantify the energy flux associated with the contractile event we are confronted with the very high 'basal' metabolism of the quiescent heart. This metabolism can be measured either as oxygen consumption or as heat production and it maybe helpful if reader remembers that when biological tissue utilizes oxygen to oxidize carbohydrate or fatty acids there is *approximately* 20 kJ of energy liberated for each litre of oxygen consumed. If a quiescent heart is said to have a basal oxygen consumption rate of $2.0\,ml\ O_2 \cdot 100g \cdot ^{-1}min^{-1}$ this is equivalent to an energy flux of $6.6\,mJ \cdot g^{-1} \cdot s^{-1}\ (mW \cdot g^{-1})$. The oxygen units will be familiar to cardiac physiologists and clinicians whereas the energy units are those most frequently used by muscle physiologists. There is no reason to believe that biochemical events in the quiescent heart are different to those in the beating heart and for that reason I consider the resting heat measurements to have initial and recovery components. For some experimental evidence on this point see Gibbs [12]. In most cardiovascular texts the quiescent metabolism of the human heart is usually estimated to be about $2.0\,ml \cdot O_2 \cdot 100\,g^{-1} \cdot min^{-1}$: the beating human heart is said to consume $8–10\,ml \cdot O_2 \cdot 100\,g^{-1} \cdot min^{-1}$ so that the basal metabolism represents 20 to 25% of the total myocardial oxygen consumption (mVO_2). I confess I have no intuitive feeling as to what the real human basal oxygen consumption rate is likely to be. The $2.0\,ml \cdot 100\,g^{-1} \cdot min^{-1}$ value is largely guessed at by extrapolation from experiments on dogs and I hope to convince you that in the dog and other animals the answer you get depends very much on how you do the experiments. The older literature on the 'arrested heart' is well reviewed by Lochner et al. [13] and I have considered more recent data in several reviews [14].

My interest in basal metabolism started with some myothermic experiments that Brian Chapman and I were doing in 1973 where we noticed that during the course of a day resting heat rate progressively fell without any concurrent decline in mechanical activity [9] and in those same series of experiments it was shown, as predicted from the fluorescent experiments of Chapman [15], that basal metabolism was markedly substrate dependent being about 70% higher with pyruvate present rather than glucose. In 1979 Denis Loiselle and I showed that the temporal decline of heat production was seen across species and that there were large species differences in the magnitude of the basal metabolism; the rat has a very high resting heat rate [16]. Subsequent myothermic studies have always confirmed the temporal decay and to a reasonable approximation the decay occurs experimentally with a half time close to 2 h. At 27° C the basal heat rate of the rabbit papillary muscle measured about 2 h after cardiectomy is close to $2.5\,mW \cdot g^{-1}$ suggesting that prior to excision the rate must be about $5\,mW \cdot g^{-1}$. In an attempt to look at this phenomenon with another technique I have tried polarographic experiments using superfused papillary muscles only to discover that the magnitude of the quiescent oxygen consumption often predicts an energy flux rate 50 to 100% higher than indicated by the heat studies (the experiments are not directly comparable in terms of oxygen tension or end product build up since in the polarographic studies the muscles are superfused whereas in myothermic experiments the muscles are out of solution). In 1979 I was fortunate enough to spend a sabbatical leave with Mark Noble, Angela Drake and Dimitri Papadoyannis [17], and we looked at the basal metabolism of KCl arrested, blood perfused dog hearts on cardiopulmonary bypass. In these experiments at 37° C the arrested O_2 consumption rate was $1.7\,ml \cdot min^{-1} \cdot 100\,g^{-1}$ in experiments where coronary flow was maintained close to its value in the normally beating heart [17] and there was no temporal decay for arrest periods as long as 1 h. The only worry I have about these experiments is that the recordings were obtained after 2–3 h of anaesthesia and the arrest periods were preceded by a 30 min period when the hearts were beating but non-working. Naturally these data raise doubts as to the physiological importance of the time-decay curves seen in isolated preparations. Two additional interesting observations were made. If we switched from blood perfusion to perfusion with Krebs solution within 10 minutes the basal mVO_2 was only $1.2\,ml \cdot 100\,g^{-1} \cdot min^{-1}$ ($\sim 4\,mW \cdot g^{-1}$) and if at the same time perfusion pressure was dropped to about 1/3 normal then the mean basal mVO_2 was only $0.55\,ml \cdot O_2 \cdot 100\,g^{-1}$.

When I returned to Monash I decided to pursue the problem further using both isolated Langendorff hearts and papillary muscles and I was assisted by Denis Loiselle who in fact has subsequently carried out some meticulous myothermic studies on both rabbit and rat papillary muscles and more recently has started collecting data on Langendorff perfused guinea pig hearts. The most surprising finding to come out of these subsequent studies is that the basal or resting heat rate has an unexpectedly low Q_{10} 1.3 to 1.4 [16, 18, 19]. Other authors have reported similar results [13, 20]. As Loiselle [19] has indicated 'A low Q_{10} may arise from a combination of metabolic reactions whose Q_{10} values are high with diffusion processes whose Q_{10} values are low, or from purely metabolic processes whose energies of activation are inherently low ... the relative temperature insensitivity of cardiac basal metabolism in vitro may be due to both factors.'

Loiselle [18] has shown that in rat papillary muscles the rate of basal metabolism is increased by passive stretch although the effect is highly variable from muscle to muscle, see also Gibbs et al. [21] it is only moderately sensitive to oxygen partial pressure and is insensitive to the presence of amino acids in the bathing medium. Using the Langendorff perfused rabbit heart Kotsanas & Gibbs have shown that at $27°\,C$ the basal metabolism is strongly dependent upon the method of arrest. If coronary flow is maintained using a high K^+ low Ca^{++} solution the basal mVO_2 declines rapidly for 15 to 3 minutes and then stabilizes at a value of $1.3\,ml \cdot 100\,g^{-1} \cdot min^{-1}$ ($4.3\,mW \cdot g^{-1}$). If only KCl (20 mM) is used (high K^+) to arrest the hearts then a value as low as $0.5\,ml \cdot 100\,g^{-1} \cdot min^{-1}$ ($1.7\,mW \cdot g^{-1}$) can be obtained. This data is consistent with the rat data of Penpargkul and Scheuer [23]. We have also been able to show the subtrate effect in the isolated perfused heart. Interestingly, we can show a linear dependence of basal mVO_2 on coronary blood flow and that there is a difference in the slope of this dependency with perfusion fluid. Nonetheless, whether we use Krebs solution or perfuse with an erythrocyte enriched Krebs solution, containing albumin [24] the zero flow intercept obtained by back extrapolation is practically identical for all the cardioplegic solutions, and is about $0.42\,ml \cdot O_2 \cdot 100\,g^{-1} \cdot min^{-1}$ ($1.4\,mW \cdot g^{-1}$), a value which is below the myothermic estimates made at a similar time after cardiectomy. Figure 6-1 is a summary diagram of recent myothermic, polarographic and whole heart data.

It is possible to draw up a list of the factors that have been found to alter the magnitude of basal metabolism, see Table 6-1. At the present time we do not know to what extent the different factors interact eg. the size of the heart is influenced by both the end-diastolic volume and the coronary flow rate; coronary

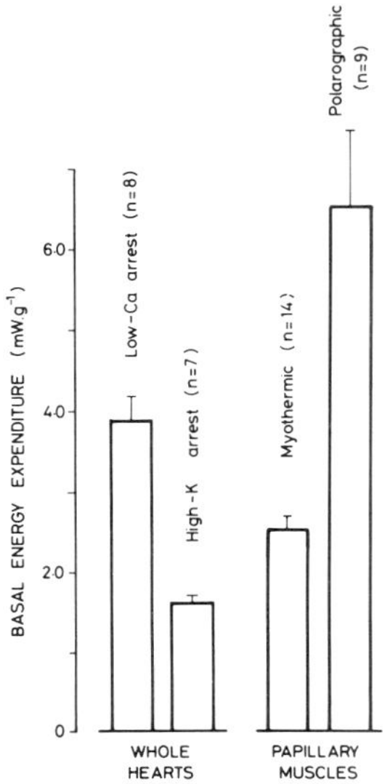

Figure 6-1. Comparison of mean basal energy expenditure in perfused hearts and in papillary muscle preparations at 27° C. In the whole heart experiments n = 8 (low Ca^{++} arrest) and n = 7 (high K^+ arrest). With the papillary muscles n = 14 (myothermic) and n = 9 (polarographic). Oxygen consumption of arrested hearts has been converted to energy units assuming 1 litre O_2 consumed liberates approximately 20 kJ. Unpublished data Kotsanas and Gibbs.

flow rate and perfusion pressure are usually interdependent.

The metabolic basis of the high basal metabolism remains to be established. If we only had to account for the zero flow energy rate of about 1.4 mW/g then this could be done largely in terms of the cost of (i) the Na^+ pump and (ii) protein synthesis, which is not inhibited during cardiac arrest [25]. I have made some calculations about the likely energetic cost [14]. To account for the much higher values that probably occur in vivo we need to consider other possibilities eg. futile cross-bridge cycling, Ca^{++} pump activity, non-phosphorylating respiration [26], futile enzymatic cycles [27]. It seems apparent that a good part of the high basal

Table 1. Factors that alter basal metabolism.

	References
1) Muscle length (EDV)	28, 44, 45
2) Substrate availability	8, 28, 30
3) Perfusion pressure	17, 30
4) Perfusion flow rate	17, 28, 30, 54
5) Oxygen tension	28, 46, 49
6) Activity prior to arrest	44
7) Time after arrest	8, 28, 30, 45, 46, 47, 48, 49
8) Temperature	4, 44, 47, 48, 49
9) Species	44, 48

74

metabolism recorded in rat heart is caused by spontaneous intracellular Ca^{++} oscillations [28].

In myothermic experiments the basal metabolism is the baseline above which active heat measurements are made and for this reason its constancy over the recording time is obviously important. Sometimes it is not possible to assess whether the energy contribution of an identified process such as the Na^+ pump, is to basal or active metabolism. eg. the Na^+-K^+-ATPase is normally continuously active to maintain the electrochemical status quo in the face of the passive influx of Na^+ ions down their concentration gradient but when a preparation is repetitively stimulated it is obvious that the Na^+ load will be increased by the repeated membrane depolarisations and the energy flux could now be considered to be part of the active metabolism [29]. It also is not clear whether this increased influx will be handled within a cardiac cycle or be compensated for much more gradually and hence raise the apparent subsequent basal metabolism. In this regard Lochner et al. [13], report that the level of cardiac activity prior to arrest markedly alters the measured basal metabolism at least in the short term and this would be consistent with a higher Na^+ pump activity.

Active metabolism

It is convenient to discuss active energy flux in terms of isometric (isovolumetric) and isotonic (auxobaric) responses. In the first full-length paper I published on cardiac heat production [21] the energy output of rabbit papillary muscle was altered by varying muscle length. It was obvious in these experiments that there was a curvilinear to linear relationship between isometric heat production and peak developed stress (force/cross sectional area). The curvature of the relationship is more evident at lower temperatures and within certain limits it can be linearized by plotting heat production against total peak stress i.e. active + passive stress.

In Figure 6-2 I show such a relation and the important thing to note is that if a preparation is shortened down to a point on its length: tension relationship where it cannot develop any active force there is still heat production. Following Hill [30] I labelled this component the activation or stress-independent heat component and suggested that it would relate to the cost of the Ca^{++} release and retrieval cycle. Subsequently it was shown that the magnitude of this component was sensitive to the extracellular Ca^{++} concentration and temperature [31] and could be greatly altered (2–3 fold) by various inotropic agents (for review see Gibbs [32]).

This method of measuring the activation heat has certain problems and indeed has been, over the years a source of joy to some referees. In the early 1970's the two most frequent criticisms were that in a shortened down muscle there would still be internal shortening, leading to shortening heat [30, 33] or there would be

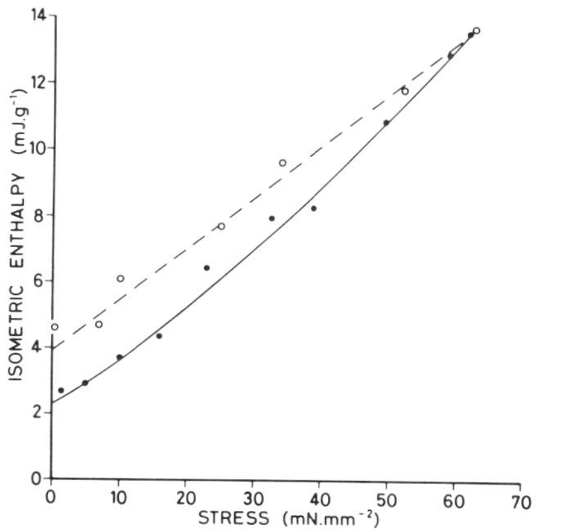

Figure 6-2. Heat:stress relationship obtained by shortening muscle down its length:tension relation (solid line) and by the latency release technique (dashed line). Muscle weighed 3.5 mg and had an l_{max} length of 6.1 mm. Data are averages of 30 contractions @ 1.0 Hz and 27° C.

work against an internal load, cf. Gordon, Huxley & Julian [34]. By the late 70's when the detailed effects of muscle length on activation mechanisms were being sorted out, see Jewell [35] and recent reviews by Stephenson & Wendt [36] and Allen & Kentish [37], the converse and to my mind more valid criticism was made that Ca^{++} release was being inactivated.

Over the last few years Mulieri and Alpert [38], again following a Hill protocol, have used mannitol to make hyperosmotic ($2.5 \times$ N) physiological saline which gradually decreases the mechanical response. Their activation heat values, now measured at l_{max}, are very similar to those obtained in my laboratory but I take no great comfort from this since when I use the mannitol technique and the stimulus frequency used by Alpert & Mulieri (0.2 Hz) I get the same result but when I increase the stimulus frequency to the one I customarily use (1.0 Hz) I get a contracture type response of varying magnitude: the resulting energy flux can then be quite high. I take this to mean that cross bridge activity is certainly not abolished. Recently I have attempted to get around some of these problems by employing a rapid release technique during the latency period following a stimulus. Experimentally a preparation is held at l_{max} for 10–15 msec after a stimulus and is then rapidly (30 mm/s) released to a shorter length where no active force development occurs (see Fig. 6-3). When this is done the measured activation heat increases by about 70% [39]. A similar increment was reported in some polarographic studies by Cooper [40]. This latency release technique can also be used to establish an enthalpy: stress relationship as shown in Fig. 6-2 (dashed line).

It is possible with the latency release techniques estimating activation heat to show that there is a correlation between the magnitude of the activation heat (AH) and peak developed stress (S). If we have a preparation developing a peak stress (force/CSA) of 60 mN/mm² we can predict an activation heat, as measured

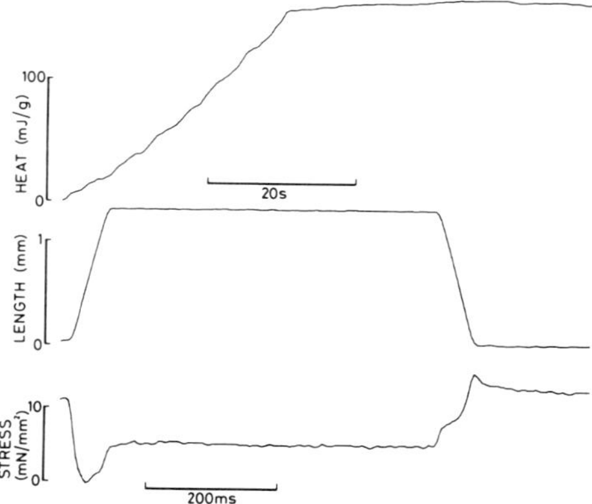

Figure 6-3. Heat and mechanical traces recorded during the latency release method of determining activation heat (see text). Note that there are different time scales. The heat trace shows the total heat in 30 contractions whereas the mechanical traces represent the force and length changes occurring during one contraction in the train. The length step is imposed by an ergometer.

by the latency release method, of $4.1\,mJ \cdot g^{-1}$. The one reservation that I have about this technique is that it gives activation heat magnitudes that are surprisingly high and would require about 100 nanomoles or more Ca^{++}/g tissue to be released per beat in preparations developing $60\,mN/mm^2$ (assuming a Ca^{++} pump stoichiometry of $2\ Ca^{++}/ATP^2$. This result, however, would be consistent with evidence presented by Pierce, Philipson and Langer [41] who suggest that even to achieve half maximal myofibrillar activation a total Ca^{++} release well in excess of 100 nanomoles/g wet weight is required in the intact cardiac cell.

In another set of release experiments the protocol was changed such that the release time throughout a twitch was varied but the release distance was kept constant and was of such a magnitude that there was no redevelopment of active force. The energy flux was measured at each time interval and a correction was made for the internal work removed by the ergometer, for details see Hill [42]. In confirmation of work carried out in whole hearts by Monroe [43] and more recent studies by Elzinga and colleagues it was found that by the peak of a contraction about 84% of the total twitch energy had been committed, a result which is similar to that reported for skeletal muscle by Hill [33]. This result reinforces a view put forward sometime ago by McDonald [44] and ourselves [45, 46] that peak developed tension is a better mechanical predictor of oxygen usage per beat than tension-time integral. Indeed on the basis of our experiments over recent years the total heat production (H_T) in an isometric contraction can be quite accurately predicted by a simple equation of the form:

$$H_T = AH + bS$$
where S = stress (mN/mm^2)

and H_T and AH are in mJ/g. The coefficient b has a value close to 0.16 and is independent of temperature: the exact value depends upon the method used to establish the active heat: stress relationships, see Fig. 6-2, and it can range between 0.12 and 0.2. To follow through the example given before in a twitch contraction developing a peak stress of $60\,mN/mm^2$ the H_T will be

$$H_T = 4.1 + 9.6 = 13.7\,mJ/g.$$

Please note that for isolated muscles or trabeculae there is an inverse relationship between peak stress and CSA. The literature has been summarized in a paper by Delbridge & Loiselle [47] and my only observation is that this inverse relationship has nothing to do with an anoxic core [48] but probably a good deal to do with geometry. My only plea is that when people make across laboratory comparisons they compare the energy output at equivalent stress levels and similar cross-sectional areas; it must also be realised that there is considerable variability in both AH and the coefficient 'b'.

Isotonic experiments

It was recognized early this century that cardiac oxygen consumption increases if the arterial pressure is raised and Sarnoff et al. [49], in one of the classic papers on cardiac energetics showed that myocardial oxygen consumption could not be related in any simple way to the external work of the heart. They also concluded that pressure work was much more costly than volume work. It was therefore, not, surprising to me in my first myothermic experiments on afterloaded rabbit papillary muscles to find that the total energy output per beat increased with afterload [21, 45, 46]. A typical example is shown in Fig. 6-4. About the same time Coleman [50, 51] reported essentially the same result using a polarographic technique, the experiments were done on cat papillary muscles. Following Hill and colleagues, see Hill [7] and Mommaerts [52], I subdivided the energy production into work, activation and stress-dependent heat terms. I have already explained how the heat: stress relationship was obtained and how the activation heat was measured, see Fig. 6-2. In my first paper [21] on cardiac energetics I subtracted out the activation heat, external work, and tension-dependent heat and found that there was energy left over. I was prepared, following Hill's skeletal muscle analysis, to suggest that this surplus heat was associated with shortening. By 1970 I was regretting this conclusion [45, 46] as I realized that I had not allowed for the recovery heat counterpart of the work term. When this type of correction was made it was apparent particularly, over the medium to high afterload range, that there was scarcely any energy surplus.

If my recent experiments upon the activation heat have some validity then there is scarcely any surplus at even the low load levels. I make this statement on

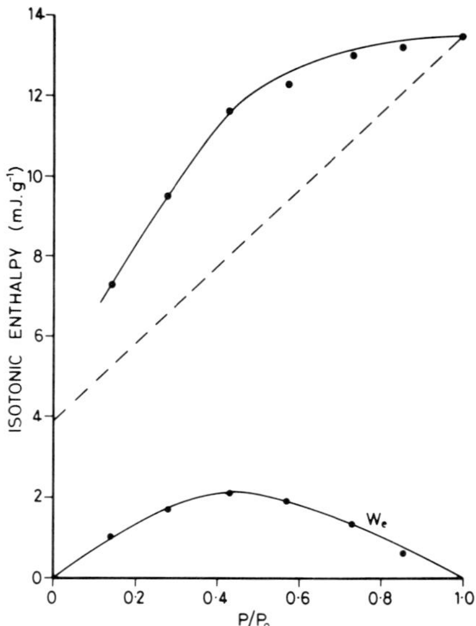

Figure 6-4. The enthalpy:load relationship recorded in a series of afterloaded contractions. All loads expressed as a fraction of the peak isometric force. The data is obtained from the same muscle used in Fig. 6-2. The external work is plotted against load and the isometric enthalpy:stress relationship has been superimposed.

the basis of taking the recovery:initial energy ratio to be 0.72% [9]. Now although current evidence suggests that there is no shortening heat component in cardiac muscle let me make it clear that energy flux does go up when cardiac muscle shortens but the 'extra' energy liberated appears to occur almost solely as the work term and its associated recovery heat. My colleague Brian Chapman would argue, however, that the phenomenological separation of energy output into shortening heat and stress-dependent heat etc. is thermodynamically misleading [3] and can lock us into the idea that work is being performed at almost 100% efficiency, see also Mommaerts [52]. It should always be remembered that in cardiac muscle there is considerable internal shortening even in isometric contractions so one probably should not be too dogmatic about there being no cardiac counterpart of skeletal muscle shortening heat.

On a more practical level it is well established that we have, in cardiac muscle, peak mechanical efficiencies that average about 20% (range 15 to 25%) over the 0.2 to 0.4 P_o load level. These values exclude consideration of basal metabolism and are higher than can be obtained in amphibian sartorius muscles over the complete initial and recovery cycles without special lever systems. These high efficiency values have always worried me somewhat so I was delighted to see that Elzinga and Westerhof, using their working cat heart preparation, also report peak stroke work mechanical efficiencies in the 20 to low 30% range [53]. These high values are obtainable because of the rapid fall off in total enthalpy (heat + work) output at medium to low load levels. At the present time we have no clear understanding as to why this dramatic fall occurs in cardiac muscle but not in skeletal muscle, see Rall [54] for details. Consideration of these mechanical efficiency data set the scene for the final aspect of myocardial energetics that I wish to cover.

Myocardial energetics and the PVA concept

In recent years there has been renewed interest in the pressure-volume relationship of the functioning heart. Results obtained in a variety of species and for both the left and right ventricular chambers show that cardiac mechanical performance can be described by considering it to have time-dependent elastance [55]. When a heart is operating in a stable inotropic state, it has been found that the end-systolic pressure-volume points of each work cycle fall on a straight line regardless of the size of the afterload or preload (end-diastolic pressure) [56].

This result is shown schematically in Fig. 6-5. Of even more interest to those of us interested in cardiac energetics is the demonstration by Suga an colleagues [57] that cardiac oxygen consumption per beat is linearly related to the ventricular systolic pressure volume area (PVA). This area is that bounded by the end-systolic line (V_dDA) and the systolic segment (ABC) of the pressure-volume loop. It emerges that PVA is the sum of (i) the stroke (external) work and (ii) a term that Suga calls the end-systolic potential energy. In an isovolumetric contraction oxygen consumption is maximal and is predicted by the potential energy term alone. Suga has shown that the slope of the relationship between oxygen consumption and PVA is independent of the afterload. If contractility is increased the slope of the PVA: mVO_2 relationship is not changed but there is a parallel shift up the mVO_2 axis [58]. The most remarkable feature of Suga's data is that when the basal and activation components are subtracted from the per beat oxygen consumption all data, regardless of the afterload level, fall on an isoefficiency line, i.e. PVA divided by 'corrected' mVO_2 is constant. The slope of the isoefficiency line is independent of afterload, preload and contractile state and averages close to 40% across different hearts. The implications of this remarkable result have been discussed in some detail recently [55] and here I will briefly reiterate how Dr Suga's data can be reconciled with the existing myothermic and polarographic data shown in Fig. 6-4.

The question that is really being asked is why is the relationship between enthalpy (mVO_2) per beat and afterload curvilinear (energy cost declining as afterload falls) yet the relationship between mVO_2 per beat and PVA is linear. It can be shown that when PVA is plotted against the mean ejection pressure (afterload) for the prevailing physiological conditions the relationship has a curvature that closely resembles that seen in the enthalpy:load diagram of Fig. 6-4

80

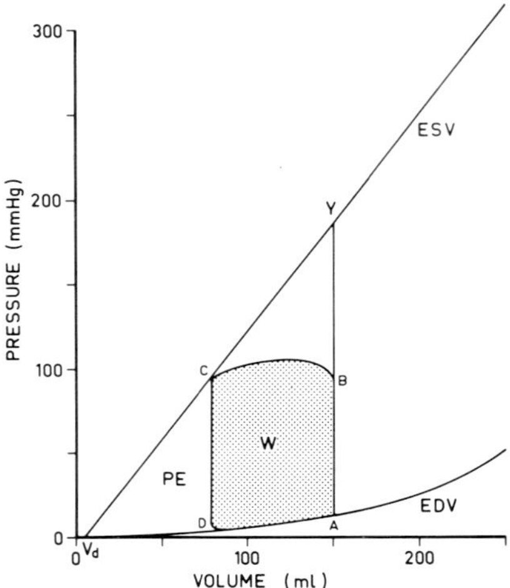

Figure 6-5. Schematic pressure-volume diagram for a human left ventricle. End-systolic pressure-volume line (V_dCY) joins nonzero volume intercept (V_d) to the upper left-hand corner of pressure-volume loop (C). In a totally isovolumetric contraction, peak pressure (Y) would be generated, and V_d, C, and Y lie on the same line under stable inotropic conditions. Pressure-volume area (PVA) in an ejecting contraction is given by sum of stroke work (area labeled W) and potential energy (area labeled PE). In an isovolumetric contraction PVA is given by the entire area enclosed by path V ABYC. This figure is taken from Gibbs and Chapman [60].

[59]. It is then possible to construct an enthalpy: load curve. We measured PVA and then made use of the constant efficiency value to predict *intial* enthalpy and then multiplied that value by 1.71 to get the *total* energy output. In our recent paper [59] I actually constructed an enthalpy: load relationship using an isoefficiency value of 56% when I should have used a value of 68% (I used the thermodynamic efficiency over the initial cycle and this value is somewhat lower, see Chapman [31]). This error on my part does not alter our argument nor the shape of the enthalpy:load curve but it would have decreased the apparent mechanical efficiency (SW/mVO_2).

All the above arguments seemed to suggest agreement between the two quite different sets of experimental results but it seemed worthwhile to make a direct test. For this reason in several recent myothermic experiments with rabbit papillary muscles I have used the Suga analysis to calculate the potential energy term and have then summed the potential energy and external work terms to calculate PVA. I have then removed the cost of the activation heat term from the total enthalpy recorded at the different afterload levels. This analysis then allows one to calculate the PVA efficiency (i.e. PVA energy/total enthalpy-activation heat). The calculated efficiency values are shown in Fig. 6-6 for a typical papillary muscle.

So far the results are in reasonable agreement with Suga's whole heart data i.e. the PVA efficiency is reasonably constant for any given heart. If should be

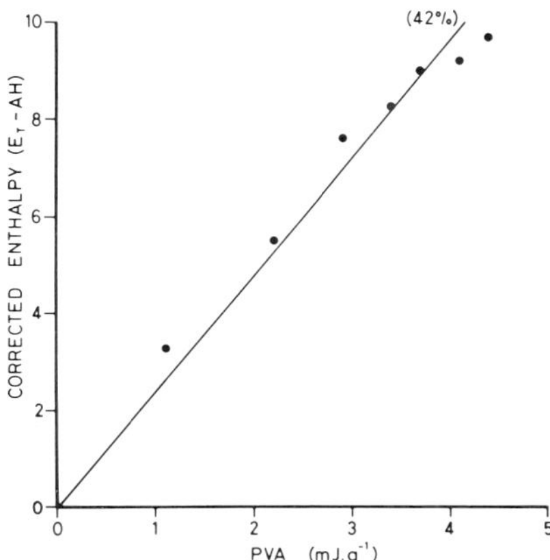

Figure 6-6. Corrected enthalpy (E_T-AH) plotted against PVA. The solid line was fitted by eye and represents a PVA efficiency of 42%. Data for the same preparation used in Figs 6-2 and 6-4.

emphasized however, that this agreement is made possible by using the latency release estimate of the activation heat magnitude. If the real activation heat magnitude is much lower then the PVA efficiency will be far from constant at light afterloads. In all the hearts I have analysed in this way the mean PVA efficiency has ranged from values in the low 30's to values in the high 40's. The mean value will be close to 40%. There is a clear tendency, however, for the PVA efficiency values to be constant over the 0.5 to 1.0 P_o afterload range but to fall off somewhat at afterload levels in the 0.1 to 0.2 P_o load range. This means that in experimental terms we have a slightly higher energy output under the lightest afterloads than the whole heart oxygen consumption data would predict.

Now both Brian Chapman and I believe that the contractile unit in cardiac muscle is not greatly different to the contractile unit skeletal muscle yet as we have attempted to show elsewhere [60] this type of data which implies that there is a stoichiometric relation between ATP consumption and the manifestation of pressure-volume potential energy raises some quite difficult problems for current muscle models.

It is clear that the Suga analysis will not work on most published amphibian skeletal muscle data because there is far too much enthalpy production in the light to medium afterload range. The tortoise data obtained by Woledge [60] may be an exception but these were obtained in tetanic contractions. The Suga analysis can account for the skeletal muscle isometric energy production, with the important proviso that the potential energy must be calculated from the experimentally determined *twitch* length:tension relationship as deduced from afterloaded isotonic shortening. If the tetanic length:tension relationship is used to calculate PVA there is far too much enthalpy predicted! The statements made above about skeletal muscle are based on a reanalysis of data, see Fig. 6-7, obtained on

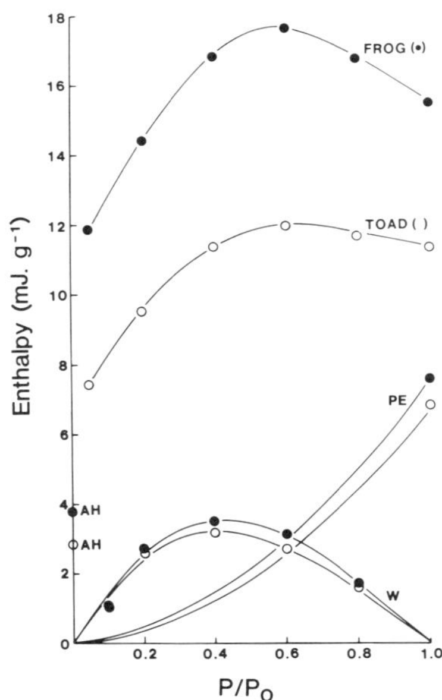

Figure 6-7. Enthalpy versus load relationships recorded in amphibian skeletal muscle at 10° C. Data taken from Tables I and II of Gibbs and Chapman [62]. The potential energy term, PE, has been calculated from the length:load relationship in afterloaded isotonic twitch contractions. If the work term, W, and the PE term are summed it gives an 'equivalent' PVA. The PVA efficiency can be calculated provided the activation heat is subtracted from the initial enthalpy. Activation heat estimates are provided on the enthalpy axis.

amphibian (frog and toad) sartorius muscles at 10° C by Brian Chapman and me [61].

Figure 6-7 shows not only the initial enthalpy at different load levels but also the external work and the calculated potential energy: the assumed activation heat magnitudes are also indicated. The calculated PVA efficiency for the isometric case (both muscles) is close to 70% (only the initial energy was being measured in these experiments). It really does appear as if in the shortening skeletal muscle there is some internal load being encountered. This means that more ATP molecules have to be hydrolysed as the velocity of shortening increases. Whether this internal load is just physical e.g., a frictional force, or whether it can be accounted for in crossbridge terms by say having the detachment rate constant, g_2, in the Huxley model [62] set at much lower levels relative to the attachment rate constant, f, (skeletal compared to cardiac) I cannot say but I do believe that Suga's observations are very important and it is essential that his data be reconcilable with current crossbridge models.

Summary

The energy output of cardiac muscle is best understood in terms of biochemical criteria (specific ATPases) but certain operational definitions can be used to partition the energy flux. This chapter reviewed some of the uncertainties that exist at the present time in subdividing the myocardial energy output. The total energy flux can classically be divided into an initial term (usage of stored high energy phosphates, HEP's) and a recovery term (oxidative and glycolytic re-synthesis of HEP's from available substrate). My colleagues and I believe that there is some temporal overlap of these two components, even at $20°$ C, and that the recovery to initial energy ratio is about: this view is perhaps not universally accepted. A large fraction of the heart's energy output, perhaps 25%, is still seen in an arrested heart. This 'basal' metabolism is affected by a variety of factors that include end-diastolic volume, substrate availability, perfusion pressure and flow, activity prior to arrest, time after arrest, temperature and species: its biochemical and physiological basis is poorly understood. The active metabolism per beat can be interpreted in terms of (i) a stress-independent or activation heat component that is largely but not completely identified with the calcium release and retrieval cycle, and (ii) a work and stress-dependent heat term which are associated with actomyosin ATPase activity (cross bridge turnover). A brief consideration was presented of how both the activation and crossbridge terms change with alterations in contractility. Existing methods of measuring the activation heat were outlined, their drawbacks discussed and a new method for measuring this component was described. The energetic cost of work and/or stress-development were examined in both isometric and isotonic contractions. It was shown that the afterload regulates the per beat enthalpy production (the Fenn effect) and that the peak mechanical efficiency is in the 20 to 30% range and is achieved at relatively low afterloads. Existing myothermic and polarographic data were reconciled with Suga's pressure-volume area (PVA) concept and it was shown that if the basal and activation components are subtracted out rabbit papillary muscles function at constant PVA efficiency except perhaps at light loads $(0-0.2 P_0.)$. The PVA concept cannot account for the enthalpy output of amphibian skeletal muscles (twitch response) except at high loads $(\sim1.0 P_0.)$: nonetheless the maximal calculated PVA efficiency is similar to that determined for cardiac muscle.

References

1. Gibbs, C.L.: Cardiac energetics. Physiol. Rev. 58: 174–254, 1978.
2. Gibbs, C.L. and Chapman, L.B.: Cardiac energetics. In: Handbook of Physiology. The Cardiovascular System I., pp 775–804, Berne, R.M., N. Sperelakis, and S.R. Geiger (Eds.) American Physiological Society, Bethesda, Md, 1979.

3. Chapman, J.B: Heat production. In: Cardiac metabolism pp 239–256, Drake-Holland, A.J. & Noble, M.I.M. (Eds), Wiley, 1983.

4. Jacobus, W.E., and Lehninger, A.L.: Creatine kinase of rat heart mitochondria. Coupling of creatine phosphorylation to electron transport. J. Biol. Chem. 248, 4803–4810, 1973.

5. Curtin, N.A. and Woledge, R.C.: Energy changes and muscular contraction Physiol. Rev. 58: 690–761, 1978.

6. Homsher, E. and Kean, C.J.: Skeletal muscle energetics and metabolism. Ann. Rev. Physiol. 40: 93–131, 1978.

7. Hill, A.V.: Trails and Trials in Physiology. London Arnold, 1965.

8. Hartree, W. and Hill, A.V.: The recovery heat production of muscle. J. Physiol. Lond. 56: 367–381, 1922.

9. Chapman, J.B. and Gibbs, C.L.: The effect of metabolic substrate on mechanical activity and heat production in papillary muscle. Cardiovasc. Res. 8: 656–667, 1974.

10. Alpert, N.R. and Mulieri, L.A.: Increased myothermal economy of isometric force generation in compensated cardiac hypertrophy induced by pulmonary artery constriction in rabbit. A characterization of heat liberation in normal and hypertrophied right ventricular papillary muscles. Circ. Res. 50: 491–500.

11. Holubarsch, Ch., Alpert, N.R., Goulette, R. and Mulieri, L.A.: Heat production during hypoxfcic contracture of rat myocardium. Circ. Res. 51: 777–786, 1982.

12. Gibbs, C.L.: The energy output of normal and anoxic cardiac muscle. In: Comparative Physiology of the Heart: Current Trends, pp 78–92, McCann, F.V. (Ed.) Birkhauser Verlag, Basel, 1969.

13. Lochner, W., Arnold, G. and Muller-Ruchholtz, E.R.: Metabolism of the artificially arrested and gas-perfused heart. Am. J. Cardiol. 22, 299–311, 1968.

14. Gibbs, C.L.: Thermodynamics and cardiac energetics. In: Microvascular, rheological, metabolic and heat transfer aspects of the heart: relation to ischemia and thrombosis. p 259–270.

15. Chapman, J.B.: Fluorometric studies of oxidative metabolism in isolated papillary muscle of the rabbit. J. Gen. Physiol. 59: 135–154, 1972.

16. Loiselle, D.S. and Gibbs, C.L.: Factors affecting the metabolism of resting rabbit papillary muscle. Pflugers Arch. 396: 285–291, 1983.

17. Gibbs, C.L., Papadoyannis, D.E., Drake, A.J. and Noble, M.I.M.: Oxygen consumption of the nonworking and potassium chloride-arrested dog heart. Circ. Res. 47: 408–417, 1980.

18. Loiselle, D.S.: The rate of resting heat production of rat papillary muscle. Pflugers Arch. 405: 155–162, 1985a.

19. Penpargkul, S. and Scheuer, J.: Metabolic comparisons between hearts arrested by calcium deprivation or potassium excess. Am. J. Physiol. 217: 1405–1412, 1969.

20. Bretschneider, H.J., Hubner, G., Knoll, D., Lohr, B., Nordbeck, H. and Spieckermann, P.G.: Myocardial resistance and tolerance to ischemia:physiological and biochemical basis. J. Cardiovasc. Surg. 16: 241–260, 1975.

21. Gibbs, C., Mommaerts, W.F.H.M. and Ricchiuti, N.V.: Energetics of cardiac contractions. J. Physiol. 191, 25–46, 1967.

22. Kotsanas, G. and Gibbs, C.L.: Factors regulating basal metabolism of the isolated perfused rabbit heart. Am. J. Physiol. (In press) 1986.

23. Penpargkul, S. and Scheuer, J.: Metabolic comparisons between hearts arrested by calcium deprivation or potassium excess. Am. J. Physiol. 217: 1405–1412, 1969.

24. Bergmann, S.R., Clark, R.E. and Sobel, B.F.: An improved isolated heart preparation for external assessment of myocardial metabolism. Am. J. Physiol. 236: H644–H651, 1979.

25. Schreiber, S.S., Hearse, D.J., Oratz, M. and Rothschild, M.A.: Protein synthesis in prolonged cardiac arrest. J. Molec. Cell. Cardiol. 9: 87–100, 1977.

26. Challoner, D.R.:Respiration in myocardium. Nature XV 217, 78–79, 1968.

27. Scrutton, M.C. and Utter, M.F.: The regulation of glycolysis and gluconeogenesis in animal

tissues. Ann. Rev. Biochem. 37: 249–302, 1968.

28. Kort, A.A. and Lakatta, E.G.: Calcium-dependent mechanical oscillations occur spontaneously in unstimulated mammalian cardiac tissues. Circ. Res. 54: 396–404, 1984.

29. Chapman, J.B., Gibbs, C.L., and Gi Wbson, W.R.: Effects of calcium and sodium on cardiac contractility and heat production in rabbit papillary muscle. Circ. Res. 27: 601–610.

30. Hill, A.V.: The heat of activation and the heat of shortening in a muscle twitch. Proc. Roy. Soc. Lond. B 136: 195–211, 1949.

31. Gibbs, C.L. and Vaughan, P.: The effect of calcium depletion upon the tension-independent component of cardiac heat production. J. Gen. Physiol. 52: 532–549, 1968.

32. Gibbs, C.L.: Modification of the physiological determinants of cardiac energy expenditure by pharmacological agents. Pharmacology and Therapeutics 18: 133–152, 1982.

33. Hill, A.V.: The variation of total heat production in a twitch with velocity of shortening. Proc. Roy. Soc. Lond. B 159: 596–605, 1964b.

35. Jewell, B.R.: A re-examination of the influence of muscle length on myocardial performance. Circ. Res. 40: 221–230, 1977.

36. Stephenson, D.G. and Wendt, I.R.: Length dependence of changes in sarcoplasmic calcium concentration and myofibrillar calcium sensitivity in striated muscle fibres. J. Muscle Res. Cell Motil. 5: 243–272, 1984.

37. Allen, D.G. and Kentish, J.C.: The cellular basis of the length-tension relation in cardiac muscle. J. Molec. Cell. Cardiol. 17: 821–840, 1985.

38. Mulieri, L.A. and Alpert, N.R.: Activation heat and latency relaxation in relation to calcium movement in skeletal and cardiac muscle. Can. J. Physiol. Pharmacol. 60: 529–541, 1982.

39. Gibbs, C.L.: Effects of ergometer releases on the energy output of rabbit papillary muscles. Proc. Aust. Physiol. Pharmacol. Soc. 16: 183P, 1985.

40. Cooper, G.: Myocardial energetics during isometric twitch contractions of cat papillary muscles. Am. J. Physiol. 23: H244–H253, 1979.

41. Pierce, G.N., Philipson, K.D. and Langer, G.A.: Passive calcium-buffering capacity of a rabbit ventricular homogenate preparation. Am. J. Physiol. 249: C248–C255, 1985.

42. Hill, A.V.: The series elastic component of muscle. Proc. Roy. Soc. Lond. B 137: 273–280, 1950.

43. Monroe, R.G.: Myocardial oxygen consumption during ventricular contraction and relaxation. Circ. Res. 14: 294–300, 1964.

44. McDonald, R.H.: Developed tension: a major determinant of myocardial oxygen consumption. Am. J. Physiol 210: 251–256, 1966.

45. Gibbs, C.L. and Gibson, W.R.: Effect of alterations in the stimulus rate upon energy output, tension development and tension time integral of cardiac muscle in rabbits. Circ. Res. 27: 611–618, 1970a.

46. Gibbs, C.L. and Gibson, W.R.: Energy production in cardiac isotonic contractions, J. Gen. Physiol. 56: 732–750, 1970b.

47. Delbridge, L.M. and Loiselle, D.S.: An ultrastructural investigation into the size dependency of contractility of isolated cardiac muscle. Cardiovasc. Res. 15: 21–27, 1981.

48. Loiselle, D.S.: Stretch-induced increase in resting metabolism of isolated papillary muscle. Biophys. J. 38: 185–195, 1982.

49. Sarnoff, S.J., Braunwald, E., Welch, G.H., Case, R.B., Stainsby, W.N. and Macruz, R.: Hemodynamic determinants of oxygen consumption of the heart with special reference to the tension-time index. Am. J. Physiol. 192: 148–156, 1958.

50. Coleman, H.N.: Effect of alterations in shortening and external work on oxygen consumption of cat papillary muscle. Am. J. Physiol. 214: 100–106, 1968.

51. Coleman, H.N., Sonnenblick, E.H. and Braunwald, E.: Myocardial oxygen consumption associated with external work: The Fenn effect. Am. J. Physiol. 217: 291–296, 1969.

52. Mommaerts, W.F.H.M.: Energetics of muscular contraction. Physiol. Rev. 49: 427–508, 1969.

53. Elzinga, G. and Westerhof, N.: Pump function and the feline left heart: changes with heart rate

86

and its bearing on the energy balance. Cardiovasc Res. 14: 81–92, 1980.

54. Rall, J.A.: Sense and nonsense about the Fenn effect. Am. J. Physiol. 242: H1–H6, 1982.

55. Suga, H., Sagawa, K. and Shoukas, A.A.: Load independence of the instantaneous pressure-volume ratio of the canine left ventricle and effects of epinephrine and heart rate on the ratio. Circ. Res. 32: 314–322, 1973.

56. Sunagawa, K. and Sagawa, K.: Models of ventricular contraction based on time-varying elastance. CRC Crit. Rev. Biomed. Eng. 7: 193–228, 1982.

57. Suga, H., Hayashi, T. and Shirahata, M.: Ventricular systolic pressure-volume area as predictor of cardiac oxygen consumption. Am. J. Physiol., 240 (Heart Circ. Physiol. 9): H30–H44, 1981.

58. Suga, H., Hisano, R., Goto, Y., Yamada, O. and Igashari, Y.: Effect of positive inotropic agents on the relation between oxygen consumption and systolic pressure volume area in canine left ventricle. Circ. Res. 53: 306–318, 1983.

59. Gibbs, C.L. and Chapman, J.B.: The effect of stimulus conditions and temperature upon the energy output of frog and toad sartorii. Am. J. Physiol. 227: 964–971, 1974.

60. Woledge, R.C.: The energetics of tortoise muscle. J. Physiol. (London) 197: 685–707.

61. Gibbs, C.L. and Chapman, J.B.: Cardiac mechanics and energetics: chemomechanical transduction in cardiac muscle. Am. J. Physiol. 249: H199–H206, 1985.

62. Huxley, A.F.: Muscle structure and theories of contraction. Prog. Biophys. Biophys. Chem. 7: 255–318, 1957.

7. Energetics of the heart

MARK I.M. NOBLE

Introduction

Dr. Gibbs' presentation once again demonstrates his large and unique contributions to the field of cardiac energetics. Apart from some studies of myocardial oxygen consumption, this is a field in which I have worked very little.

Initial and recovery energy flux

Dr. Gibbs did not include the evidence that these fluxes are reflected in the concentrations of ATP and phosphocreatine present in the heart. Initial excitement about the possibility of cyclical changes in these compounds during the cardiac cycle (using NMR) has not been sustained. In my reading, I have not come across any solid published study establishing this fact. Nor have I encountered any such studies showing that increased heart activity (e.g. sudden increase in heart rate) leads to a temporary fall in these compounds. This is of considerable interest in relation to the question of control of ATP synthesis to exactly match ATP utilisation rate. It appears to be commonly assumed that this is a simple negative feedback control mediated by a change in [ATP], [ADP]/[ATP] ratio, phosphocreatine, inorganic phosphate or some combination of this group of molecules. In an intact heart, which is now amenable to study by NMR techniques, it should be possible to settle this question. No definitive study of this type has been published to my knowledge.

While this is the most obvious hypothesis, I suspect that doubt is creeping into the mind of some cardiac energeticists. I have the impression that mean intracellular calcium is now being postulated in some quarters (e.g. Paul England at the 1985 Spring Meeting of the Cardiac Muscle Research Group in Edinburgh) as the mediator of the matching mechanism. In the paced non-working blood perfused dog heart [1] the linear relationship between myocardial oxygen consumption and heart rate may readily be explained on the basis of such a hypothesis. With increasing numbers of calcium release an uptake cycles, mean cytoplasmic calcium ion concentration will rise and this will increase the ATP synthesis rate of mitochondria. However, this component of myocardial oxygen consumption corresponds to the first component of active metabolism discussed by Dr. Gibbs, namely 'a stress-independent or activation heat component that is largely but not completely identified with the calcium release and retrieval cycle.' The hypothesis must fall down however when one makes the heart generate pressure, this gives a corresponding increase in oxygen consumption, but as far as we know from isolated muscle work, no corresponding increase in intracellular calcium ion concentration.

The initial 'burst of energy liberation'

Monroe showed many years ago (and it has recently been confirmed by Elzinga [2] that 90% plus of the oxygen consumption of the heart is consumed in the first part of systole involved in generating pressure and accelerating blood. During the remainder of systole the heart 'free-wheels.'

In skeletal muscle tetani there is more energy in terms of heat liberated to 'start up' tension initially than to maintain it. This phenomenon in heart cannot be explained by calcium pumping which occurs during *relaxation* or by sodium pumping which occurs during diastole. The explosive release of calcium internally upon depolarisation should not be exothermic. In the case of skeletal muscle, calcium pumping continues throughout the tetanus in which maintenance heat is much lower than initial heat. In my opinion, no adequate explanation has been given for this 'start up' phenomenon other than that of Iwazumi, which depends on the assumption of an electrostatic mechanism of muscle contraction [3]. His explanation, which I heard at an earlier meeting, is that there is a reversible entropy change due to reorientation of muscle water during myosin activation. Water is normally polarised in multilayers with alternation of polarity of adjacent dipole molecule [4]. Myosin activation caused a larger electric field which orients all the molecules to the same polarity, analogous to the formation of ice, ie exothermal entropy change.

The PVA concept

Most of the correlations between left ventricular pressure, (integrated in one way or another) plus/or work (including PVA), and oxygen consumption give quite reasonable correlation coefficients [2]. However, they may all give a false impression in view of the finding, by Monroe in the early 60s, that most of the oxygen consumed in a single beat occurs in the first 50 msec during pressure development and acceleration of blood. If he was right, most of the pressure (included in the various integrations that are correlated with oxygen consumption) is not contributing at all. Using other critical ways of looking at these haemodynamic predictors of oxygen consumption, Elzinga concluded '... differences in prediction between indices which have been claimed to be very reliable measures of cardiac oxygen consumption shows that our ignorance in heart muscle is comparable to that of frog skeletal muscle ...'

Effect of perfusion pressure and flow and substrate availability

We have recently carried out studies in beating hearts (as opposed to the arrested hearts mentioned in Gibbs' chapter) which show, in our opinion, that perfusion pressure and flow are not true determinants of oxygen consumption, but merely act indirectly via changes in the mechanics of the ventricular wall (e.g. garden hose or erectile effect) [5]. Older studies [6], showed no effect of changing substrate, in contrast to the effect found by Gibbs on basal metabolism.

References

1. Gibbs, C.L., Papadoyannis, D.E., Drake, A.J. and Noble, M.I.M.: Oxygen consumption of the non-working and potassium chloride-arrested dog heart. Circulation Res 47: 408–417, 1980.
2. Iwzumi, T.: A new field theory of muscle contraction. University Microfilms, Ann Arbor, Michigan, 1970.
3. Ling, G.N.: In Search of the Physical Basis of Life. Plenum Press, 1985.
4. Elzinga, G.: Cardiac oxygen consumption and the production of heat and work. In Cardiac Metabolism, Ed. AJ Drake-Holland and MIM Noble, J Wiley, New York, 173–194, 1983.
5. Drake-Holland, A.J., Elzinga, G., Noble, M.I.M., ter Keurs, H.E.D.J. and Wempe, F.N.: The effect of palmitate and lactate on mechanical performance and metabolism of cat and rat myocardium. J. Physiol. 339: 1–15, 1983.
6. Vergroesen, I., Noble, M.I.M., Wieringa, P.A., Spaan, J.A.E.: Quantification of oxygen-consumption and arterial pressure as independent determinants of coronary flow. Amer. J. Physiol. (H) in press, 1986.

General discussion of the energetics of cardiac muscle

It was underlined that one needs understanding of the basic mechanism of energy turnover at a cellular level before the energetics of the structurally complex heart interacting with the vascular system can be understood fully. This is for example relevant during a contraction of the ventricle in which energy is accumulated in the elastic structures that serves as the driving energy for rapid filling.

8. On the force-length relation in myocardium

HENK E.D.J. TER KEURS, JONATHAN C. KENTISH
and JEROEN J.J. BUCX

Introduction

The enigma that puzzles those who study cardiac pump function is 'what controls
the force of the heartbeat?' Classical work of Ringer [1], Frank [2], Starling [3],
Bowditch [4], Sarnoff [5] and Barany [6] unraveled the main determinants of
contraction of the myocardium:
- Composition of the extracellular milieu [1]
- Interval between the heartbeats [4]
- Intrinsic properties of the crossbridges [6]
- Neurohumoral control mechanisms [5] and
- muscle length [2, 3]

In this chapter we will review some of our studies that pertain to the mechanism
that underlies the relation between muscle length and force development. We
will present evidence that the force generated by cardiac muscle varies with cell
length because of the effect of varied overlap between the contractile filaments of
the sarcomeres on the sensitivity of the contractile system to activator Ca^{2+}. The
results are pertinent to different species and can be recognized in the endsystolic
pressure volume relations found in the intact heart [7].

Methods

Sarcomere length (SL) in the central part of trabeculae from rat, ferret and sheep
heart was measured by laser diffraction, as described previously [7]. In short, the
intensity distribution of the first order diffraction pattern was monitored by a
photodiode array which was scanned electronically every 0.5 ms. The median SL
was computed electronically after a correction had been made for the contribution of light scattered from the zeroth order. Muscle length was measured and
controlled with a servo motor with a capacitive length transducer. The force
transducer was a semiconductor strain gauge with a short carbon fiber extension

arm. The muscles were superfused at 2 ml/min with an oxygenated saline [7] containing various Ca^{2+} concentrations and were stimulated at 0.2 Hz. After a 30 min period for stabilization of the muscles, the force–SL relations were determined as follows. First the muscle length was set to give a resting SL of 2.10–2.15 μm. After 6 control contractions muscle length was altered for four beats. The resting force and resting SL were measured just before the fourth beat and the total force and active SL were measured at peak force during the fourth beat (Fig. 8-1). Active force in the muscle was calculated as the total force at the SL at the peak of contraction minus the resting force at the same SL; this assumes that the parallel elastic elements are in or in parallel with the sarcomere alone [7].

The muscle was then skinned (cell membranes destroyed) by a 30 minute superfusion with 'relaxing solution' (see ref. 8 for details of solutions) to which 1% Triton X-100 had been added. This 'skinning solution' and all subsequent solutions were pumped through the bath at 1 ml/min. The skinned muscle was then bathed in solutions containing 1 nM to 200 μM free Ca^{2+}. The method used to establish the relationships between force and SL at a given Ca^{2+} concentration is illustrated in Fig. 8-1B. First a 'reference' contracture was produced by changing from the relaxing solution (free Ca^{2+} = 0.3 μM) to an 'activating solution' containing 4.3 μM free Ca^{2+} (Fig. 8-1B Panel A). During the reference contracture the SL was maintained at 2.1 μm by stretching the muscle. The muscle was then relaxed for 2 min and was activated with an activating solution of the desired [Ca^{2+}] (up to 200 μM) for 2 or 3 minutes. In the last minute, by which time force and SL were steady (Fig. 8-1B) muscle length changes were imposed for about 5 s. Force and SL were measured when they had reached new steady values during each stretch or release. After the series of length changes shown in Fig. 8-1B the muscle was returned to relaxing solution and the reference contracture was repeated (Fig. 8-1B Panel C). The forces in the first and second reference contractures were used to correct for the loss of contractile force in the skinned preparations. The protocol shown in Fig. 8-1B was repeated for a range of Ca^{2+} concentrations from 1 nM to 200 μM.

Results

Force–sarcomere length relations in intact muscle of rat

Force–sarcomere length relations, derived from a typical trabecula with a protocol as in Fig. 1A at extracellular Ca^{2+} concentrations that were varied between 0.3 and 2.5 mM are shown in Fig. 8-2. The mean resting force, which was the same in all Ca^{2+} concentrations, was negligible between 'slack' sarcomere length (about 1.9 μm) and a SL of 2.2 μm and increased nearexponentially as the SL was increased above this sarcomere length (results not shown [9]). Above a SL of about 2.2 μm further stretch of the muscle produced little increase in the length of

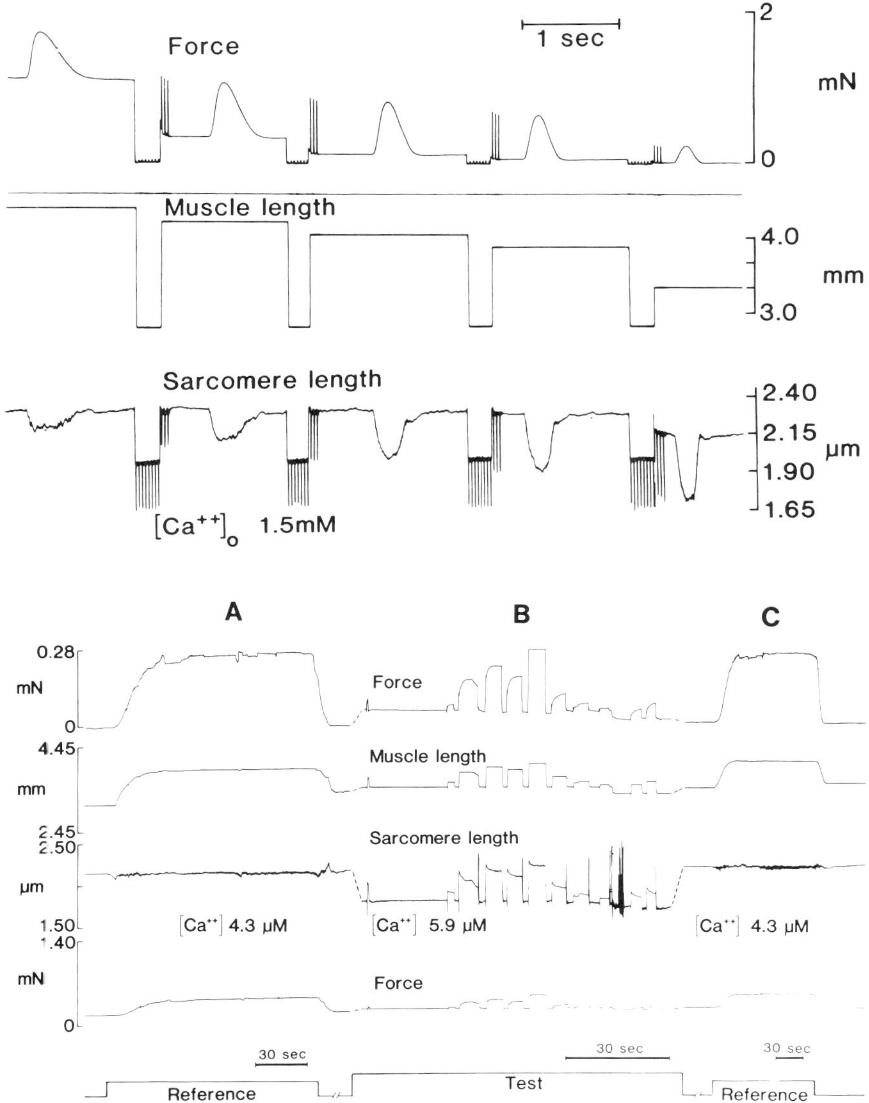

Figure 8-1. A. Experimental protocol used to establish the force–sarcomere length relations in the intact trabecula. In the example shown the bathing $[Ca^{2+}]$ was 1.5 mM. The muscle was stimulated at 0.2 Hz and stretched to different lengths for four beats. Note the different chart speeds. Considerable sarcomere shortening was seen during contraction. B. The protocol for the determination of the force–sarcomere length relations in the skinned muscle. The muscle was activated for 2 or 3 min. by a known concentration of Ca^{2+} in the test solution (5.9 µM in this case) and in the last minute the muscle was stretched transiently to different lengths (panel B). To correct for any deterioration in the contractile performance of the muscles during this protocol, the muscle was bathed in a 'reference' solution of 4.3 µM Ca^{2+} before and after the test solution (panels A and C) (from ref. [9] with permission).

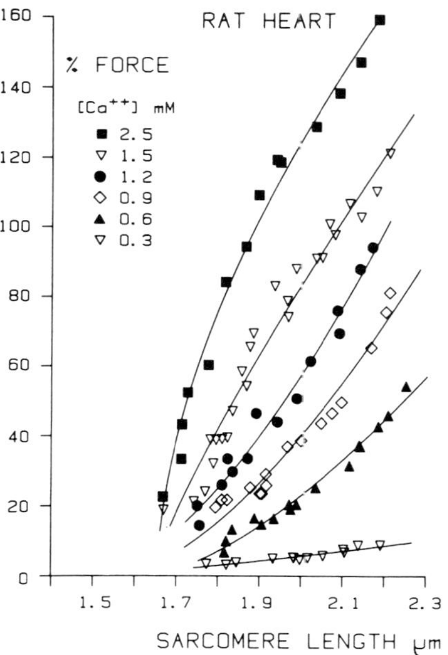

Figure 8-2. Force–sarcomere length relations of an intact trabecula from rat heart. A shows active force taken as total force at a peak of contraction minus the resting force borne at the sarcomere length measured at peak contraction. The concentration of Ca^{2+} was 2.5 (■), 1.5 (∇), 1.2 (●), 0.9 ($\triangle$), 0.6 (▲) or 0.3 (∇) mM.

the sarcomeres in the centre of the resting muscle. This behavior indicates that the elastic elements in parallel with the sarcomeres were extremely stiff (viz. 7).

As in the resting muscle, in the actively contracting muscle sarcomere lengths above about 2.35 μm were never seen, even if the muscle was highly stretched. No active force was developed below a SL of 1.5 μm–1.6 μm. The force (F)–sarcomere length (SL) relations were fitted to $F = a . (SL-SL_o)^c$ by nonlinear least squares analysis [10]. The relationship between force and SL was curved away from the SL axis at Ca_o^{2+} higher than 1 mM and curved toward the SL axis at lower Ca_o^{2+}.

Force development and force–sarcomere length relations in skinned muscle

Considerable internal shortening occurred during contraction of the skinned muscles. Fig. 8-1B shows force development of a skinned trabecula superfused with an activating solution of $Ca^{2+} = 4.3\,\mu$M and held at constant sarcomere length. It can be seen that 7–20% stretch of the muscle was needed to keep sarcomere length constant.

Force and SL measured from recordings at various Ca^{2+} concentrations (Fig.

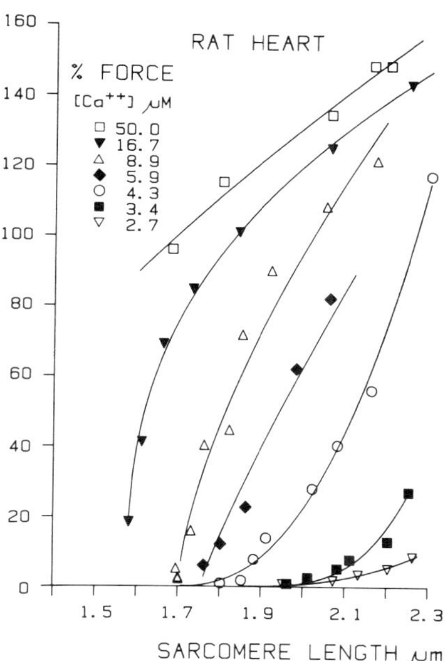

Figure 8-3. shows active force in a trabecula after skinning at seven Ca^{2+} concentrations between the threshold and the saturating concentration.

8-1) were used to plot a family of force–SL relations at Ca^{2+} concentrations from 1 nM to 50 µM. Ca^{2+} concentrations from 1 nM to 0.7 µM did not produce activation of the skinned muscles. As the SL was increased above 2.0 µm the passive force increased from zero, but this increase was less steep than in the same muscles before they had been skinned (results not shown).

At Ca^{2+} concentrations above 0.7 µM active force was developed (Fig. 8-3). The absolute force at SL = 2.00 µm in the skinned preparations at 8.9 µM was about 15% higher than in the intact trabeculae at Ca_o^{2+}. Note the similarity of the force-sarcomere length relations shown in Fig. 2 and 3 which are taken from different trabeculae (see also ref. [9]).

We compared force–SL relations in same muscles before and after they had been skinned [8]. Variables as the external geometry of the preparation and the number of myofibrils were constant throughout in this comparison. It is clear (Fig. 8-3) that the shape of the force–SL relation depended largely on the $[Ca^{2+}]$. The curves for Ca^{2+} concentrations up to 8.9 µM were similar in shape to, though slightly steeper than, those for the unskinned muscles at extracellular Ca^{2+} concentrations of 1.5 mM (cf. Figs. 8-2 and 8-3). At maximally activating Ca^{2+} concentrations the relation was approximately straight and at SL = 1.6 µm considerably more force was generated than in the intact muscles. Data at such high Ca^{2+} concentrations were obtained relatively infrequently because of partial or complete loss of the diffraction pattern that was irreversible in some muscles, particularly at high sarcomere lengths.

The Force–[Ca^{2+}] relations of skinned muscles

The force–[Ca^{2+}] relations, derived from the force-sarcomere length relations in the skinned muscles [8] were approximated by sigmoid on a semi logarithmic scale (Fig. 8-4A). These curves showed that increases in SL shifted the Ca^{2+}-activation curves to the left i.e. to lower Ca^{2+} concentrtions. This increase in Ca^{2+}-sensitivity with SL appeared to be present at all sarcomere lengths in the range 1.7–2.3 μm.

The curves were fitted by non-linear least squares analysis [10] to the modified Hill equation:

$$F = F_{MAX} \frac{[Ca^{2+}]^n \times 100\%}{K^* + [Ca^{2+}]^n}$$

where:

F = developed force,
n = the Hill coefficient, (cf. Table II)
K* = a compound affinity constant
F$_{MAX}$ = maximal F at that sarcomere length

The [Ca^{2+}] for 50% activation was then given by:

$$\log[Ca^{2+}] = (\log 10 K^*)/n.$$

or

$$pCa = -(\log_{10} K^*)/n.$$

The [Ca^{++}] for 50% activation decreased from 9.53 μM to 3.77 $\pm$ 0.32 (mean $\pm$ SEM) in proportion to an increase in sarcomere length between 1.65 and 2.15 μm. The Hill coefficient increased slightly from 2.82 $\pm$ 0.23 to 4.54 $\pm$ 0.74 (n = 6 $\pm$ SEM; cf: [9]) but significantly (p<0.02, as determined by linear regression) with increasing sarcomere length between 1.75 and 2.15 μm.

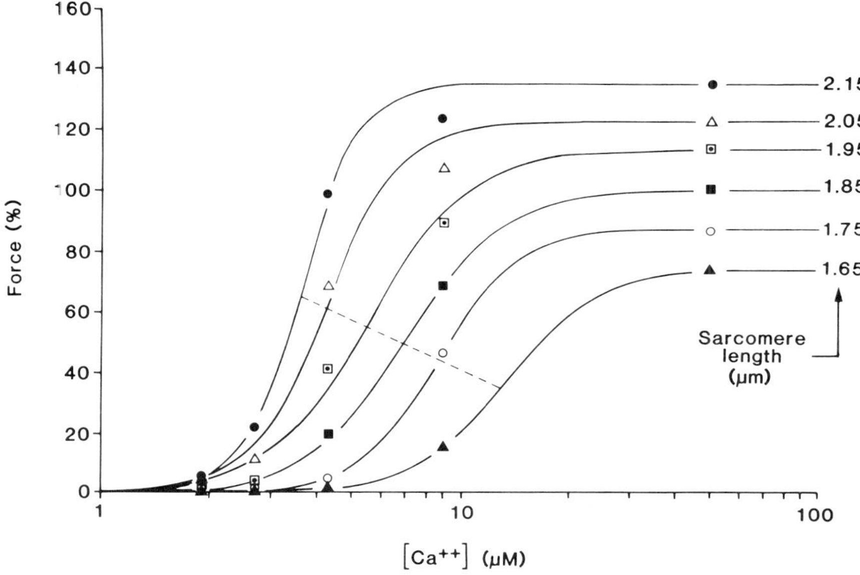

Figure 8-4. Force–[Ca^{2+}] relations at selected sarcomere lengths (shown in μm next to the appropriate curves). These relations were obtained by replotting the force–sarcomere length relations of 6 preparations. The solid lines show sigmoidal curves drawn according to the modified Hill equation. The slope of the curves given by the Hill coefficient n increased in the averaged $F - [Ca^{2+}]$ relations from 3.28 ± 0.29 at SL = $1.65\,\mu$m to 5.37 ± 0.82 at SL = $2.15\,\mu$m. The Ca^{2+} concentration at which 50% of F_{max} was developed decreased (dashed line) from $13.4\,\mu$M ± 0.54 uM at SL = 1.65 um to $3.59\,\mu$M 0.14 uM at SL = $2.15\,\mu$m (from Kentish et al., Circ. Res., 1986, 58: 755–768; with permission).

Ferret and sheep heart

As the force – length relations described above could be considered unique to the rat we compared the results with those obtained in ferret and sheep trabeculae. The results are shown in Fig. 8-5. As in rat, force increased in these muscles with increasing sarcomere length between $1.6\,\mu$m and $2.4\,\mu$m. The relations between force and sarcomere length were convex toward the ordinate at high Ca^{2+} and convex toward the abscissa at low Ca^{2+} concentrations at intermediate Ca^{2+} concentrations the relation was linear. At intermediate Ca^{2+} concentration the relation was linear.

The latter Ca^{2+} was 2.0 mM for ferret and sheep whereas it was only 0.5 mM for rat trabeculae. Moreover, force increased in ferret and sheep muscles with Ca^{2+} up to 6.0 mM whereas it saturated at 2.5 mM in the rat trabeculae (cf. also Fig. 8-2).

Twitch force in cardiac muscle is limited at high Ca^{++} by the capacity of the sarcoplasmic reticulum to store and release Ca^{++}. Addition of Sr^{++} to the

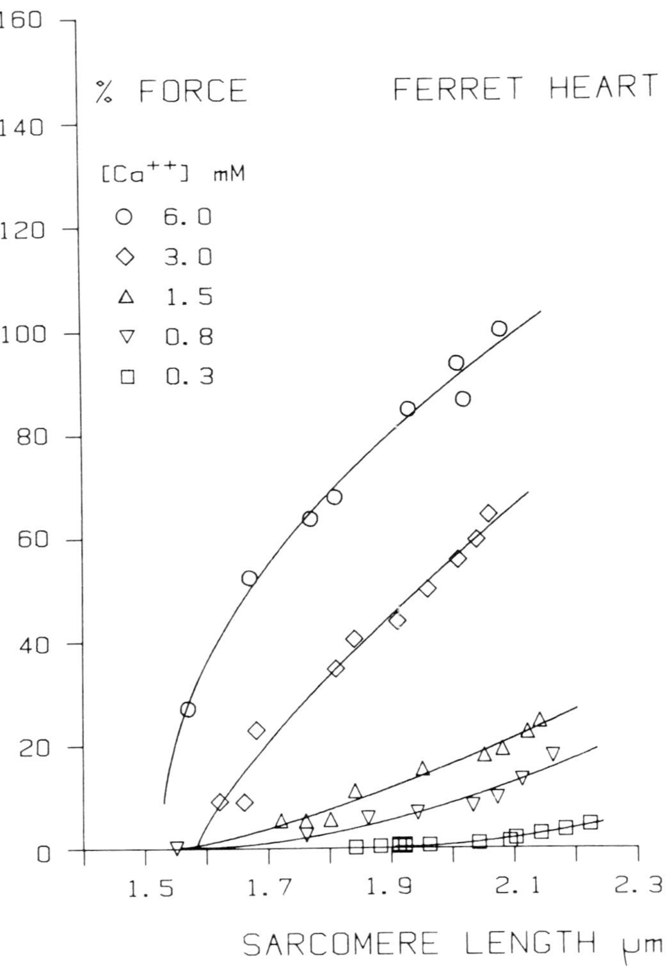

Figure 8-5. shows the force–sarcomere length relation for ferret and sheep trabeculae at extracellular Ca^{2+} concentrations that were varied between 0.5 and 6.0 mM. Note the similarity between these relations and those found in rat trabeculae. Note also that the sensitivity to external Ca^{2+} is less than in rat. Maximal force was attained in potentiated contractions after a series of extrasystoles (ES) (PES; potentiated contractions after 10 ES at 1 Hz; PESM after 10 ES at 2 Hz).

extracellular fluid is known to increase force about 25% above the maximal possible force in Ca^{2+}-containing solution [11]. The Sr^{2+} addition prolonged the twitch and increased peak force in rat trabeculae. Extrasystoles did not induce further potentiation in the presence of Sr^{2+}. Furthermore, it became possible to tetanize the muscles; however, the force during the plateau of the tetani did not exceed peak twitch force. The force–sarcomere length relation in the presence of 5 mM Sr^{2+} reproduced the relationship found in the skinned fiber at 16.7 μM Ca^{2+} (see Fig. 8-3.; see also Bucx et al. J. Physiol. 1986, in press).

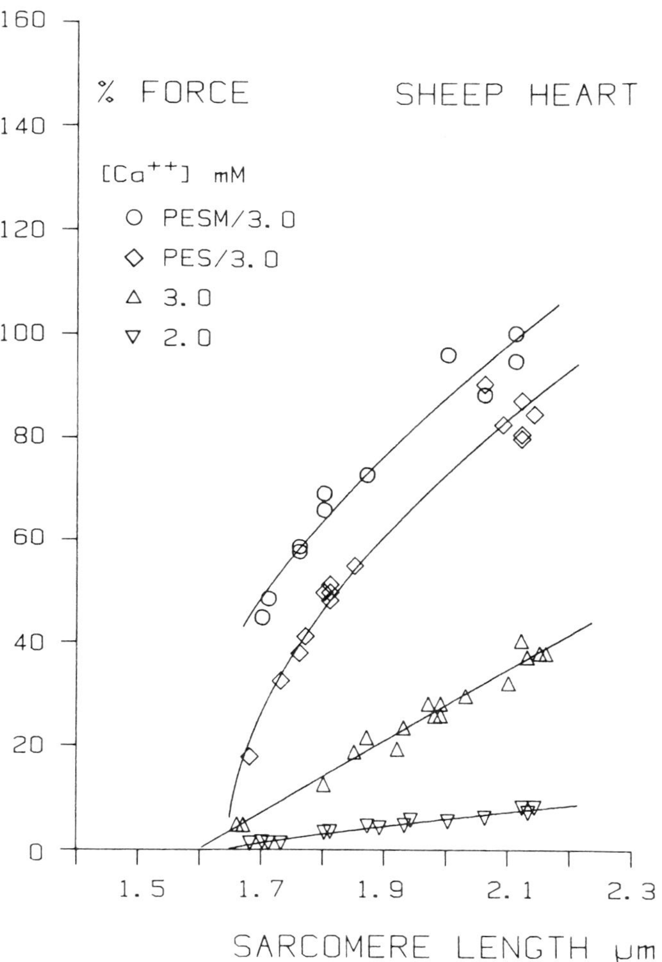

Discussion

The influence of various $[Ca^{2+}]$ on the shape of the force–sarcomere length relation has been observed in a number of studies [9] and has been interpreted as length dependent activation [12, 13, 14]. This property may be considered the response of the membranes of the cell or the sarcoplasmic reticulum to stretch, much like the membrane of a stretch receptor responds to the stimulus by a

100

change of the ion conductance of its membrane. This would lead to length dependence of the release of activator calcium in cardiac cells. Alternatively the response of the myofilaments to calcium could depend on the overlap between the actin and myosin. The latter would encompass a variation between a sarcomere length of 2.3 μm, where 'optimal' overlap between actin and myosin without double overlap between the actin filaments exists, and a sarcomere length of 1.6 μm where the two actin filaments from opposite Z-bands are in double overlap over 40–50% of their length and myosin touches the Z-band.

Species differences

The influence of [Ca]$^{2+}$ on the shape of the force–sarcomere length relation in rat trabeculae is similar to the effect of [Ca]$^{2+}$ on cat and ferret papillary muscle [15, 33]. This correspondence is further confirmed by the observed properties of the force–sarcomere length relations in sheep and ferret trabeculae (Fig. 8-5.) suggesting that also in these species the force–sarcomere length relation depends on Ca^{2+} concentration and can be accounted for by length dependent activation. It is likely that differences in the excitation–contraction coupling process between the species cause the differences in force development by the cardiac muscle at a particular sarcomere length and at a given Ca^{++} concentration.

Contribution of excitation–contraction coupling

We have previously shown that the effect of varied Ca^{++} can be mimicked by the effect of postextrasystolic potentiation [7]. This suggested that the force, that can be developed during the cardiac beat, depends on the intracellular calcium level which is determined both by the extracellular calcium concentration and by the interval between the heart beats. The similarity of the effect of these two interventions on the force–sarcomere length relation suggests that the final step that causes length dependent activation is the same. In the discussion below we will see that this final step is probably a length dependence of the contractile filaments to calcium, which implies that calcium supply to the myofilaments by the excitation contraction coupling process plays only a minor role in this phenomenon. However the capacity of the sarcoplasmic reticulum to release activating calcium ions probably imposes a limit on the maximal force of the myocardium. The ability of the sarcoplasmic reticulum to release divalent cations has been shown to increase in the presence of Sr^{++} ions [16]. The observations reported here suggest, indeed, that by addition of strontium ions to the extracellular medium, a level of activating divalent cations can be reached in the cell that is close to the saturating level for the contractile filaments (see below). The effect of added Sr^{++} ions to allow the intact trabeculae to generate as much force as the skinned muscles at a high activating Ca^{2+} suggests that intact cardiac cells operate at suboptimal Ca^{2+} concentrations as a result of limited Ca^{2+} release [16].

The role of passive elastic elements

The observation that the passive skinned muscles still revealed considerable stiffness is an important one as it probably indicates that the elastic elements which are composed of: i) elastin [17], ii) connecting filaments in the sarcomere [18] and iii) collagen fibers are still present in the skinned trabeculae [9]. This implies that shortening of sarcomeres below slack length must have caused the development of a restoring force of which the magnitude is as yet unknown. The presence of restoring forces must have caused us to underestimate the active force developed by the myofilaments alone in both intact and in skinned muscle. This particularly pertains to the highest activating Ca^{2+} concentrations in the skinned muscles in which considerably more shortening took place than at suboptimal Ca^{2+} concentrations or in the intact muscles.

Active force and sarcomere length

The force–SL relations for the intact muscle and for the skinned muscle have the same basic shape (Figs. 8-2 and 8-3). The only major difference was that, whereas in the intact muscles force development was zero at a SL of 1.6 μm and below, in the skinned muscle a considerable force could be produced at these sarcomere lengths if the $[Ca^{2+}]$ was raised to 50 μM (Figs. 8-2 and 8-3). A considerable force has also been observed in maximally activated fragments of single skinned cells from rat ventricle at sarcomere lengths as low as 1.2 μm [19]. The force–SL relation at maximal activation was however steeper for the trabeculae than for fragments of skinned single cells; extrapolation of the data in Fig. 8-6 indicates that zero force would have occurred at a sarcomere length of about 1.2 μm, whereas force in fragments of single cells at this SL was 60% of maximum [19]. This difference was not due to incomplete activation of the myofibrils at the lowest sarcomere lengths in our experiments, because the force was not increased if the $[Ca^{2+}]$ was raised further to 280 μM. The apparent discrepancy probably represents a true difference between the two types of preparation: trabeculae, unlike single cells, contain intercellular connections [17] and extracellular connective tissue [20] that could produce forces that oppose shortening at the shorter sarcomere lengths.

The similarity of the force–sarcomere length relations in intact and skinned muscles suggests that the properties of the relation in intact myocardium can be accounted for by the inherent properties of the myofibrils (and elastic components responsible for the restoring forces see above).

102

If the inherent properties of the myofibrils in the intact and skinned muscle are similar [9] one may conclude that length dependence of calcium release by the excitation-contraction coupling process [19] is small, as has been concluded from aequorin experiments [21].

Length dependent sensitivity of the myofilaments to calcium

Figure 8-4 shows that the shape of the force–sarcomere length relations at varied Ca^{2+} is a consequence of length-dependent Ca^{2+} sensitivity of the contractile system, as has previously been suggested by Fabiato [22] for cell fragments and by Hibberd and Jewell [23] for detergent skinned trabeculae in which sarcomere length in the relaxed muscle was measured.

The results of this study show that the length-dependence of myofibrillar Ca^{2+}-sensitivity occurs over the entire range of active sarcomere lengths (1.6–$2.3\,\mu$m) that corresponds to the ascending limb of the length–tension relationship in the working heart [24, 25, 26]. Thus it is likely that this phenomenon contributes to the Frank-Starling relation under all physiological conditions.

Our experiments provide no clue as to the mechanism of the length dependence of Ca^{2+}-sensitivity. One plausible mechanism is that the affinity of troponin for Ca^{2+} increases with SL. Recent experiments using skinned muscles loaded with photoproteins [27, 28] (see Kentish and Allen, this volume) support this hypothesis.

The force–[Ca^{2+}] relation at all sarcomere lengths is too steep to be explained by positive cooperativity between the three Ca^{2+}-binding sites on cardiac troponin, especially since there is evidence that only one of these sites is directly involved in Ca^{2+}-regulation of contraction [29]. On the other hand interactions between adjacent tropomyosin molecules could explain positive cooperativity (see also 23), or an increase of the sarcomere length could increase the number of possible crossbridges and, by virtue of a cooperative process, increase both steepness and affinity [30]. This hypothesis implies that maximal force at high Ca^{2+} depends mainly on the number of crossbridges that can attach to actin, while the tacit assumption is that the contribution of restoring forces to the decline of force at optimal Ca^{2+} and at short sarcomere lengths would be minimal. It is unknown as yet to what extent the decrease of force with decreasing sarcomere length below slack length is due to a decrease of the number of crossbridges or to an increase of the restoring force that is set up in the elastic structures of the cardiac cell. This question awaits further research.

Implications for the cardiac endsystolic pressure–volume relation

We have previously shown that internal shortening in experiments at this temperature does not affect the resulting force–sarcomere length relation [31, 7]. This corresponds to the observation that the contractile behavior of the intact ventricles, as expressed by the endsystolic pressure–volume relation, is independent of the ejection pattern prior to the end of systole. The fact that fundamentally the same force–SL relations have been found in different species (Figs. 8-2 and 8-5) suggests that they reveal a basic property of myocardium, which one would then also expect to encounter in the endsystolic pressure–volume relations of the cardiac chambers (of course after the appropriate corrections for the geometry of the chambers). That this expectation is justified was recently shown by a study in the laboratory of Dr. Sagawa [32], in which it was found that both at low and at high contractility canine left ventricular endsystolic pressure–volume relations deviate from linearity in a manner that can be predicted on the basis of force–sarcomere length relations of isolated muscle preparations.

This argues strongly against the principle that the heart operates simply as a structure with a compliance that varies in time [34], or equivalently, as a body with a time-varying elastic constant, as has been assumed in the earlier concepts of viscoelastic behavior of muscle in general. Instead, the comparison of the cardiac muscle and cardiac chamber properties reveals that properties of the heart as a pump can be explained by length dependence of force generation by the cardiac sarcomeres.

Acknowledgements

Supported by grants from the: Alberta Heritage Foundation for Medical Research of which Dr. ter Keurs is Medical Scientist and; Netherlands Heart Foundation (74022, 77086). We thank Ms. Anna V. Tyberg and Peter de Tombe for their assistance with the preparation of the manuscript.

References

1. Ringer, S.: A further contribution regarding the influence of different constituents of the blood on the contraction of the heart. J. Physiol. (London) 4: 29–42, 1883.
2. Frank, O.: Zur Dynamik des Herzmuskels. Z. Biol. 32: 370–447, 1895.
3. Starling, E.H.: The Linacre lecture on the law of the heart, given at Cambridge, 1915. London: Longmans, Green, 1918.
4. Bowditch, H.P.: Uber die Eigenthuemlichkeiten der Reizbarkeit, welche die Muskelfasern des Herzens zeigen. Ber K saeschs. Ges. Wissenschaften. Math. Phys. Klasse 652–689, 1871.
5. Sarnoff, S.J., Brockman, S.K., Gilmore, J.P., Linden, R.J. and Mitchell, J.H.: Regulation of ventricular contraction: Influence of cardiac sympathetic and vagal nerve stimulation on atrial and ventricular dynamics. Circ. Res. 8: 1108–1122, 1960.
6. Barany, M.: ATPase activity of myosin correlated with speed of muscle shortening. J. Gen. Physiol 50: 197–216, 1967.
7. ter Keurs, H.E.D.J., Rijnsburger, W.H., van Heuningen, R. and Nagelsmit, M.J.: Tension

development and sarcomere length in rat cardiac trabeculae; Evidence of length-dependent activation. Circ. Res. 46: 703–714, 1980.

8. Kentish, J.C.: The inhibitory effects of monovalent ions on force development in detergent-skinned ventricular muscle from guinea pig. J Physiol (London) 352: 353–374, 1984.

9. Kentish, J.C., ter Keurs, H.E.D.J., Ricciardi, L., Bucx, J.J.J. and Noble, M.I.M.: Comparison between the sarcomere length-force relations of intact and skinned trabeculae from rat right ventricle. Circ Res 58: 755–768, 1986.

10. Snedecor, G.W. and Cochran, W.G.: Statistical methods. Ames, Iowa, Iowa State University Press, 1973.

11. Schouten, V.J.A.: Excitation-contraction coupling in heart muscle. Thesis, University of Leiden, The Netherlands, 1985.

12. Jewell, B.R.: A reexamination of the influence of muscle length on myocardial performance. Circ. Res. 40: 221–230, 1977.

13. Parmley, W.W. and Chuck, L.: Length-dependent changes in myocardial contractile state. Am. J. Physiol. 224: 1195–1199, 1973.

14. Lakatta, E.G. and Jewell, B.R.: Length-dependent activation. Effect on the length-tension relation in cat ventricular muscle. Circ Res 40: 251–257, 1977.

15. Allen, D.G., Jewell, B.R., Murray, J.W.: The contribution of activation processes to the length-tension relation of cardiac muscle. Nature 248: 606–607, 1974.

16. Fabiato, A.: Appraisal of the hypothesis of the 'Depolarization-induced' release of calcium from the sarcoplasmic reticulum in skinned cardiac cells from the rat or pigeon ventricle. In: Structure and Function of Sarcoplasmic Reticulum, Eds S Fleischer and Y Tonomura. Florida, Academic Press, 1986.

17. Winegrad, S. and Robinson, T.J.: Force-generation among cells in the relaxed heart. Eur. J. Cardiol. 7 [Suppl]: 63–70, 1978.

18. Magid, A., Ting-Beall, H.P., Carvell, M., Kontis, T. and Lucaveche, C.: Connecting filaments, core filaments and side struts: A proposal to add three load-bearing structures in the sliding filament model. In: Contractile Mechanism in Muscle, eds GH Pollack, H Sugi. New York, Plenum Press, pp. 307–323, 1984.

19. Fabiato, A. and Fabiato, F.: Dependence of the contractile activation of skinned cardiac cells on the sarcomere length. Nature 256: 54–56, 1975.

20. Kentish, J.C.: The influence of monovalent cations on myofibrillar function. PhD Thesis. University of London, England, 1982.

21. Allen, D.G. and Kurihara, S.: The effects of muscle length on intracellular calcium transients in mammalian cardiac muscle. J. Physiol. (London) 327: 79–94, 1982.

22. Fabiato, A.: Sarcomere length dependence of calcium release from the sarcoplasmic reticulum of skinned cardiac cells demonstrated by differential microspectrophotometry with Arsenazo III (abstr) J. Gen. Physiol. 76: 15a, 1980.

23. Hibberd, M.G. and Jewell, B.R.: Calcium- and length-dependent force production in rat ventricular muscle. J. Physiol. (London) 329: 527–540, 1982.

24. Page, S.G.: Measurements of structural parameters in cardiac muscle. In: The physiological basis of Starling's Law of the Heart. Ciba Found Symp 24:13–25, 1974.

25. Sonnenblick, E.H. and Skelton, C.L.: Reconsideration of the ultrastructural basis of cardiac length–tension relations. Circ Res 35: 517–526, 1974.

26. ter Keurs, H.E.D.J.: Calcium and Contractility. In: Cardiac Metabolism, eds AJ Drake-Holland and MIM Noble. New York, J Wiley and Sons, pp. 73–99, 1983.

27. Allen, D.G. and Kentish, J.C.: The effects of length changes on the myoplasmic calcium concentration in skinned ferret ventricular muscle. J. Physiol. (London) 366: 67p, 1985.

28. Stephenson, D.G. and Wendt, I.T.: Length dependence of changes in sarcoplasmic calcium concentration and myofibrillar calcium sensitivity in striated muscle fibres. J. Muscle Res. Cell. Motil. 5: 243–272, 1984.

29. Holroyde, M.J., Robertson, S.P., Johnson, J.D., Solaro, R.J. and Potter, J.D.: The calcium and magnesium binding sites on cardiac troponin and their role in the regulation of myofibrillar adenosine triphosphatase. J. Biol. Chem. 225: 11688–11693, 1980.

30. Brandt, P.W., Cox, R.N. and Kawai, M.: Can the binding of Ca^{2+} to two regulatory sites on troponin C determine the steep pCa–tension relationship of skeletal muscle? Proc. Nat. Acad. Sci. USA 77: 4717–4720, 1980.

31. Pollack, G.H. and Krueger, J.W.: Sarcomere dynamics in intact cardiac muscle. Eur. J. Cardiol. 4 [Suppl]: 53–65, 1976.

32. Sagawa, K., Maughan, L.W., Burkhoff, D., and Yue, D.: The similarity between pressure–volume relation and muscle force–length relation. Cardiovasc. Res. 19: 523, 1985.

33. Martyn, D.A., Rondinone, J.F., and Huntsman, L.L.: The dependence of force and velocity on calcium and length in cardiac muscle segments. Adv. Exp. Med. Biol. 170: 821–836, 1984.

34. Suga, H., Sagawa, K. and Shoukas, A.A.: Load independence of the instantaneous pressure–volume ratio of the canine left ventricle and effects of epinephrine and heart rate on the ratio. Circ. Res. 32: 314–322, 1973.

9. Segment length mechanics of cardiac muscle; force, velocity and stiffness in cardiac muscle vary with length and calcium

LEE L. HUNTSMAN and DONALD A. MARTYN

Introduction

Data we have obtained from studies of isolated ferret papillary muscles are pertinent to two of the major issues Dr. ter Keurs has pointed out. All of our observations have been made using the area sense coil technique for segment length measurement [1].

Segment length and calcium effects

Force–segment length relations from intact ferret papillary muscles are remarkably consistent with those from skinned rat preparations. Replotting the F-pCa data shown in Fig. 8-4 of Dr. ter Keurs' paper yields the F–SL relations indicated by dashed lines in Fig. 9-1. Assuming maximum segment length (100%) to occur at a sarcomere length of 2.35 μm, the F–SL relation for maximally activated ferret papillary muscle is as shown by the solid line [2]. It is noteworthy that, even when plotted on the same stress scale, our data fall exactly in that region of the data from rat muscle which would yield a similar linear response. Ferret data at lower calcium concentrations yield curved F–SL relations which are also similar to results from skinned rat preparations.

This congruence of data from intact and skinned preparations, of different species, suggests that the filament behavior described by the F-pCa data is of fundamental importance. As Dr. ter Keurs points out, the filament response seems to account for observed mechanical behavior. The mechanisms which underlie this response are not at all clear, however, and it is important to note that at least two mechanisms, a sensitivity shift and a magnitude shift, seem to be involved in the length effect.

Unloaded shortening velocity (V_o) also exhibits a strong dependence on length and calcium [3]. Typical results in our preparation are shown in Fig. 9-2. This dependence is very similar to that seen for force and suggests that a common

108

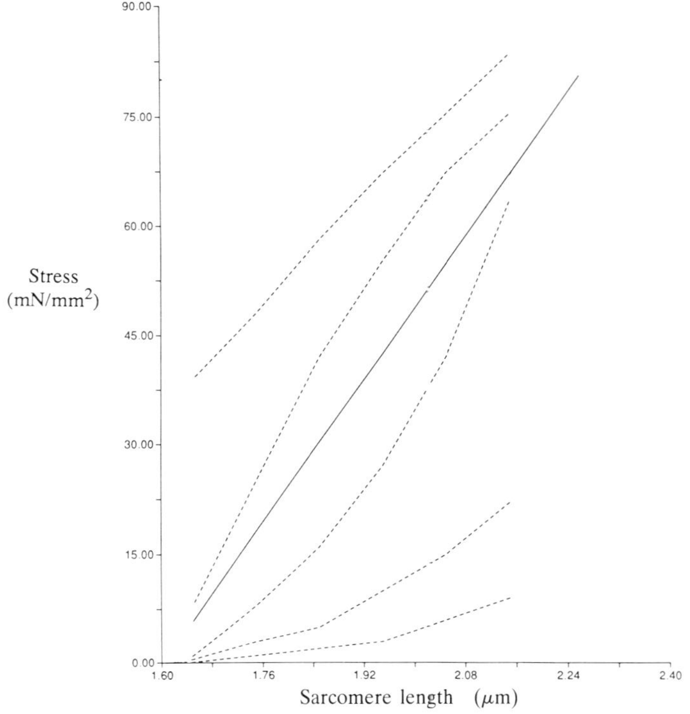

Figure 9-1. Force-length data from intact ferret papillaries (solid line) compare remarkably well with results from skinned rat muscle (dashed lines). The dashed lines are calculated from the data in Figure 8-4 of Dr. ter Keurs' paper. The solid line is for maximal activation, scaled based on the assumption that 100% SL corresponds to 2.35 μm sarcomere length.

mechanism may account for the way length and activation control contraction.

Restoring forces

If, as Dr. ter Keurs suggests, restoring forces are sufficiently large to create a substantial difference between filament mechanics and measured behavior, it would be expected that: 1) F–SL and V_o–SL relations should show an inflection in the range of 1.85–1.90 μm sarcomere length (80% SL_{max}); 2) unloaded contractions should be actually auxotonic at the filaments and, consequently, V_o should have a different time course at different lengths, becoming more like F(t) at short lengths; and 3) measured stiffness, which is dominated by the very high stiffness associated with actin–myosin interactions, should be high at all lengths even though measured force drops at short lengths.

None of these predictions is borne out in our data. Force and velocity vary smoothly with length [2, 3]. V_o has a very different time course than force, but

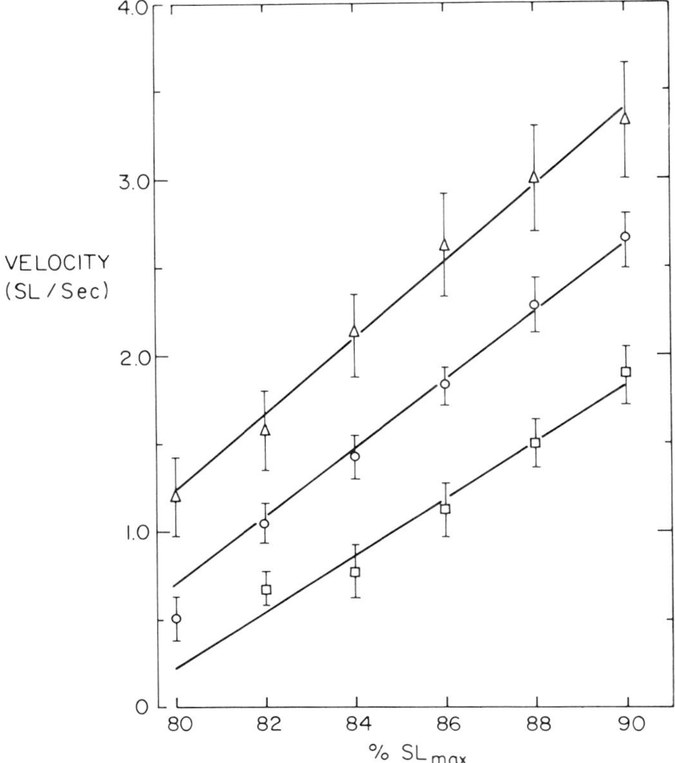

Figure 9-2. Unloaded velocity of shortening (V_o) varies strongly with segment length and extracellular calcium concentration (1.125 mM, __; 2.25 mM, O; and 4.5 mM, __).

that course does not change with length (Fig. 9-3). Imposition of even a small afterload alters the time course to be more like that of force. Stiffness has been found to be high, much like that observed in skeletal muscle preparations, and proportional to force. This proportionality holds at all lengths, as shown in Fig. 9-4.

Restoring forces are obviously present in cardiac muscle. Based on our observations, however, it appears unlikely that they are large enough to materially affect the mechanical properties which are measured during contraction.

Summary

Our findings, therefore, support the idea that the filament response to sarcomere length and calcium is sufficient to explain the effects of those factors on the mechanical properties of intact preparations. The data do not, however, seem to

110

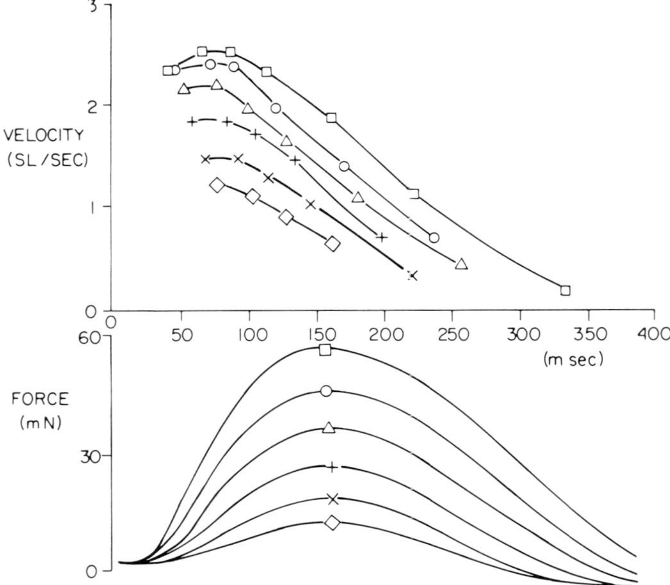

Figure 9-3. The time course of unloaded velocity (top panel) is different from that of force (lower panel). The differences are consistent over a range of lengths (90%, □; 88%, ○; 86%, △; 84%, +; 82%, ×, and 80%, ◇).

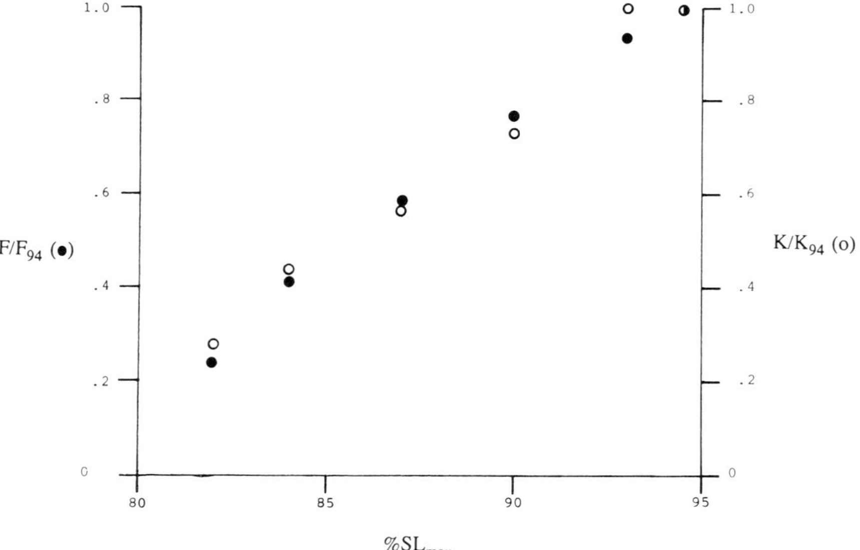

Figure 9-4. Stiffness (○), measured by high speed releases, varies with length as does force (●).

support the notion that restoring forces are significant in the determination of force, velocity, and stiffness.

References

1. Huntsman, L.L., Joseph, D.S., Nichols, G.L. and Oiye, M.Y.: Auxotonic contractions in cardiac muscle segments. Am. J. Physiol. 237: H131–H138, 1979.
2. Huntsman, L.L., Rondinone, J.F. and Martyn, D.A.: Force–length relations in cardiac muscle segments. Am. J. Physiol. 244: H701–H707, 1983.
3. Martyn, D.A., Rondinone, J.F. and Huntsman, L.L.: Myocardial segment velocity at a low load: time, length and calcium dependence. Am. J. Physiol. 244: H708–H714, 1983.

General discussion of the cardiac force–sarcomere length relation

While there was general agreement, – during a discussion of the apparent linearity of the end-systolic pressure–volume relationship – that the curve must flatten at high pressures the adequacy of the linear model at low pressures was debated with the reminder that the interest in proposing the model was only to provide a useful, empirical, first approximation of the behavior of the heart. Dr. Sagawa underlined the comparability of the behaviour of the pressure–volume relation in the ventricle at varied contractility to that of force–sarcomere length relation in isolated muscle in vitro. Possible effects of nonuniformity of sarcomere lengths are expected in the latter relation. However, sarcomere nonuniformity was observed mainly during activation with high calcium concentrations and at long sarcomere lengths, whereas the diffraction patterns suggested uniformity at lengths (1.6–2.15 μm) and at calcium concentrations that are presumed to occur in the intact cell.

It is as yet unknown how large restoring forces in isolated cardiac muscle are and where they originate. Study of these forces at cellular level is required to identify the responsible structures and to assess their magnitude. Even so, restoring forces in the intact ventricle may exceed those in isolated muscle if shear force is generated.

The role of calmodulin was discussed. Because of its close link to the thick filament calmodulin might be involved in length dependent sensitivity. Presently no data suggest this mechanism of control. It is also known that calmodulin dependent kinases are virtually continually active (cf. Dr. Solaro's chapter), while the effect of length changes is instantaneous.

10. Regulation of the actin-myosin interaction by calcium; the troponin tropomyosin complex

WILLIAM D. MCCUBBIN, DAVID M. BEYERS and CYRIL M. KAY

Introduction

Muscle contraction is regulated by the free Ca^{2+} from storage vesicles (the sarcoplasmic reticulum) and the Ca^{2+} concentration changes from 10^{-8} to 10^{-5} M. In vertebrate striated muscle (skeletal and cardiac), Ca^{2+} binds to troponin on the thin filament reversing the inhibition of the troponin-tropomyosin complex, and allowing myosin and actin to interact, with ensuing contraction of the muscle.

Some twenty three years ago, Ebashi [1] proposed that Ca^{2+} regulation in skeletal muscle is controlled by a thin filament protein complex, which was subsequently shown to be composed of two proteins, tropomyosin and troponin. It was later found that troponin could also be isolated from bovine cardiac muscle [2]. It is now well established that both skeletal and cardiac troponin consists of three non-identical subunits, TN-C (the Ca^{2+}-binding subunit), TN-I (the inhibitory subunit) and TN-T (the tropomyosin-binding subunit) [3]. The structure of the thin filament of striated muscle is shown diagrammatically in Fig. 10-1. It is made up of a two-stranded beaded helical structure composed of actin monomers, along with two strands of two chain a-helical tropomyosin molecules, which run along the two grooves of the actin helix, lying end to end beaded helical structure composed of actin monomers, along with two strands of two chain a-helical tropomyosin molecules, which and overlapping slightly. Individual tropomyosin molecules are about 40 nm long and each is associated with a single troponin complex. The stoichiometry of the major structural proteins in skeletal and cardiac muscle is thought to be 7:1:1:1:1:1 (actin : myosin : tropomyosin : TN-I : Tn-T) [4].

Over the past decade, the most popular theory of thin filament regulation has been the steric blocking hypothesis, proposed on the basis of X-ray diffraction, and electron microscopic studies on relaxed and contracting muscle [5, 6], in which actin-myosin interaction is physically blocked in the resting state by tropomyosin, perhaps anchored in this 'off' position by the binding of TN-I to actin. Contraction is signalled by the binding of Ca^{2+} to TN-C, followed by a con-

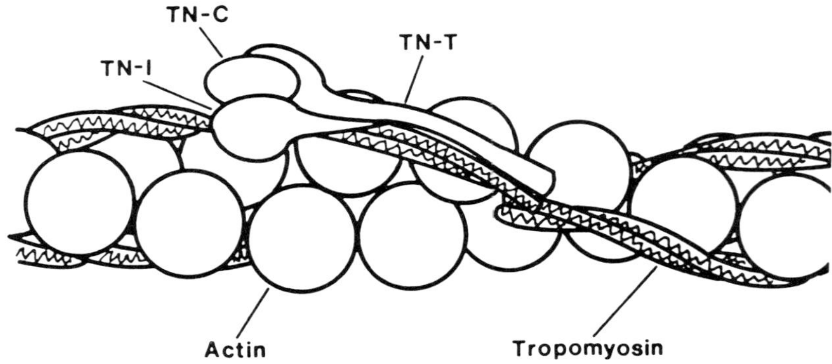

Figure 10-1. Proposed model for the structure of the thin filament of striated muscle (from Mak and Smillie (1980) [48] after Ebashi et al. (1969) [48]).

formational change in troponin, which removes the inhibition produced by TN-I and permits tropomyosin to move to the 'on' position and thus allow cross bridge attachment to the thin filament. This sequence of events is illustrated schematically in Fig. 10-2. This simple steric blocking model has been challenged by a variety of structural and chemical observations. The most recent thinking suggests a role for the troponin-tropomyosin complex in regulating a kinetic step in the actin-activated ATPase pathway, perhaps the release of inorganic phosphate from the actomyosin complex following ATP hydrolysis [7]. This relatively slow step is believed to be accompanied by a change in the angle of attachment of the S-1 head of myosin to actin, from 90° to 45°. This rotation of the myosin crossbridge could be blocked by the regulatory proteins in the absence of calcium.

Cardiac troponin subunits

A great deal of attention has focused on individual troponin subunits after it was realized that these proteins retain their basic functional properties in solution and that they could be reconstituted to a biologically active complex. Cardiac troponin is believed to operate in a similar fashion to its skeletal counterpart. The isolation of purified cardiac troponin subunits [8] has demonstrated that these proteins are qualitatively similar to the skeletal ones in size, amino acid composition and biological properties. It has also been shown that hybrid troponin complexes, formed from various skeletal and cardiac subunit combinations are generally capable of regulating actomyosin in vitro [9].

Important differences do exist though between skeletal and cardiac muscle; e.g. skeletal muscle must contract or relax rapidly, whereas cardiac muscle contracts in a continuous rhythmical manner, with no opportunity for rest. A growing body of evidence suggests that these altered regulatory requirements are

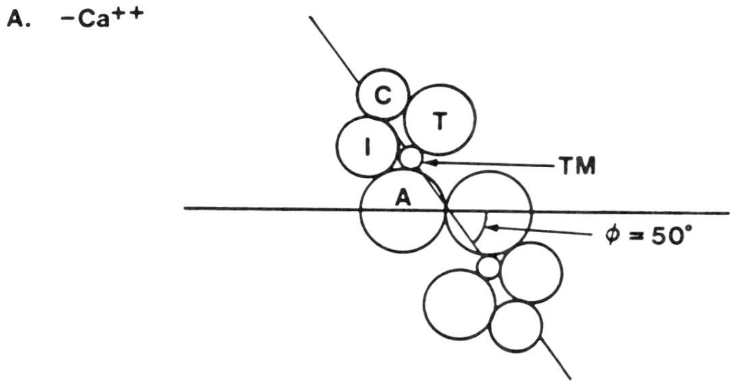

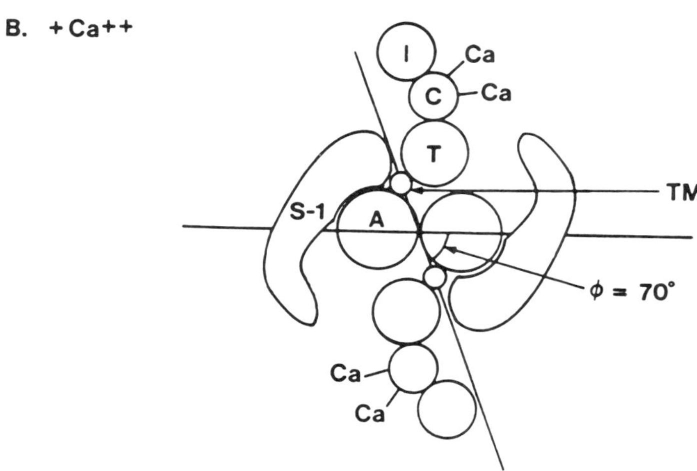

Figure 10-2. Steric model for the regulation of striated muscle contraction. The view looking down the thin filament axis towards the Z-line is schematically depicted. The proteins represented are: A (actin), TM (tropomyosin), C (TN-C), I (TN-I), T (TN-T), S-1 (myosin subfragment S-1). (A) depicts relaxed muscle, $[Ca^{2+}] \sim 10^{-8}$ M. (B) represents contracting muscle $[Ca^{2+}] \sim 1 - ^{-5}$ M (from Potter and Gergely (1974) [49]).

in fact reflected at the level of the troponin subunits. It is pertinent at this state to review the chemical, physical and biological properties of the cardiac troponin system.

Purification of cardiac troponin subunits

Methodology for isolation of the troponin subunits from cardiac muscle has been in a state of flux over the past several years. Recently we have turned to the excellent resolving powers of high performance liquid chromatographic procedures to aid us in this task [10]. In Fig. 10-3, we show the results of chromatography with the strong anion exchange resin, Synchropak Q300, in the presence of urea, which has produced successful resolution of troponin into pure subunits. Additionally the TN-T component has been resolved into several peaks corresponding to isoforms differing in amino acid composition and sequence.

Cardiac TN-C

The amino acid sequence of this protein indicates that the molecular weight is 18,459, a figure confirmed by SDS/PAGE as well as sedimentation equilibrium measurements. The protein is acidic (pI 4, I-4.3), has a high phe : tyr ratio (3 : 9), lacks tryptophan, and has 2 free sulfhydryl groups. The high phe : tyr ratio shows up clearly in the characteristic 'saw-toothed' absorption spectrum, as well as the aromatic CD profile, where one sees negative bands at 259 and 265 nm, positions suggestive of phe, by analogy with the CD spectrum of acetyl-L-phenyl-alanine-ethyl ester.

Equilibrium dialysis showed that cardiac TN-C has two Ca^{2+}/Mg^{2+} sites, $K_{Ca2+} = 1.4 \times 10^7 M^{-1}$, $K_{Mg2+} = 3.5 \times 10^3 M^{-1}$ [11]. In the TN-C-TN-I complex or in whole troponin, the Ca^{2+}-affinity of each class of binding site is increased by one order of magnitude. The possibility exists that the presence of actin may also influence the Ca^{2+}-binding properties of TN-C [12].

Conformational probes

In the early '70's, we showed that numerous spectroscopic and hydrodynamic changes occur upon binding of Ca^{2+} to cardiac TN-C. Perhaps the most dramatic effect observed is the increase in the amount of ordered secondary structure in the presence of Ca^{2+}.

(a) Circular dichroism.
Circular dichroism (CD) studies have indicated that Ca^{2+} binding increases the a-helical content by some 50% in bovine cardiac TN-C [13]. Representative spectra showing the associated increase in negative ellipticity with Ca^{2+} addition are shown in Fig. 10-4.

(b) Fluorescence.
It is possible to use the intrinsic fluorescence of TN-C to follow the Ca^{2+}-induced conformational change in this protein. As we have seen, TN-C lacks tryptophan so the emission spectrum will be a reflection of the three tyrosines present. Upon excitation at 276 nm one observed an emission maximum near 307 nm which undergoes an approximately 60% increase in intensity as Ca^{2+} is added [14]. In the

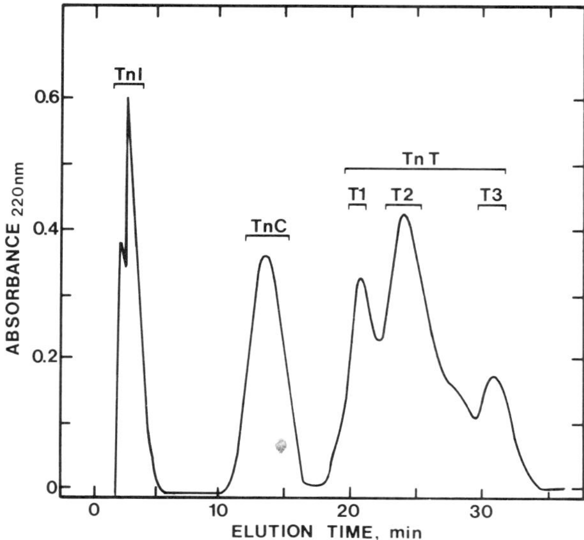

Figure 10-3. Separation of bovine cardiac troponin on an analytical SynChropak Q-300 strong anio-exchange column. Column: 250 × 4.1 mm I.D. Conditions: A – B gradient, the basic buffer consisted of 8 M urea, 50 mM Tris HCl, 2 mM EGTA, 0.5 mM EGTA, 0.5 mM DTT, pH 7.5; buffer A was the basic buffer with no KCl, while buffer B consisted of the basic buffer containing 1 M KCl. A linear KCl gradient with the KCl increasing at a rate of 5 mM/min and a flow rate of 1 ml/min was applied with the following compositions at the times indicated. Time 0 min, 80% A – 20% B, time 40 min, 60% A – 40% B. Sample 2.5 mg troponin per 200 μl of starting buffer. Chart speed 12 in./h. Absorbance was measured at 220 nm, 10 mM cells [10].

apo state, the relatively large number of carboxylate residues induces a partial quenching of the tyrosine emission. As Ca^{2+} is added, some of these carboxylates are neutralized, particularly ones close to the tyrosyl chromophores, the quenching mechanism is released, and the emission is enhanced.

(c) Difference UV absorption spectroscopy.
This technique has proved useful to study the Ca^{2+}-induced conformational change in cardiac TN-C [8]. A typical spectrum is shown in Fig. 10-5. The maxima noted near 287 and 277 nm are due to perturbations in the environment of tyrosine residue(s). Since the peaks are positive, this implies a red-shift in the absorption spectrum consistent with the environment around one or more tyrosine residues becoming more non-polar. A charge neutralization rather than a complete burying of the chromophore is also consistent with the relatively small value for the difference maxima. The fine structure noted near 269, 265, 259 and 253 nm may be attributed to contributions from the 9 phe residues in the protein sequence.

This concept of exposure of the tyrosine residues in cardiac TN-C in the presence and absence of Ca^{2+} may be further explored using solvent perturbation

118

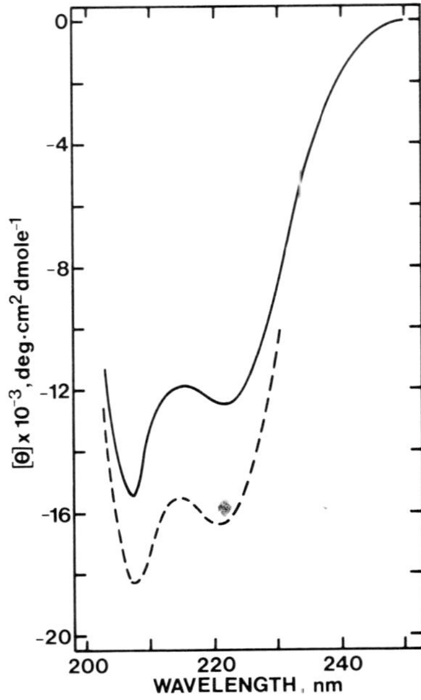

Figure 10-4. Far UV CD spectra of cardiac TN-C in the presence and absence of calcium. TN-C was dissolved in 0.15 M KCl, 50 mM Tris HCl, pH 7.5, 1 mM EGTA. (——), 'minus Ca^{2+}'; (---), 'plus Ca^{2+}' [49].

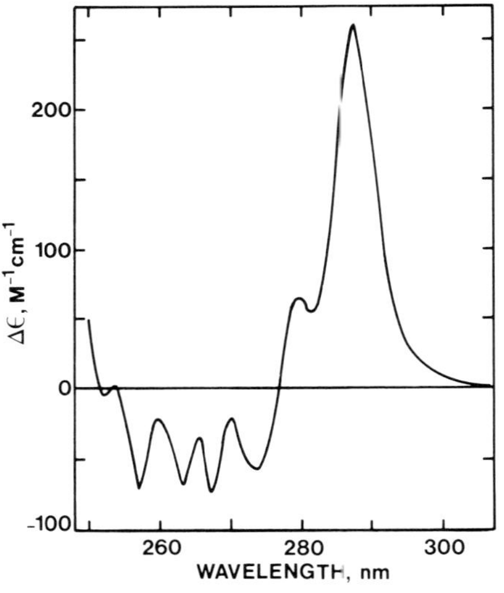

Figure 10-5. This figure shows a typical Ca^{2+}-induced UV difference spectrum for cardiac TN-C. The protein was dissolved in 100 mM MOPS, 50 mM KCl, 1 mM EGTA, pH 7.11. To the solution in the sample beam, an aliquot of 0.1 M $CaCl_2$ was added such that the pCa^{2+} was 4.2. To the solution in the reference beam an equal volume of water was added [8].

spectroscopy in the presence of 20% inert organic solvents [15]. This technique can distinguish buried from exposed chromophores. We find that all 3 tyrosines are solvated by dimethyl sulfoxide (DMSO) and are therefore exposed in the apo state while addition of Ca^{2+} apparently buries one residue. This is in line with other data, e.g. all 3 tyr residues in the apo protein exhibit a single pKa of 10.5 which, although somewhat higher than normal, suggests a basically exposed nature. As well, proton NMR studies (Fig. 10-6) demonstrated that in Ca^{2+}-saturated cardiac TN-C, tyr 150 located in binding site IV, is buried in the hydrophobic core of the protein [10]. Additional laser photo CIDNP data was also in accord with this conclusion [17].

(d) Hydrodynamics.
The results of hydrodynamic studies indicate that the binding of Ca^{2+} affects the overall shape of cardiac TN-C. The observed decrease in Stokes radius and viscosity, as well as an increase in sedimentation coefficient, at constant molecular weight, suggest a conformational change to a more globular shape: the frictional ratio (f/f_{min}) going from 1.52 in the absence of Ca^{2+} to 1.40 in the presence of this cation [18].

Carboxyls as Ca^{2+}-liganding groups

From the known preference of Ca^{2+} for oxygen containing liganding groups it was clear that prime candidates for binding residues would be carboxyl moieties. We showed in an early study on skeletal TN-C, that conversion of 2/3 of the Ca_2H groups to neutral amides almost abolished the responsiveness of the structure to Ca^{2+}, presumably because some of the key carboxyls involved normally in Ca^{2+}-binding are blocked. We would expect a similar situation to hold for the cardiac analogue [19].

To learn more about the microenvironment of these carboxyl groups, we carried out conformational studies on the cardiac TN-C system as a function of pH [20]. As Fig. 10-7 reveals, protons can induce a similar conformational change as does Ca^{2+}, in terms of the far ultraviolet circular dichroic ellipticity (cf. Fig. 10-4) and the ultraviolet difference absorption spectrum (cf. Fig. 10-5). From the mid-points of these titration curves, we deduced that protonation of groups (presumably carboxyls) with pKa values of 6 were producing the considerable increase in all parameters. Such high pKa values for carboxyl groups have been reported previously, e.g. glu 35 in lysozyme [21]; they are usually associated with carboxyls located in regions containing adjacent carboxyls, particularly if the environment is somewhat hydrophobic. Some of the carboxyls could be hydrogen bonded to nearby tyrosines. Both situations apply in cardiac TN-C.

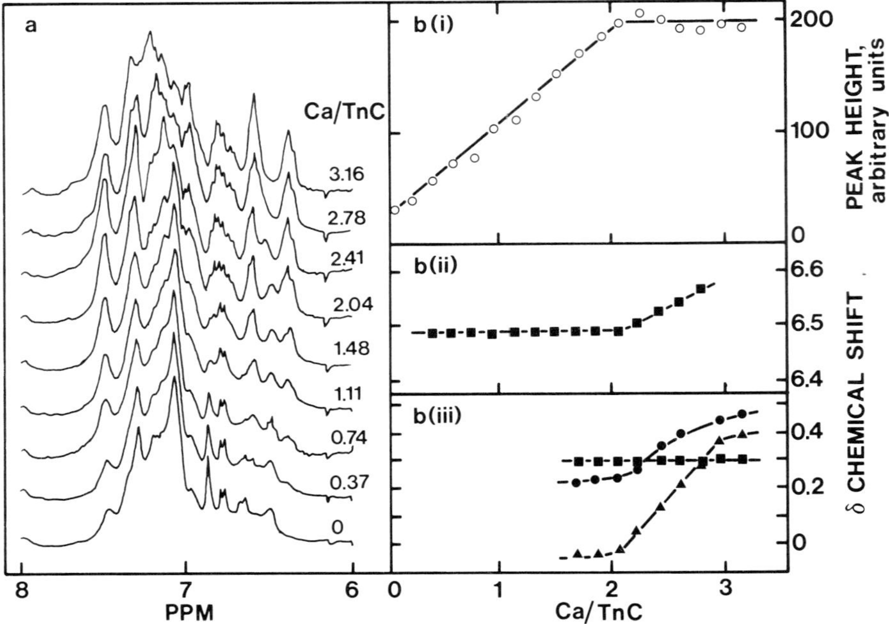

Figure 10-6. (A). NMR spectra during Calcium binding to apocardiac TN-C. The protein (1.07 mM) in 0.15 M KCl and 25 mM MOPS was titrated with Ca^{2+}. The aromatic region of the NMR spectrum is presented as a function of increasing Ca^{2+}/TN-C.
(B) (i). Plot of the height of the proton resonance of 150 meta plus Ca^{2+}-tyrosine as a function of Ca^{2+} added. In (ii) and (iii), several chemical shifts are also plotted as a function of added Ca^{2+} [16].

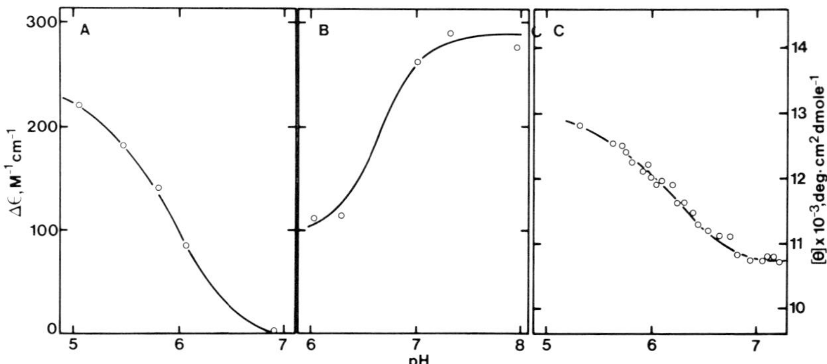

Figure 10-7. This figure shows the effect of changes in pH on (A) the magnitude of the acid-produced tyrosine difference peak near 287, (B) the magnitude of the Ca^{2+}-induced tyrosine difference spectrum at 287 nm, and (C) the ellipticity at 220 nm of cardiac TN-C (modified from [20]).

Transmission of the energy of the Ca^{2+}-induced refolding of TN-C to the other thin filament proteins

If TN-C is to act as a trigger in the regulatory mechanism of muscle contraction, then it is essential that the information and/or energy produced by the Ca^{2+}-induced conformational change in this protein is transmitted, initially to the other TN subunits and subsequently to the whole thin filament complex. Initially, we combined subunits of cardiac troponin in a 1 : 1 : 1 mole ratio and observed that the resulting complex behaved like the native undissociated troponin, in among other things, conferring Ca^{2+} sensitivity on the ATPase activity of a synthetic actomyosin preparation. We extended these observations to include an examination of their far UV CD spectra in the presence and absence of Ca^{2+} (Fig. 10-8). The reconstituted complexes were sensitive to Ca^{2+} and a conformational change, analogous to that induced initially in TN-C could still be involved by this cation [8]. Also, the binding constants obtained for Ca^{2+} were higher than those obtained for TN-C alone under similar conditions. Ca^{2+} also stabilized the various complexes against thermal denaturation.

Inclusion of the tropomyosin moiety to which the troponin complex is linked via the TN-T member, allowed us to demonstrate that the Ca^{2+}-induced change in TN-C was still effective in a fully reconstituted relaxing system containing all the troponin subunits and tropomyosin. These facts are all consistent with the molecular model presented in Fig. 10-2.

An important finding that came out of these studies on synthetic cardiac troponin complexes was the necessity to maintain the -SH groups of the various members of the troponin complex, particularly TN-I, in the reduced state. Using CD spectroscopy as a ruler of complex formation, we could only detect viable interactions when thiols were maintained intact. Unless -SH groups are protected, it is conceivable that non-physiological disulfide formation (both intra- and intermolecular) of the various members of the troponin complex may result when attempts are made to reconstitute such a complex from individual subunits, or even when dealing with native troponin. Such misassembled complexes may possess a degree of rigidity not permitting normal responsiveness to Ca^{2+} [22].

The shape of cardiac troponin and its subunits

Most of what is known about the size and shape of cardiac whole troponin has been gleaned from hydrodynamic measurements [23]. Fig. 10-9 illustrates the results of such a study. From the limiting value of the Stokes radius of 5.2 nm corresponding to monomeric troponin with $Mr = 78,000$ (radius of equivalent sphere = 2.8 nm), the translational frictional ratio (f/f_{min}) is calculated to be 1.85, which is considerably larger than the range (1.15–1.30) found for most globular proteins, thus indicating that troponin is an unusually asymmetric molecule. The

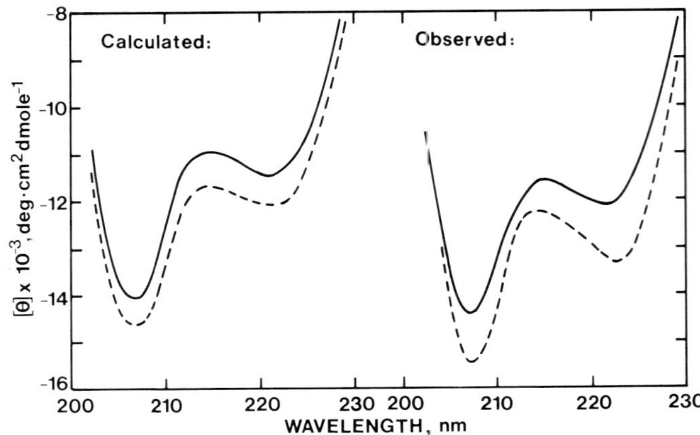

Figure 10-8. Calculated and observed CD spectra of reconstituted cardiac troponin in the presence (– – –) and absence (———) of calcium. The cardiac troponin subunits were dissolved in 0.5 M KCl, 50 mM Tris HCl, pH 7.5, 1 mM EGTA and mixed in an equimolar ratio [8].

relatively high reduced viscosity of troponin (>10 ml/g) is considerably larger than the values (3–5 ml/g) normally exhibited by globular proteins supporting the idea of asymmetry of troponin.

What about the shapes of the constituent subunits? The TN-C component has been shown to be globular (axial ratio of the equivalent elipsoid being no greater than 3 or 4:1). Similar studies suggested a moderate asymmetry for the TN-1 entity [24]. Hydrodynamic studies are rather difficult to perform on cardiac TN-T because of the tendency to aggregation; however, results suggest that TN-I forms highly asymmetric aggregates in solution [24]. These data imply that the overall shape of the troponin complex may well be dominated by the TN-T subunit. An electron microscopic investigation of the skeletal protein [25] showed that TN-T corresponds to the tail section of rotary-shadowed troponin, a long rod-like molecule with a length of -16.5 nm.

It has been demonstrated by immunoelectron microscopy [26], affinity chromatography [27] and cross-linking studies [28] that the C-terminal half of skeletal TN-T can interact with tropomyosin. This section of TN-T is probably located close to TN-C and TN-I, about 13.0 nm from the tropomyosin overlap region. It has also been shown that a highly-helical region in the N-terminal half of TN-T has been implicated in an additional interaction with the C-terminal region of tropomyosin [29, 30]. Thus the evidence points to skeletal TN-T as an elongated molecule with several distinct domains, which are involved in interactions with other thin filament components. Such detailed information is lacking as yet on cardiac TN-T but very recently chicken cardiac TN-T has been sequenced and some interesting speculations put forward [31]. These authors find substantial sequence conservation (as well as similar hydrophobicity/hydrophilicity domains), between the C-terminal 212 amino acids of cardiac and skeletal TN-T.

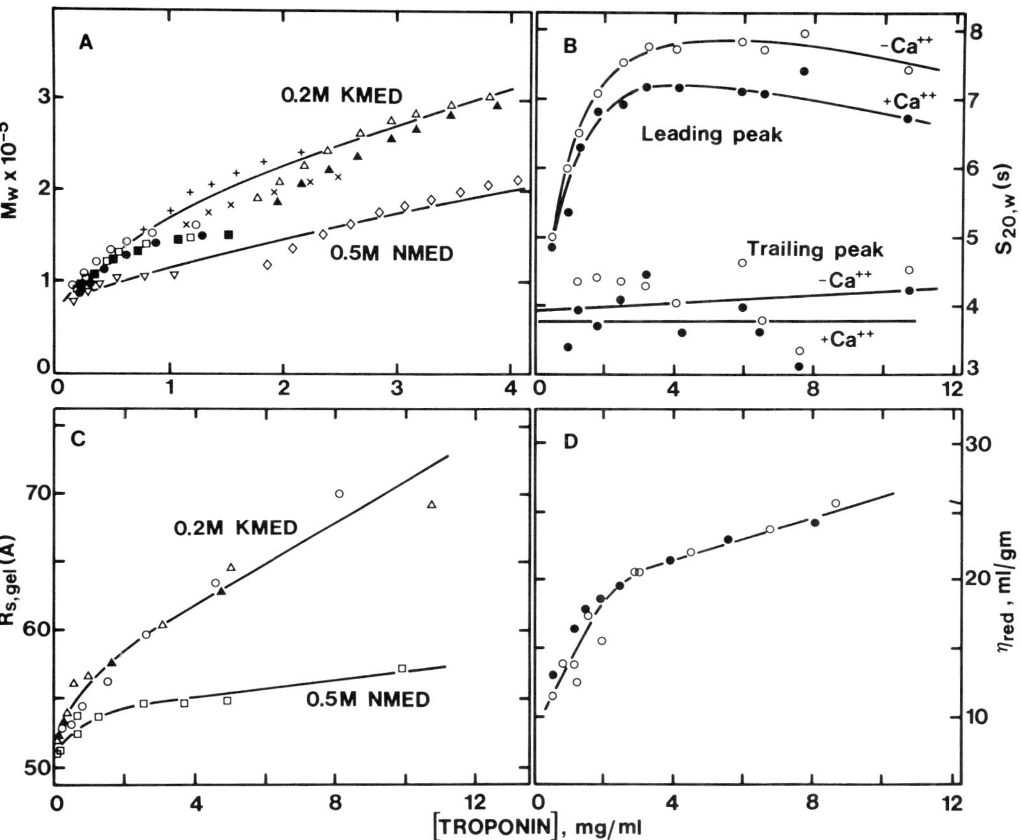

Figure 10-9. (A). Effect of protein concentration on the molecular weight of cardiac troponin. Conventional and meniscus depletion sedimentation equilibrium experiments were performed on samples of cardiac troponin in 0.2 M KMED or 0.5 M NMED at pH 7.2. Most runs were recorded with interference optics although two scanner experiments in 0.2 M KMED ($-Ca^{2+}$) are also included ($+$, $\times$). the solid lines were visually drawn through the data. Initial protein concentrations mg/ml and equilibrium rotor speeds rpm were ($\bigcirc$, $\bullet$) 0.58, 16,000; ($\square$, $\blacksquare$) 1.1, 14,000; ($\triangle$) 2.53, 3600; ($\blacktriangle$) 2.78, 3600; ($+$) 1.35, 4800; ($\times$) 2.0, 4800; ($\triangledown$) 0.98, 17,000; ($\diamondsuit$) 2.8, 4800. Open symbols: $-Ca^{2+}$; closed symbols $+2$ mM Ca.

(B). Effect of protein concentration on the sedimentation coefficient of cardiac troponin. Troponin samples (0.5 ml) in 0.2 M KMED (pH 7.2) were sedimented at 60,000 rpm and Schlieren photos were taken at 16 min intervals. Double sector cells of width 12 mM were used, except at the two lowest protein concentrations (30 mm cells). Ca^{2+} concentrations were: ($\bigcirc$) No Ca^{2+}, ($\bigcirc$) 2 mM Ca^{2+}.

(C). Effect of protein concentration on the apparent Stokes radius of cardiac troponin. Two types of gel filtration columns were used: (a) Sephacryl S-300 (74×1.1 cm) in 0.2 M ($\bigcirc$) or 0.5 M ($\square$) KMED (pH 7.2). Flow rate: 15 ml/h, (b) Biogel A 1.6 M (55×0.8 cm) in 0.2 M KMED at pH 7.2 ($\triangle$, $\blacktriangle$). Flow rate 6 ml/h. Samples (300 μl) at the concentrations indicated were applied and 0.4 ml fractions were collected. Ca^{2+} concentrations were: ($\bigcirc$, $\square$, $\triangle$) no Ca^{2+}, ($\blacktriangle$) 2 mM Ca^{2+}.

(D). Viscosity of cardiac troponin in 0.2 M KMED (pH 7.2). Reduced viscosity (η red) was measured for samples (0.5 ml) in the absence ($\bigcirc$) or presence ($\bullet$) of 2 mM Ca^{2+}. Modified from data in (23).

124

Since this region of skeletal TN-T contains the binding sites for tropomyosin, TN-T and TN-C, they conclude that cardiac TN-T is probably structurally and functionally similar in this C-terminal region. An important difference noted in the sequence of the cardiac analogue is the considerably longer N-terminal domain (79 residues versus 47 in the skeletal protein) as well as a greater percentage of acidic residues (glutamic acid) in this region. Since the N-terminal region of skeletal TN-T has been shown to be involved in the interaction between adjacent tropomyosin chains or between tropomyosin and the actin filament, the authors propose that the N-terminal domain of cardiac TN-T occupies a similar position on the thin filament as that proposed for skeletal TN-T. However, the structural differences between the N-terminal region of cardiac TN-T and its skeletal counterpart suggest that the molecular details of their interaction with tropomyosin or actin differ correspondingly.

The low- and high-affinity Ca^{2+}-binding site(s) in cardiac TN-C

The Ca^{2+} binding subunit of cardiac troponin TN-C, is part of a family of homologous Ca^{2+}-binding proteins which are thought to have evolved from a common ancestral protein by gene duplication. Other members include calmodulin, parvalbumin and the regulatory light chains of myosin. The X-ray crystal structure of parvalbumin revealed that each Ca^{2+}-binding site consists of a 'helix-loop-helix' arrangement in the polypeptide chain which is folded around the bound cation. Four such regions were found in the sequence of rabbit skeletal TN-C [32] and later studies showed that this protein indeed binds 4 Ca^{2+} ions [33]. These Ca^{2+}-binding sites are usually labelled I to IV, starting from the N-terminus. Sites I and II are the low affinity Ca^{2+}-specific sites while III and IV represent the high-affinity $Ca^{2+} -Mg^{2+}$ sites [33]. It was noticed [34] that there were extensive amino acid replacements in the site I region of the bovine cardiac TN-C sequence and the suggestion was made that this protein would only be able to bind 3 Ca^{2+} ions. This prediction has been confirmed [35]. Thus cardiac TN-C has two high-affinity sites like skeletal TN-C, one low-affinity Ca^{2+}-specific site and one defunct or mutated low-affinity site.

The three-dimensional structure of the Ca^{2+}-binding sites

The three-dimensional structure of the three Ca^{2+}-binding sites in cardiac TN-C has not been determined as yet, however, it may be advantageous to examine some details of the recent X-ray structures reported for turkey [36] and chicken [37] skeletal TN-C. Figure 10-10 shows a ribbon diagram of the turkey skeletal TN-C molecule. The structure is rather unusual. It is a two-domain entity with the upper helical one in the diagram being the N-terminal region containing the two low affinity Ca^{2+}-specific regulatory sites. The lower domain contains the C-terminal portion with the two high-affinity Ca^{2+}/Mg^{2+} sites. The domains are connected by a long 9-turn a-helical portion of chain. Although Ca^{2+} was included in the crystallization medium (10 fold excess over protein) only the two high affinity sites are metalfilled; the regulatory domain is metal-free. This is undoubtedly a function of the low pH (5.0) used for crystallization and may reflect a stabilizing effect of competing hydroxonium ions. Thus the structure is similar to what one might expect for TN-C in the relaxed state of muscle.

The physiological role of the two classes of Ca^{2+}-binding sites

As has been noted earlier, binding of Ca^{2+} by cardiac TN-C induces a large conformational change. Circular dichroism studies showed that most of this change results from the occupation of the high-affinity Ca^{2+}/Mg^{2+} sites [20, 38]. On the other hand, only relatively minor conformational alterations are associated with Ca^{2+}-binding to the low-affinity Ca^{2+}-specific sites. For the cardiac subunit the changes include NMR-detected variations in phenylalanine environment [16], and a two-fold increase in the fluorescence of an external probe [39]. Additional evidence comes from a study using limited tryptic digestion to generate large fragments of cardiac TN-C. It is found that a N-terminal peptide, comprising residues 1-88 or so and containing defunct site I as well as Ca^{2+}-specific site II, binds 1 mole of Ca^{2+} with low affinity, and slows limited conformational sensitivity to the presence of this cation [40].

Nevertheless, it appears that the Ca^{2+} specific site(s) in TN-C is (are) responsible for the regulation of muscle contraction. Actomyosin ATPase is activated in the same range of free Ca^{2+} concentration that is required to saturate the two Ca^{2+}-specific sites on skeletal TN-C [33], or the single site on cardiac TN-C [11]. Kinetic studies with skeletal TN-C also support a biologically-important role for these sites [41]. Stopped-flow fluorescence measurements with dansylaziridine-labelled TN-C indicated that Ca^{2+} removal from the Ca^{2+}-specific sites occurs with a half-life of 2–3 ms, while $t_{1/2}$ for the removal of Ca^{2+} from the Ca^{2+}/Mg^{2+} sites is ~ 700 ms. Similar results were observed for cardiac TN-C [42]. Since these $t_{1/2}$ values would be even higher in native troponin, because of the increased affinity for Ca^{2+} in the complex, Ca^{2+}-exchange in the Ca^{2+}/Mg^{2+} sites is clearly too slow to participate in a rapid switching mechanism where contraction-relaxation events must be complete within about 50 ms of excitation [43]. In any case, the intracellular concentrations of Ca^{2+} ($\sim 10^{-8}$ M) and Mg^{2+} (a few millimolar) are sufficiently high that the Ca^{2+}/Mg^{2+} sites would be occupied even under relaxing conditions [44]. Recent studies have suggested that these sites stabilize the structure of the protein to maintain it in a receptive conformation for the regulatory event of Ca^{2+} exchange with the low-affinity Ca^{2+}-specific regulatory sites(s) [45].

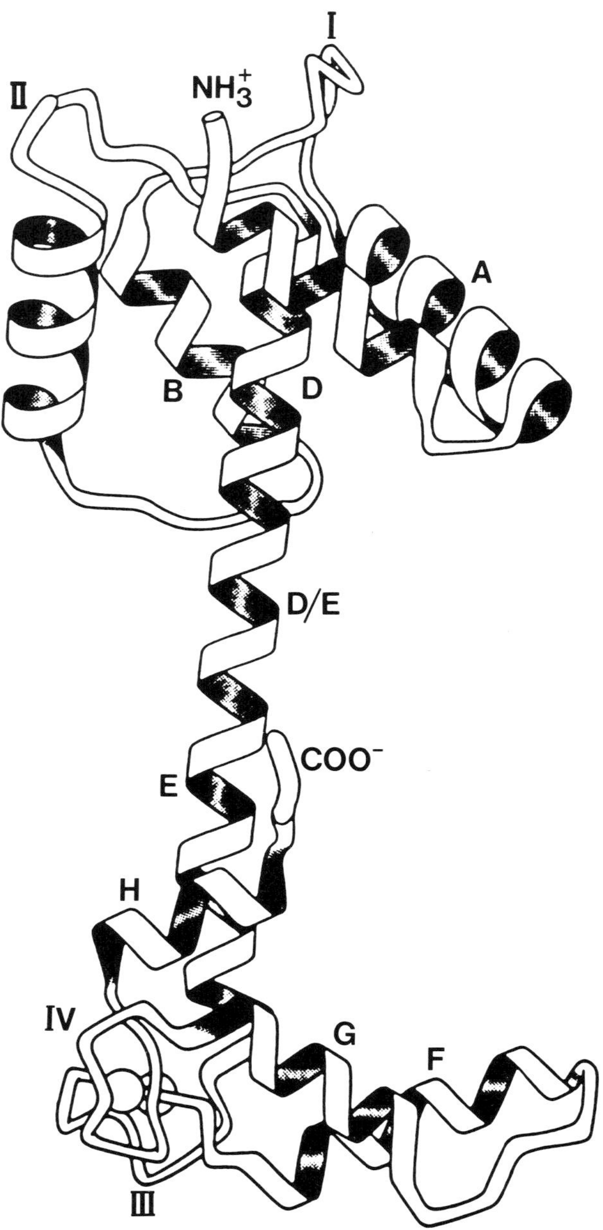

Figure 10-10. A ribbon representation of the polypeptide chain of turkey skeletal muscle troponin C. The upper domain is the calcium regulatory domain (N-domain), while the lower domain is the high-affinity Ca^{2+}/Mg^{2+} binding domain (C-domain). The eight helices involved in the four supersecondary helix-loop-helix motifs are labeled A-H sequentially. There is an additional helical segment at the beginning of the N-domain sequence. The segments of polypeptide chain forming the Ca^{2+} binding loops are labeled I to IV sequentially. Ca^{2+} ions are found in the crystal structure only in sites III and IV (46).

It is worthwhile at this point to return to the X-ray structure of turkey skeletal TN-C to inquire into the nature of the Ca^{2+}-induced conformational change. It has been suggested that the binding of the two Ca^{2+} ions at the Ca^{2+}-specific sites causes the N-terminal regulatory domain to undergo a conformational change such that it is very similar to the C-terminal region which always is filled with Ca^{2+} or Mg^{2+} under physiological conditions. The majority of this change is found in movement and reorientation of the B and C helices and the helical peptide connecting the two domains [46] (cf. Fig. 10-10). Cardiac TN-C, on the other hand, has only one Ca^{2+}-specific site (site II) and it is conceivable that the changes induced by Ca^{2+} binding are somewhat diminished. Certainly, shape estimates of whole cardiac troponin by hydrodynamic methods are essentially unchanged by the presence of Ca^{2+}, suggesting that the Ca^{2+} trigger on the cardiac thin filament involves a relatively minor conformational alteration, perhaps with subtle altera-tions occurring at regions of the protein surface that interact with other subunits, e.g. generation of a hydrophobic hatch on helix B could be a possible binding site for TN-I, considered to be between residues 49–80 on TN-C.

How can the observed structural insensitivity of these proteins to Ca^{2+} be reconciled with a control mechanism, such as the steric blocking hypothesis, in which fairly large protein motions are presumed to occur? In fact, there may be no discrepancy at all. Since troponin contains sites which interact with both tropomyosin and actin, it is conceivable that a rather small Ca^{2+}-induced con-formational change within the troponin complex would be amplified when re-layed to these other proteins. For example, a slight rotation of one troponin subunit relative to the others might escape detection by hydrodynamic techniques while still causing a substantial change in the orientation of these interaction sites. Alternatively, one or more interaction sites (i.e. between TN-I and actin) could be strengthened or weakened in a Ca^{2+}-dependent manner, thus allowing tro-ponin to move relative to tropomyosin and/or actin.

Future considerations

Some of the basic points pertaining to the Ca^{2+} regulation of cardiac muscle contraction-relaxation have been outlined in protein chemistry terms. A number of questions remain unanswered and it is anticipated that future research efforts will be directed to some of the more important ones. For example, are the actin filamentous structures (or the G-actin constituent monomers) modified in any way by the 2.0 nm or so movement of troponin across the actin surface in response to the Ca^{2+}-signal? As well, establishment of the X-ray structure of cardiac TN-C will be extremely important as it will yield valuable information regarding the effect that the mutation of Ca^{2+}-binding site I has on the overall shape/flexibility of this N-terminal domain. In the final analysis, all possible mechanistic models for contraction-relaxation will have to be analyzed within a framework of chemical equilibrium and cooperativity along the thin filament. This cooperativity between adjacent troponin-tropomyosin units has become very interesting in light of the present knowledge that TN-T extends to the tropomyosin overlap region.

Acknowledgements

The work described in the authors' laboratory was generally supported by the Medical Research Council of Canada, the Alberta Heart Foundation and the Alberta Heritage Foundation for Medical Research. They are also indebted to their technical support staff, K. Oikasa, V. Ledsham and A. Keri.

References

1. Ebashi, S.: Third component participating in the superprecipitation of natural actomyosin. Nature 200: 1010, 1963.
2. Ebashi, S., Ebashi, F. and Kodama, A.: Troponin as the calcium receptive protein in the contractile system. J. Biochem. (Tokyo) 62: 137–138, 1967.
3. Greaser, M.L. and Gergely, J.: Purification and properties of the components from troponin. J. Biol. Chem. 248: 2125–2133, 1973.
4. Potter, J.D.: The content of troponin, tropomyosin, actin and myosin in rabbit skeletal muscle myofibrils. Arch. Biochem. Biophys. 162: 436–441, 1974.
5. Huxley, H.E.: Structural changes in the actin and myosin containing filaments during contraction. Cold Spring Harb. Symp. Quant. Biol. 37: 361–376, 1972.
6. Parry, D.A.D. and Squire, J.M.: Structural role of tropomyosin in muscle regulation: analysis of the X-ray diffraction patterns from relaxed and contracting muscles. J. Mol. Biol. 75: 33–55, 1973.
7. Chalovich, J.M., Eisenberg, E.: Inhibition of actomyosin ATPase activity by troponin tropomyosin without blocking the binding of myosin to actin. J. Biol. Chem. 257: 2432–2437, 1983.
8. Burtnich, L.D.: This isolation of characterization of the components of bovine cardiac troponin. Ph. D. Thesis, University of Alberta, 1977.
9. Hincke, M.T., McCubbin, W.D. and Kay, C.M.: A circular dichroism and biological activity study on the hybrid species formed from bovine cardiac and rabbit skeletal troponin subunits. FEBS Lett. 83: 131–136, 1977.
10. Cachia, P.J., Van Eyk, J. McCubbin, W.D., Kay, C.M. and Hodges, R.S.: Ion – exchange high performance liquid chromatographic purification of bovine cardiac and rabbit skeletal muscle troponin subunits. J. Chromatog. 343: 315, 1985.
11. Holroyde, M.J., Robertson, S.P., Johnson, J.D., Solaro, R.J. and Potter, J.D.: The calcium and magnesium binding sites on cardiac troponin and their role in the regulation of myofibrillar adenosine triphosphatase. J. Biol. Chem. 255: 11688–11693, 1980.
12. Potter, J.D. and Zot, H.G.: The role of actin in modulating Ca^{2+} binding to troponin. Biophys. J. 37: 43a, 1982.
13. Burtnick, L.D., McCubbin, W.D. and Kay, C.M.: Molecular and biological studies on cardiac muscle calcium binding protein (TN-C). Can. J. Biochem. 53: 15–20, 1975.
14. Szynkiewicz, S., Stepkowski, D., Breyeska, H. and Drabikowski, W.: Cardiac troponin C: A rapid and effective method of purification. FEBS Lett. 181: 281–285, 1985.
15. McCubbin, W.D., Oikawa, K., Sykes, B.D. and Kay, C.M.: Purification and characterization of

troponin C from pike muscle: A comparative spectroscopic study with rabbit skeletal troponin C. Biochemistry 21: 5948–5956, 1982.

16. Hincke, M.T., Sykes, B.D. and Kay, C.M.: Hydrogen-1 NMR investigation of bovine cardiac troponin C. Comparison of tyrosyl assignments and calcium induced structural changes to rabbit skeletal TN-C and bovine brain calmodulin. Biochemistry 20: 3286–3294, 1981.

17. Hincke, M.T., Sykes, B.D. and Kay, C.M.: Laser photochemically induced dynamic nuclear polarization proton NMR studies on three homologous calcium binding proteins: cardiac troponin C, skeletal troponin C and ca-modulin. Biochemistry 20: 4185–4193, 1981.

18. Byers, D.M. and Kay, C.M.: Hydrodynamic properties of bovine cardiac troponin-C. Biochemistry 21: 229–233, 1982.

19. McCubbin, W.D. and Kay, C.M.: Physico-chemical and biological studies on the metal-induced conformational change in troponin A. Implication of carboxyl groups in the binding of calcium ions. Biochemistry 12: 4228–4232, 1973.

20. Hincke, M.T., McCubbin, W.D. and Kay, C.M.: Calcium binding properties of cardiac and skeletal troponin C as determined by circular dichroism and ultra-violet difference spectroscopy. Can. J. Biochem. 56: 384–395, 1978.

21. Nozaki, Y., Bunville, L.C. and Tanford, C.: Hydrogen ion titration curves of beta-lactoglobulin. J. Am. Chem. Soc. 81: 5523, 1959.

22. Hincke, M.T., McCubbin, W.D. and Kay, C.M.: The interaction between beef cardiac troponin T and troponin I as determined by UV difference spectroscopy, circular dichroism and gel filtration. Can. J. Biochem. 37: 768–775, 1979.

23. Byers, D.M., McCubbin, W.D. and Kay, C.M.: Hydrodynamic properties of bovine cardiac troponin. FEBS Lett. 104: 106–110, 1979.

24. Byers, D.M. and Kay, C.M.: Hydrodynamic properties of bovine cardiac troponin I and Troponin T. J. Biol. Chem. 258: 2951, 1985.

25. Flicker, P.F., Phillips, G.N. and Cohen, C.: Structure of troponin and its interaction with tropomyosin. Biophys. J. 37: 266a, 1982.

26. Ohtsuki, I.: Molecular arrangement of troponin-T in the thin filament. J. biochem. (Tokyo) 86: 491–497, 1979.

27. Pearlstone, J.R. and Smillie, L.B.: Identification of a second binding region on rabbit skeletal troponin T for alphatropomyosin: FEBS Lett. 128: 119–122, 1981.

28. Chong, P.C.S. and Hodges, R.S.: Proximity of sulfhydryl groups to the sites of interaction between components of the troponin complex from rabbit skeletal muscle. J. Biol. Chem. 257: 2549–2555, 1982.

29. Jackson, P., Amphlett, G.W. and Perry, S.V.: The primary structure of troponin T and the interaction with tropomyosin. Biochem. J. 151: 85–97, 1975.

30. Pearlstone, J.R. and Smillie, L.B.: The binding site of rabbit skeletal alpha-tropomyosin on troponin-T. Can. J. Biochem. 55: 1032–1038, 1977.

31. Cooper, T.A. and Ordahl, C.P.: A single cardiac troponin T gene generates embryonic and adult isoforms via developmentally regulated alternate splicing. J. Biol. Chem. 260: 11140–11148, 1985.

32. Collins, J.H., Potter, J.D., Horn, M.J., Wilshire, G. and Jackson, N.: The amino acid sequence of rabbit skeletal muscle troponin-C: Gene replication and homology with calcium binding proteins from carp and hake muscle. FEBS Lett. 36: 268–272, 1973.

33. Potter, J.D. and Gergely, J.: The calcium and magnesium binding sites on troponin and their role in the regulation of myofibrillar adenosine triphosphatase. J. Biol. Chem. 250: 4628–4633, 1975.

34. Van Eerd, J.-P. and Takahashi, K.: The amino acid sequence of bovine cardiac troponin-C: Comparison with rabbit skeletal troponin-C. Biochem. Biophys. Res. Comm. 64: 122–127, 1975.

35. Burtnick, L.D. and Kay, C.M.: The calcium-binding properties of bovine cardiac troponin-C.: FEBS Lett. 75: 105–110, 1977.

36. Herzberg, O. and James, M.N.G.: Structure of the calcium regulatory muscle troponin-C at angstrom resolution. Nature 313: 653–659, 1985.

130

37. Sundaralingam, M., Bergstrom, R., Strasberg, G. Rao, S.T., Roychowdhury, P., Greaser, M. and Wang, B.C.: Molecular structure of troponin C from chicken skeletal muscle at 3~ angstrom resolution. Science 227: 945–948, 1985.

38. Johnson, J.P. and Potter, J.D.: Detection of two classes of Ca binding sites in troponin C with circular dichroism and tyrosine fluorescence. J. Biol. Chem. 253: 3775–3777, 1978.

39. Johnson, J.D., Collins, J.H., Robertson, S.P. and Potter, J.D.: A fluorescent probe study of and Ca binding to the Ca specific sites of cardiac troponin and troponin-C. J. Biol. Chem. 255: 9635–9640, 1980.

40. McCubbin, W.D. and Kay, C.M.: Trypsin digestion of bovine cardiac troponin-C in the presence and absence of calcium. Can. J. Biochem. Cell. Biol. 63: 812–823, 1985.

41. Johnson, J.D., Charlton, S.C. and Potter, J.D.: A fluorescence stopped flow analysis of Ca exchange with troponin C. J. Biol. Chem. 254: 3497–3502, 1979.

42. Johnson, J.D., Collins, J.H., Robertson, S.P. and Potter, J.D.: A fluorescent probe study of &Ca exchange with Ca-specific site of cardiac troponin-C: Circulation 58: 11–71, 1978.

43. Carlson, F.D. and Wilkie, D.R.: Muscle Physiology, Prentice-Hall, New Jersey, 1974.

44. Potter, J.D., Robertson, S.P. and Johnson, J.D.: Magnesium and the regulation of muscle contraction. Fed. Proc. 40: 2653–2656, 1981.

45. Zot, H.G. and Potter, J.D.: A structural role of the Ca-Mg sites on troponin-C in the regulation of muscle contraction. J. Biol. Chem. 257: 7678–7683, 1982.

46. Herzberg, O., Moult, J. and James, M.N.G.: A model of the calcium induced conformation transition of troponin-C. J. Biol. Chem. 261: 2638–2644, 1986.

47. Mak, A.S. and Smillie, L.B.: Structural interpretation of the two-site binding of troponin of the muscle thin filament. J. Mol. Biol. 149: 541–550, 1981.

48. Ebashi, S., Endo, M. and Ohtsuki, I.: Control of muscle contraction. Quart. Rev. Biophys. 2: 351–384, 1969.

49. Potter, J.D. and Gergely, J.: Troponin, tropo-myosin and actin interactions in the calcium regulation of muscle contraction. Biochemistry 13: 2697–2703, 1974.

Abbreviations

ATPase, adenosine triphosphatase; CD, circular dichroism; photo CIDNP, photochemically induced dynamic nuclear polarization; EGTA, ethyleneglycolbis (B-aminoethylene) N, N'-tetraacetic acid; DMSO, dimethyl sulfoxide; NMR, nuclear magnetic resonance; SDS, sodium dodecyl sulfate; PAGE, polyacrylamide gel electrophoresis; UV, ultraviolet; pCa^{2+}, negative logarithm of the free Ca^{2+} concentration; MOPS, morpholinopropane sulfonic acid. XM KMED (or NMED) analytical buffer consisting of XM KCl (or NaCl), 50 mM MOPS, 1 mM EGTA and DTT.

11. Evidence that a decrease in sarcomere length reduces the Ca^{++} affinity of troponin in the intact cardiac myofibril

JONATHAN C. KENTISH and DAVID G. ALLEN

Introduction

Biochemical studies on troponin (TN), such as those described by Dr. Kay, have been invaluable in defining the number and affinity of the Ca^{2+}-binding sites in the molecule. Such studies have usually been performed using isolated TN in solution. However, there is indirect evidence that the Ca^{2+}-affinity of TN in the intact myofibril may be different from that in the isolated protein and may be altered by processes and constraints involved in the production of force (for review, see [1]). We have been particularly interested in whether the Ca^{2+}-affinity of cardiac TN is reduced at shorter sarcomere lengths (SL). If this is so, it could explain such phenomena as (i) the SL-dependence of myofibrillar Ca^{2+}-sensitivity [2, 3, 4] and Chapter 6 by ter Keurs et al. in this volume and (ii) the small 'bump' on the decay of the Ca^{2+} transient that is seen if an aequorin-injected papillary muscle is rapidly shortened (Allen and Kurihara [5]); this bump was attributed to Ca^{2+} release from troponin because of a reduced Ca^{2+}-affinity at the shorter SL, though it could equally well have been due to Ca^{2+} release from the sarcoplasmic reticulum or from mitochondria.

To try to establish whether or not the Ca^{2+}-affinity of cardiac troponin is indeed lower at short SL, we [5] have used skinned cardiac muscles (trabeculae from rat or ferret) in which all cellular membranes were destroyed by 1–24 hr treatment of the muscle with the detergent Triton X-100; this 'skinning' procedure leaves TN as the major site of Ca^{2+} binding in these muscles. Our approach was to partially activate these skinned muscles with Ca^{2+} (in an artificial cytosol), and then rapidly reduce their length. We reasoned that if the Ca^{2+}-affinity of TN were reduced at the shorter length, some Ca^{2+} should be released from TN by this procedure and should be detectable. Alternatively, if the Ca^{2+}-affinity of TN was insensitive to SL, no Ca^{2+} release would occur. We loaded the muscles with the Ca^{2+}-sensitive bioluminescent protein, aequorin, to check for any Ca^{2+} release.

We found that when the skinned muscles were activated to about 80% of maximum force (with ~15 μM Ca^{2+}) and then released by 10% of the initial

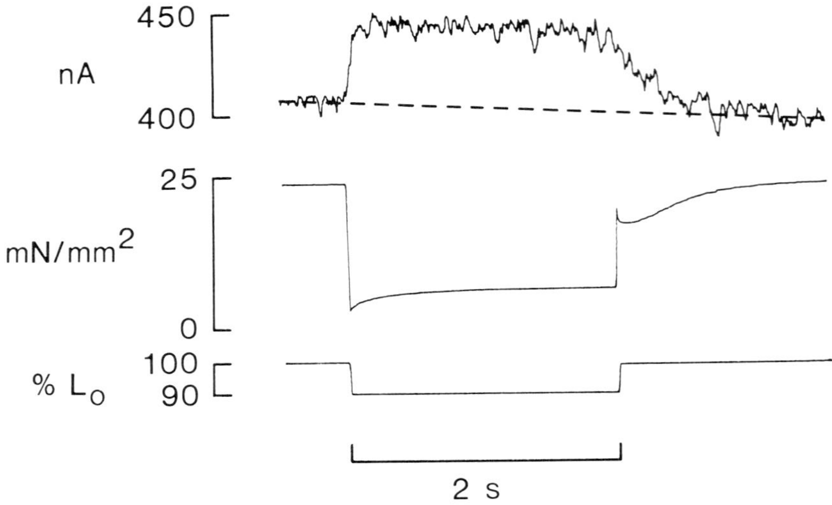

Figure 11-1. Chart records of aequorin light emission (top), muscle force (middle), and muscle length (bottom) in a detergent-skinned trabecula from ferret ventricle. The muscle was bathed in an activating solution containing 15 uM free Ca^{2+}, which was weakly buffered with 100 uM EGTA. Note that the reduction in muscle length caused aequorin light to increase, and that after the muscle was restretched the fall in light had a relatively slow time-course, similar to that of force redevelopment. The dashed line indicates the slow fall of light that resulted from the consumption of aequorin or its diffusion out of the muscle. Averaged records from 16 muscle releases. 22° C. Taken from Allen and Kentish [6] with permission.

length, force production fell considerably and the light emission from aequorin rose (Fig. 11-1). The increase in light indicated that the $[Ca^{2+}]$ in the myofibrillar space of the muscle had risen. Almost certainly, the extra Ca^{2+} was released from TN. These experiments therefore support the idea that the Ca^{2+}-affinity of TN is not constant, but is reduced at shorter SL.

The Ca^{2+}-affinity of TN could have been directly influenced either by muscle length or by force production, as both were reduced by muscle release. However, when the muscle was restretched rapidly (in 10 ms) to its original length, there was a slow decrease of light (presumably as Ca^{2+} rebound to TN) and a slow increase of force (Fig. 11-1). Thus the timecourse of the light response was similar to that of force redevelopment and very different from that of the length increase. From this it would appear that the Ca^{2+}-affinity of TN is more closely related to force production than to SL itself. It could be that the association between Ca^{2+}-affinity and force is due to a slow increase in the number of myosin crossbridges bound to actin after the restretch of the muscle; these crossbridges would not only generate force but also could directly increase the Ca^{2+}-affinity of TN, as originally suggested by Bremel and Weber [7] for crossbridge attachment at much lower (μM) concentrations of MgATP (rigor attachment).

The conclusion from these studies is that the Ca^{2+} affinity of TN in the intact myofibril decreases if the SL is reduced. This effect can at least partly account for the observed fall of myofibrillar Ca^{2+}-sensitivity at shorter SL [2, 3, 4]. In addition, we have obtained some evidence that the effect of a change of SL upon the Ca^{2+}-affinity of TN may be mediated via changes in the number of myosin crossbridges attached to actin. This illustrates that the properties of TN are influenced by protein interactions within the working myofibril. Consequently, a complete understanding of the role of TN in excitation-contraction coupling will require the characterization of TN in the intact myofibril as well as in solution.

References

1. Allen, D.G. and Kentish, J.C.: The cellular basis of the length-tension relationship in cardiac muscle. Journal of Molecular and Cellular Cardiology 17: 821–840, 1985a.
2. Fabiato, A. and Fabiato, F.: Myofilament-generated tension oscillations during partial calcium activation and activation dependence of the sarcomere length-tension relation of skinned cardiac cells. Journal of General Physiology 72: 667–699, 1978.
3. Hibberd, M.G. and Jewell, B.R.: Calcium- and length-dependent force production in rat ventricular muscle. Journal of Physiology 329: 527–540 1982.
4. Kentish, J.C., ter Keurs, H.E.D.J., Ricciardi, L., Bucx, J.J. and Noble, M.I.M.: Comparison between the sarcomere length-force relations of intact and skinned trabeculae from rat right ventricle. Influence of calcium concentrations on these relations. Circ. Res. 58: 755–768, 1986.
5. Allen, D.G. and Kurihara, S.: The effects of muscle length on intracellular calcium transients in mammalian cardiac muscle. Journal of Physiology 327: 79–94, 1986.
6. Allen, D.G. and Kentish, J.C.: The effects of length changes on myoplasmic calcium concentration in skinned ferret ventricular muscle. Journal of Physiology, 366: 67P, 1985b.
7. Bremel, R.D. and Weber, A.: Cooperation within actin filament in vertebrate skeletal muscle. Nature, New Biology 238: 97–101, 1972.

General discussion of the physicochemistry of contractile proteins

It was discussed that a lack of exact correspondence between results on calcium binding to troponin in physicochemical studies and of studies in muscle with a preserved structure probably relates to the effects of intermolecular interactions in the intact structure. This is, for example, suggested by experiments in which the effect of activation of skeletal myofibrils by strontium ions was determined by the presence of either skeletal troponin-C or cardiac troponin-C. In the case of optical studies of the physicochemical properties of the contractile proteins the constraints are evidently imposed by the development of optical artefacts in the presence of complex solutions.

Length dependence of force development can not simply be related to variation of the number of active cross bridges with variation of length as the ATPase activity of skinned muscle is largely independent of sarcomere length at maximal calciumactivation (Kentish unpublished observations). This suggests that restoring forces may be important to the shape of the force length relation.

12. Mechanics of cardiac contraction and the phosphorylation of sarcotubular and myofilament proteins

R. JOHN SOLARO, STEPHEN T. RAPUNDALO, J. LEE GARVEY, EVANGELIA G. KRANIAS

Introduction

Ca²⁺, protein phosphorylation and cardiac dynamics

Acute changes in the time course and intensity of cardiac ventricular contraction occur physiologically on a beat-to-beat basis according to the particular hemodynamic 'load' on the cardiovascular system. Although these changes are related to a variety of factors, a main controller is the intensity of activity of parasympathetic and sympathetic nervous activity reaching the heart. Variations in autonomic nervous system activity alter the amplitude and rate of contraction as well as the overall time of the contraction-relaxation cycle. Examples of the altered mechanical dynamics of heart muscle preparations that occur with varying levels of adrenergic and cholinergic stimulation and with changes in the frequency of beating are depicted schematically in Fig. 1. A challenge to cardiac physiologists and biochemists is the understanding of the cellular mechanisms responsible for the alterations in the mechanical properties of the sort shown in Fig. 12-1.

This understanding must begin with an analysis of how the various perturbations shown in Fig. 12-1 are ultimately related to the activation and deactivation of the contractile machine and to the movements of Ca^{2+} ion to and from the myofilaments. The main process involved in these flows and actions of Ca^{2+} ion in cardiac cells are summarized in the scheme shown in Fig. 12-2. Contraction is stimulated by Ca^{2+}-binding to the thin filament receptor, troponin (Tn), which activates the reaction of myosin heads with actin. Relaxation results from the reversal of this activation by removal of Tn-bound Ca^{2+} into sinks for Ca^{2+}. Although the route of Ca^{2+} during relaxation involves mainly pumping in the SR, rate limiting processes in shutting down of myofilament contractile activity are not yet clear. The route of Ca^{2+} ions flowing to the myofilaments include movements across both the sarcolemma and the sarcoplasmic reticulum depending on the particular species and the conditions of activation [1]. Generally though, under physiological rates of stimulation in mammalian hearts with well

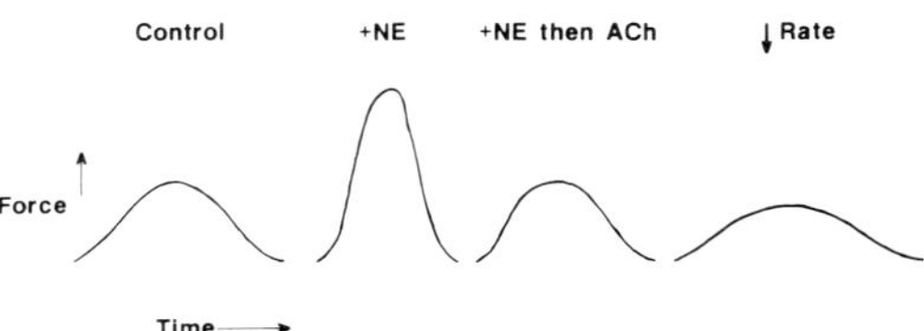

Figure 12-1. Idealized effects of various inotropic interventions on the dynamics of isometric twitch force of mammalian ventricular muscle preparations.

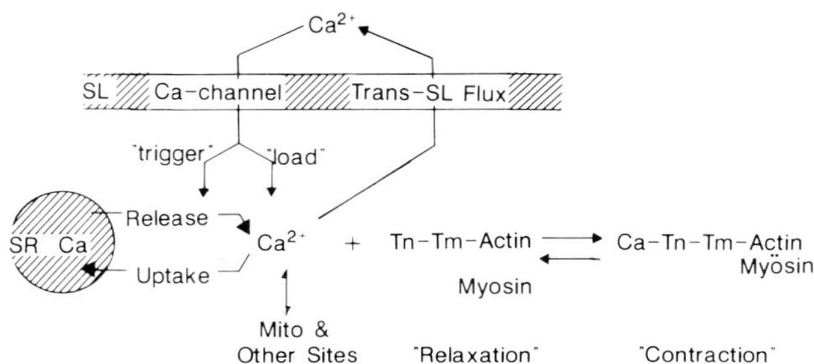

Figure 12-2. Scheme depicting intracellular Ca^{2+} flows and their relation to activation and relaxation of contractile activity in a myocardial cell. See text for description.

developed internal membranes, the sarcoplasmic reticulum (SR) most likely provides the bulk of Ca^{2+} ions activating the myofilaments. It follows that the amount of Ca^{2+} in the releasable pool of the SR is an important determinant of contractile state. The size of this reservoir of activating Ca^{2+} ions depends on the ability of the Ca^{2+}-pump of the SR to compete with other cellular sinks for Ca^{2+}, such as the mitochondria, intracellular Ca-binding proteins and extrusion through the Na^+/Ca^{2+} exchanger and through the Ca^{2+}-pump of the sarcolemma [2]. The amount of Ca^{2+} in the SR is also related to trans-sarcolemmal 'Ca^{2+}-loading' associated with a slow phase of the Ca-current [2]. It is also apparent from the studies of Fabiato and Baumgarten [2], that gating of SR Ca^{2+}-release channels is related to the fast phase of the Ca^{2+}-current.

Altered mechanical activities shown in Fig. 12-1 must reflect alterations in the processes by which Ca^{2+} is supplied and removed from the myofilaments on alterations in the process of activation and de-activation of the myofilaments. The sarcolemma, SR and the myofilaments contain protein components near the Ca^{2+}-binding sites that undergo reversible phosphorylation, and, it is likely that the interconversion of these proteins provides the main mechanism by which control of contraction and relaxation by Ca^{2+} is altered by extracellular signals. This chapter focuses on the regulation of the levels of phosphorylation of these proteins in the SR and in the myofilaments and on the role of these phosphorylations in the functional responses shown in Fig. 12-1. Clearly though, primary events in the intracellular signalling involving protein phosphorylation occur at the surface membrane and these are also discussed.

Figure 12-3 shows a scheme of structures that are believed to be involved in the trans-sarcolemmal signals eventually determining the levels of phosphorylation of protein in the SR and myofilaments. Ca^{2+} and cAMP are the most studied and clearly understood second messengers for neurohumoral signals generated by binding to muscarinic and adrenergic receptors. Levels of cAMP and Ca^{2+} regulate the activity of kinases and, most likely phosphatases as well, that determine the state of phosphorylation of intracellular proteins. As mentioned above net transsarcolemmal movements of Ca^{2+} into the cell are determined by the membrane potential, gating of Ca^{2+}-channels, activity of the Na^+/Ca^{2+} exchange mechanism, and a sarcolemma ATPase associated with Ca-extrusion. Intracellular levels of cAMP are determined by its synthesis from ATP by adenylate cyclase in the surface membrane and by its breakdown by phosphodiesterases. Adrenergic and muscarinic receptors are coupled to the adenylate cyclase by a cGMP dependent protein and, as shown in Fig. 12-3, regulation of cyclase activity is accomplished by complex integrated effects of adrenergic and muscarinic agonists on inhibitory and excitatory proteins [3]. Levels of cAMP in turn determine the level of activity of dependent protein kinases. Substrates for cAMP dependent protein kinase (cAMP-PK), are proteins that, depending on their level of phosphorylation, appear to regulate Ca^{2+} movements and responsiveness of the myofilaments to Ca^{2+}. These proteins in SR and myofilaments are discussed in detail below. In the case of the sarcolemma, there is indirect evidence that cAMP dependent phosphorylation of proteins near or in the Ca^{2+}-channel is an important determinant of the open state of the channel. This forms one mechanism by which the level of activity of adenylate cyclase is coupled to a regulation of trans-sarcolemmal Ca^{2+} movements. There is also evidence that phospho-proteins are associated with and regulate the activity of the Na^+/Ca^{2+} exchanger as well as the ATPase responsible for Ca-extrusion out of the cell [4]. Levels of intracellular Ca^{2+} not only activate contraction by binding to TnC, but also act to activate Ca^{2+}-dependent protein kinases. One class of these kinases is activated by a Ca^{2+}-calmodulin complex and formation of a ternary complex of Ca^{2+}-calmodulin-kinase.

Protein kinase C (Ca^{2+}/phospholipid dependent-PK) is another type of Ca^{2+} dependent kinase that also depends on phospholipid for its activation [5]. Regulation of the activity of protein kinase C by neurohumoral signals occurs by transduction at the cell surface involving breakdown of inosital phospholipids especially phosphatidyl inositol-4,5 biphosphate to inositol-1,4,5-trisphosphate (IP3) and diacylglycerol. These two breakdown products serve a second messenger function. IP3 acts to mobilize intracellular Ca^{2+} stores in diverse cell types, but its role in Ca^{2+}-release from muscle cells is in dispute. In the case of the heart

138

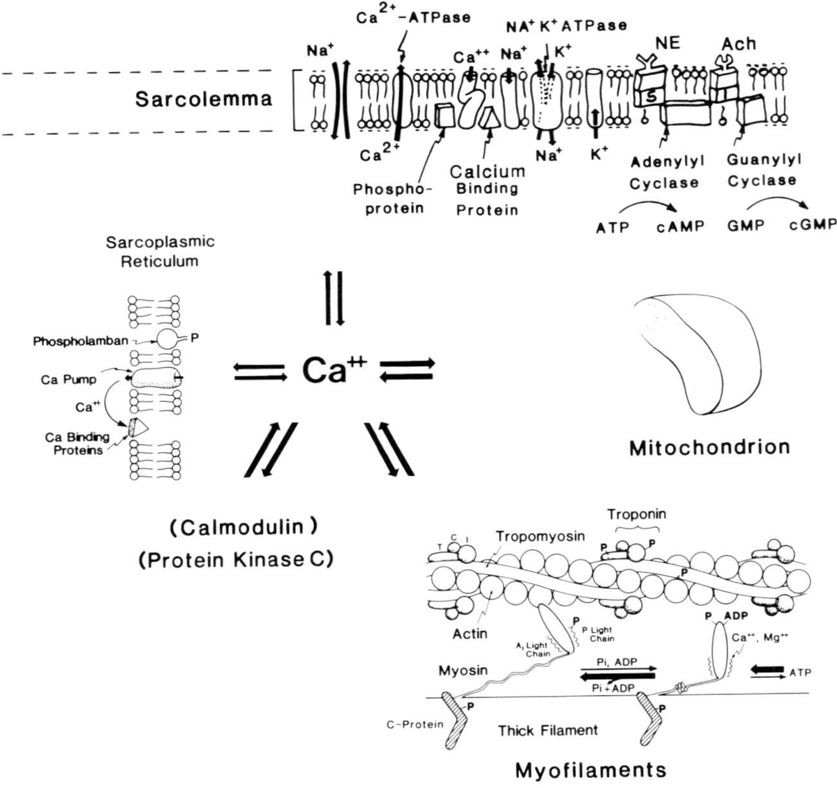

Figure 12-3. Cartoon of the sarcolemma, sarcoplasmic reticulum and myofilaments of the myocardium with emphasis on elements involved in regulation of activity by Ca^{2+} or protein phosphorylation.

IP3 appears to release Ca^{2+} from the SR, but too slowly to account for activation during the contraction-relaxation cycle [6]. The formation of diacylglycerol is related to activation of protein kinase C. This kinase is dependent on phospholipids and Ca^{2+} for its activation, and the action of diacylglycerol is to greatly enhance the affinity of the enzyme for Ca^{2+} thereby permitting its activation with no change in intracellular free Ca^{2+} concentration [5]. As discussed below, there are a number of intracellular cardiac proteins, which are in vitro substrates for Ca^{2+}/Pl-PK.

Sarcoplasmic reticulum (SR) and myofilament phosphorylation: in vitro studies

A. SR phosphorylation

The sarcoplasmic reticulum (SR) is a primary site of intracellular Ca^{2+} regulation, that acts not only to sequester myoplasmic Ca^{2+} and initiate relaxation, but also to store and release Ca^{2+} for myofilament activation. A 100,000 dalton Ca-pump is the main SR protein and couples ATP hydrolysis to transport of Ca^{2+} (Fig. 12-3). Ca^{2+} release occurs through SR channels that are poorly understood in terms of structure/function relations, but appear to be gated by the rapid phase Ca^{2+} influx forming part of the inward Ca^{2+} current during excitation [2]. In cardiac SR, a regulatory mechanism exists in which phospholamban, a specific protein component of the SR membrane serves as the major regulator of cardiac SR Ca^{2+} handling [7]. Phospholamban is a polymeric proteolipid of 22–27,000 daltons which upon boiling in sodium dodecyl sulfate, prior to gel electrophoresis, dissociates into subunits of 9-11,000 daltons [8, 9]. It appears that phospholamban contains several kinds of phosphorylatable sites that are phosphorylated by different protein kinases (Fig. 12-4) including cAMP-dependent, Ca^{2+}-calmodulin-dependent [10–14] and Ca^{2+}-phospholipid dependent enzymes [15, 16].

Cardiac SR contains primarily type II cAMP-dependent protein kinase [17], as determined by Triton X-100 solubilization and subsequent elution on a DEAE-cellulose column using histone as a substrate. The identity of the protein kinase isozyme has also been established by electrophoretic analysis of the regulatory subunits(s) after photoaffinity labelling with the cAMP analog 8-azido-[32P]-cAMP. The type II regulatory subunit was the major subunit identified.

Phosphorylation of SR by endogenous or exogenous, soluble, cAMP dependent protein kinase is associated with stimulation of the initial rates of Ca^{2+}-transport [11, 12, 18]. This stimulatory effect appears to be due to enhancement of individual steps in the Ca^{2+}-ATPase reaction sequence:

$$E \leftarrow + 2\,Ca^{2+} \rightarrow E\text{-}Ca_2 \leftarrow + ATP \rightarrow E\text{-}Ca_2\text{-}ATP \leftrightarrow$$
$$(1) \qquad\qquad (2) \qquad\qquad (3)$$

$$ADP + Ca_2\text{-}E \sim P \leftrightarrow Ca_2\text{-}E\text{-}P \leftarrow 2Ca^{2+} \rightarrow E'\text{-}Pi$$
$$(4) \qquad\qquad\qquad (5)$$

Cyclic AMP-dependent phosphorylation of phospholamban results in stimulation of the apparent initial rates of formation of the phosphorylated intermediate of the Ca^{2+}-ATPase (E~P), particularly at low (<10–7 M) free Ca^{2+} concentrations [19, 20]. Stimulation of E~P formation is associated with an increase in the affinity of the Ca^{2+} pump for calcium and a possible increase in Ca^{2+} binding sites. Cyclic AMP-dependent phosphorylation of phospholamban stimulates the initial rates of E~P decomposition, which appears to be one of the slow steps in the Ca^{2+}-ATPase reaction sequence and thus a regulatory step of the overall enzymatic activity. Therefore, alteration of the initial rates of this step may be an indication of the possible stimulatory role of cAMP-mediated phosphorylation in cardiac SR function in vivo.

Phosphorylation of phospholamban by cAMP-dependent protein kinase has

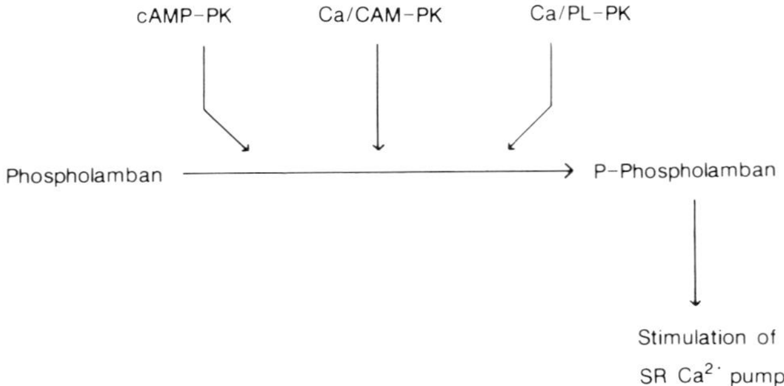

Figure 12-4. Schematic showing the sites of phosphorylation on phospholamban, which serve as subsrates for various protein kinases.

also been shown to stimulate Ca^{2+} efflux from cardiac SR [21, 22]. When cardiac SR was preincubated with cAMP-dependent protein kinase, the rate of EGTA-induced Ca^{2+} efflux from SR loaded with 45Ca^{2+} was significantly increased, and the Ca^{2+} concentration needed to attain half-maximal activation of Ca^{2+}-efflux was reduced [21, 22].

Cardiac SR also contains a calcium-sensitive, calmodulin-activated protein kinase which primarily phosphorylates phospholamban [9, 13, 21, 23, 24, 25]. Ca^{2+}/CAM-dependent phosphorylation of phospholamban does not require cAMP but it is absolutely dependent on the presence of free Ca^{2+}, over a concentration range (10^{-7} to 10^{-5} M) that corresponds to physiological levels. Exogenous calmodulin is also required for activation of the membrane bound enzyme (EC50 = 49 nM) [13]. Phosphorylation of SR vesicles by the Ca^{2+}/CAM-dependent protein kinase has been shown to be associated with a significant increase (2 to 4-fold) in the rate of Ca^{2+} transport at low calcium concentrations (<3 fM), while Ca^{2+} transport was minimally affected at higher Ca^{2+} concentrations [24]. This stimulation is due to an increase in the apparent affinity of the calcium pump for Ca^{2+}. Studies performed in vitro therefore, support a regulatory role for a Ca^{2+}/CAM-dependent protein kinase in mediating phosphorylation of SR function.

Since cardiac SR function is modulated by both cAMP-dependent and Ca^{2+}/CAM-dependent protein kinases, it becomes important to consider the interrelationship of the effects of these two kinases on the SR Ca^{2+} pump. It has been shown that cAMP-dependent stimulation of cardiac SR can occur independently of CAM-mediated effects. The regulatory effects by Ca^{2+}/CAM-dependent phosphorylation have also been demonstrated to occur independently of cAMP-stimulated phosphorylation [26]. When both phosphorylations are operating, they appear to have an additive effect. These findings indicate that cAMP-dependent and Ca^{2+}/CAM-dependent regulation of Ca^{2+} transport in cardiac SR may occur in independent and additive manners.

Calcium-activated, phospholipid-dependent protein kinase (protein kinase C) has also been shown to phosphorylate phospholamban [15, 16]. The site of phosphorylation appears to be distinct from those catalyzed by either cAMP-dependent or Ca^{2+}/CAM-dependent protein kinases [16]. Phosphorylation of phospholamban by protein kinase C resulted in stimulation of Ca^{2+} activity [15] and oxalate-supported Ca^{2+} uptake [16]. Thus pathways involving regulation of protein kinase C activity may represent another regulatory mechanism for cardiac SR function in addition to cAMP-dependent and Ca^{2+}/CAM-dependent pathways.

In addition to the protein kinases, cardiac SR appears to contain an intrinsic protein phosphatase activity, which can dephosphorylate both cAMP-dependent and Ca^{2+}/CAM-dependent sites on phospholamban [27, 28]. Dephosphorylation of SR caused a decrease in the stimulation of initial rates of calcium transport, compared to phosphorylated vesicles, and the calcium affinity of dephosphorylated SR was similar to that of non-phosphorylated vesicles [27]. However, the dephosphorylated SR vesicles could be rephosphorylated in the presence of ATP and this was accompanied with full recovery of the stimulation on calcium transport [29]. These data indicate that the calcium pump in cardiac SR may be under reversible regulation by phosphorylation/dephosphorylation processes.

B. Myofilament phosphorylation

A cartoon representing structure/function relations in the cardiac myofilament is also shown in Fig. 12-3. Activation of myofilament force and shortening is triggered by Ca^{2+} binding to troponin C (TnC), the Ca^{2+}-receptor protein of the Tn complex [30]. Ca^{2+}-TnC acts to disinhibit thin-filament-thick filament reactions. which are inactivated in the absence of Ca^{2+} by the action of the Tn-Tm complex. Tm either sterically blocks cross-bridge binding to actin or acts to regulate transitions among force-generating and relaxed states of the actin-cross bridge kinetic cycle [31]. Inhibition by Tm requires the presence of TnI, an inhibitory component, and TnT, the Tm binding component of Tn. As summarized in Table 1 [32, 33], TnT, TnI and Tm all exist as phospho-proteins, and thus there exists the potential that variations in the state of phosphorylation may influence the protein-protein interactions involved in the transduction of the Ca^{2+}-TnC signal. Thick-filament associated components, with putative regulatory functions, that also exist as phosphoproteins include C-protein and the P-light chain of myosin. P-light chains not only regulate the rate of myosin ATPase activity [34], but may also participate in thick-filament related regulation of myofilament activation [35]. C-protein is localized along the thick filaments at 43 nm intervals in two 300 nm zones on either side of the M-line (see [33] for review). Its function is not clear, although there have been suggestions based on indirect evidence that it may function in the intact sarcomere either to alter myosin ATP hydrolysis, as a 'vernier' in the filament assembly, or as a modulator of thin filament regulation.

142

Table 12-1 lists the main phosphoproteins of the cardiac thick and thin filaments and the kinases which act in vitro to phosphorylate them. Cardiac TnI and C-protein serve as excellent substrates for cAMP dependent protein kinase. In the case of TnI, this activity is tissue specific for the heart variant, which has a unique stretch of amino acids at the N-terminus containing the phosphorylation site [36, 37]. Among variants of C-protein, the cardiac form is also the best substrate for cAMP dependent protein kinase [38], indicated in Table 12-1, C-protein and TnI, as well as TnT are also substrates for the Ca^{2+} phospholipid dependent protein kinase, protein kinase C, [39, 40]. TnT is also phosphorylated by a kinase which is essentially specific for TnT, and is unaffected by Ca^{2+}-calmodulin and/or cAMP [41]. Similarly, a relatively specific Tm kinase has been isolated from muscle [42]. It is important that the in vitro phosphorylations listed in Table 12-1, have been shown to occur not only in the isolated proteins, but also in assembled cardiac Tn, Tn-Tm, thin or thick filaments, and myofibrils [43, 44, 33]. This has not been the case with some of the myofilament components of fast striated muscle. For example, fast skeletal TnI phosphorylation by cAMP PK and skeletal TnT phosphorylation by protein kinase C occur in vitro only if the substrate is the isolated protein [36].

Table 12-1 also summarizes some ideas derived from in vitro experiments as to the functional significance of the phosphorylations of the various thick and thin filament regulatory proteins. Little is known as to role of TnT and Tm phosphorylation, although the fact that the kinases for these proteins are relatively abundant in the striated muscles of animals in the perinatal period suggests that the phosphorylation may have some significance in myofilament assembly or turnover. The site of Tm phosphorylation is at a residue in the C-terminal end of the molecule that is associated with overlap with a neighboring Tm, but whether or not the phosphorylation is important in end-to-end interactions of Tm along

Table 12-1. Phosphoproteins of the cardiac myofilaments.

Protein	Kinase	Effect of Phosphorylation
Troponin T	'TnT' Kinase, Ca^{2+}/Phospholipid	(?)
Troponin I	cAMP dependent	Altered Ca^{2+}-Sensitivity
	Ca^{2+}/CAM dependent	
	Ca^{2+}/Phospholipid	
Tropomyosin	Ca^{2+}, cAMP and CAM independent	(?)
	'Tm Kinase'	
C-Protein	cAMP dependent	Deactivation
	Ca^{2+}/CAM dependent	(?)
	Ca^{2+}/Phospholipid	
Myosin	Ca^{2+}/CAM dependent	Activation at
P-light Chain	Myosin Light Chain Kinase	submaximal Ca^{2+}
		(?)

the thin filament is not clear [45]. In vitro studies have shown that phosphorylation of TnI either in reconstituted or native myofibrils results in a reduction of the concentration of Ca^{2+} required to half-maximally activate force or ATPase activity [46, 47]. Therefore, the sensitivity of cardiac myofilaments to Ca^{2+} is apparently regulated by the state of phosphorylation of TnI. The mechanism of this desensitization is a reduction of the affinity of the regulatory site of TnC for Ca^{2+}, that arises from an enhancement of the 'off rate' for Ca^{2+} with these sites [30, 48]. It has been shown that phosphorylation of C-protein by cAMP dependent protein kinase reduced its ability to activate myosin ATPase activity, when added exogenously in reconstituted preparations [49]. On the other hand, we (Garvey, Kranias and Solaro, unpublished) have found no effect of C-protein phosphorylation on the Ca^{2+}-activation of preparations reconstituted with cardiac acto-myosin, containing native C-protein and skeletal Tn-Tm (which does not phosphorylate under the conditions of the experiments).

Winegrad and colleagues (see [47] for review) have studied the functional role of myofilament protein phosphorylation using preparations that retain 'α, β- and muscarinic receptors, but are permeable to ions and nucleotides. The studies show that activation of endogenous adenylate cyclase by cAMP and inhibition by cGMP act to regulate the levels of TnI phosphorylation and determine the Ca^{2+}-sensitivity of the myofilaments. Moreover, work in Winegrad's laboratory also indicates that β-receptors may be coupled to activation of a process regulating maximum force development of the myofilaments depending on the isomyosin population. The influence of light chain phosphorylation on the activity of myosin has been a controversial topic in muscle biology owing to the different effects obtained in various laboratories studies various aspects of the question [50]. Most recent evidence [51] indicates that phosphorylation activates tension development in skinned fiber preparations at submaximally activating levels of free Ca^{2+}.

SR and myofilament phosphorylation: in vivo studies

An obvious and important question that arises from evidence obtained in vitro, is: How and when are these myofilament and membrane proteins phosphorylated in the beating heart and what does the phosphorylation do? Our approach to these questions is outlined in Fig. 12-5 in which we show an outline of experiments on isolated rabbit or guinea pig hearts perfused with 32P-Krebs buffer to label the nucleotide pool. The hearts are freeze-clamped in various inotropic states and processed for isolation of purified myofibrils and microsomal fractions enriched in SR vesicles [52, 27].

Results of gel electrophoresis and associated autoradiograms indicating covalent labelling with 32P are shown for SR in Fig. 12-6 and for myofibrils in Fig. 12-7 in an experiment in which the hearts were freeze-clamped at the peak of the response to stimulation with the beta-adrenergic agonist, isoproterenol. In the

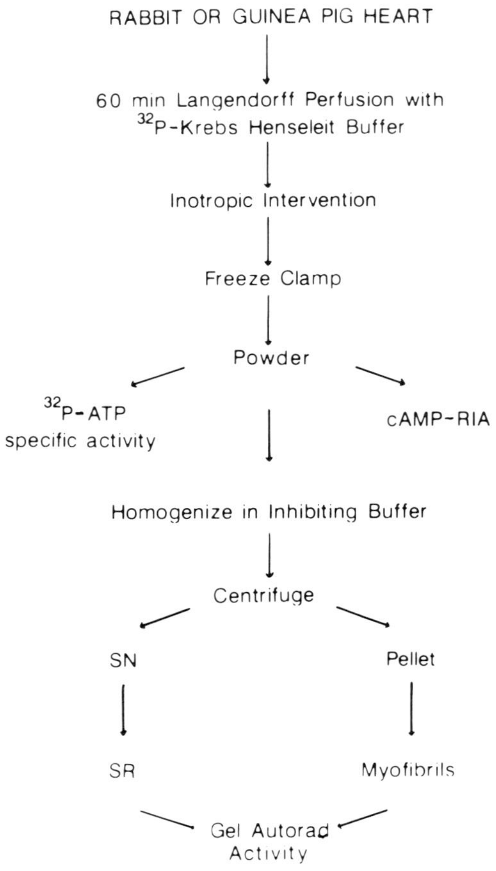

Figure 12-5. Outline of approach used to determine the levels of phosphorylation and functional alterations of SR and myofilament proteins in situ in beating hearts. The term 'inhibiting' buffer refers to preparative solutions that inhibit phosphoryl transfer during isolation procedures.

case of the SR, it is clear that beta-adrenergic stimulation was associated with the appearance of a 27,000 dalton phosphoprotein, presumably the dimeric form of phospholamban. Sometimes, 32P-incorporation also occurred in an 11,000 dalton protein, but the 27,000 and 11,000 dalton phosphoproteins appeared to be inter-convertible. In the example shown in Fig. 12-6 this interconversion occurred by boiling the sample under reducing conditions before electrophoresis. This effect of boiling is a well known property of phospholamban, when phosphorylated in vitro, and the results depicted in Fig. 12-6 show that phospholamban phosphoryl-ated in situ has this same property. This provides evidence that the protein phosphorylated in situ is indeed phospholamban and not a contaminant protein from other membranes. Further proof of this is the fact that stimulation of 32P-incorporation in cardiac SR by isoproterenol was also associated with an increase in the initial rates of Ca^{2+} transport, assayed in the presence of oxalate, using SR vesicles in either microsomal fractions or homogenates from the perfused hearts [29]. Phosphorylation of SR vesicles due to isoproterenol stimulation has also been shown to be associated with increased SR Ca^{2+}-ATPase activity [53]. Myofibrils obtained from hearts beating in the control conditions show incorporation of 32P into several proteins including C-protein, Tm, TnT, TnI and the P-light chain of myosin (Fig. 12-7). The co-valent phosphate in these proteins is therefore turning over during the course of the perfusion. This indicates that incorporation of covalent phosphate in these proteins which has been shown to occur in vitro, also occurs in situ. However, it is clear from the results shown in Fig. 12-7 that stimulation with isoproterenol does not uniformly increase the level of phosphorylation of all of the myofilament phosphoproteins. Phosphorylation of C-protein and TnI are selectively stimulated and simultaneous measurements of activation of cAMP dependent protein kinase and levels of cAMP provide strong evidence that the phosphorylations are through the beta-receptor and the adenylate cyclase pathway [27]. Indeed, stimulation of phospholamban, TnI and C-protein phosphorylation by isoproterenol is blocked in hearts pre-treated with sotalol, a beta-adrenergic blocking agent. As predicted from the in vitro studies, the relative ATPase activity of myofibrils obtained from hearts stimulated with isoproterenol and showing increased levels of TnI phosphorylation are less sensitive to Ca^{2+} than the control preparations [27].

Although dephosphorylation of phospholamban occurs during the decline of the inotropic response to catecholamines [53], it has been found in several laboratories that phosphorylation of TnI outlasts the inotropic response as measured by increased peak left ventricular pressure or -dp/dtmax [54, 32] (Garvey, Kranias and Solaro, unpublished). Moreover, we have also found that the desensitization of the myofibrils with respect to Ca^{2+}-activation also persists. On the other hand, the onset and decline of the effects of isoproterenol on phospholamban phosphorylation and Ca^{2+}-ATPase activity have been shown to be associated with the relaxation effects [53]. Rates of dephosphorylation of both TnI and SR are, however, enhanced by addition of muscarinic agonists after the catecholamine pulse [54, 55]. There is also evidence that this effect may not be due entirely to inhibition of adenylate cyclase [55]. Thus, in the case of the SR, findings from in situ studies are in agreement with in vitro results on the effects of cAMP-dependent phosphorylation on SR function and support the hypothesis that phosphorylation of phospholamban may be responsible for mediating at least part of the Ca^{2+} catecholamine effects on the mammalian myocardium. Since both phosphorylation of TnI and C-protein reduce activation at a given level of free Ca^{2+}, it has been hypothesized that these phosphorylations may be important in the 'relaxant' effect of catecholamines [52]. Clearly, the exact role of TnI and C-protein phosphorylation in the mechanical response of the myocardium to catecholamine stimulation remains to be clarified.

What is the role of the Ca^{2+}/CAM-dependent and Ca^{2+}/phospholipid depen-

146

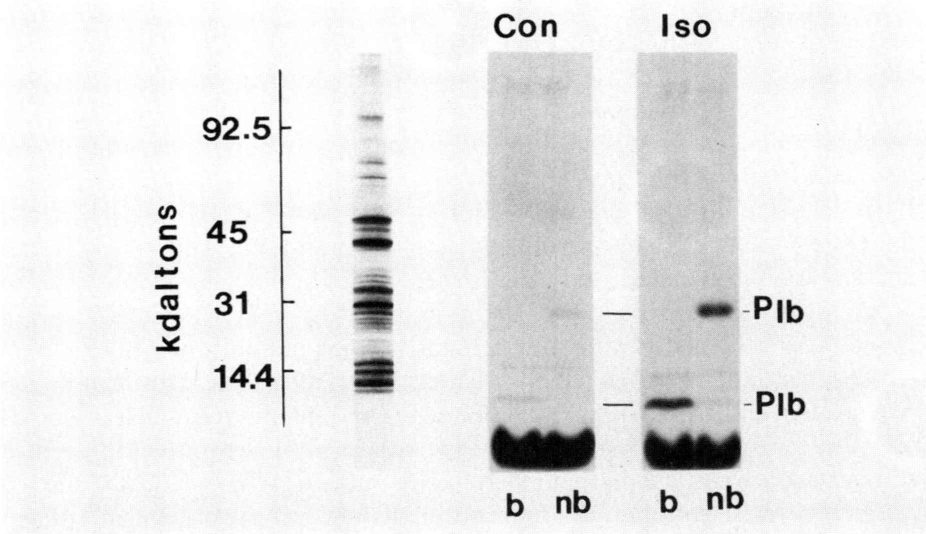

Figure 12-6. Sodium dodecyl sulfate gel electrophoresis (far left lane) and associated autoradiograms showing degree of phosphorylation of vesicles of sarcoplasmic reticulum phospholamban (Plb) in preparations from control hearts and hearts freeze-clamped at the peak of the inotropic response to perfusion with isoproterenol. Lanes loaded with non-boiled (nb) preparations demonstrate a different mobility of the phosphorylated band than gels loaded with boiled (b) protein. Plb and Plb' indicate different oligomeric forms of phospholamban. See text for details.

dent protein kinase pathways in the inotropic response to catecholamines which are, after all, certainly associated with increases intracellular free Ca^{2+}? It was shown some time ago that experimental manipulations (perfusion with elevated Ca^{2+} in the Krebs buffer or ouabain, or during paired pulse stimulation) that raise intracellular free Ca^{2+} do not affect the level of TnI phosphorylation [56]. This also appears to be the case for C-protein (Garvey, Kranias and Solaro, unpublished). Although amphibian hearts show variations in levels of P-light chain phosphorylation during the contraction/relaxation cycle, in mammalian hearts these levels appear to remain at about 0.5 mol P/mol P-light chain during a broad range of inotropic interventions [57, 58, 59]. In vivo studies on the effect of Ca^{2+}/CAM-dependent phosphorylation of phospholamban do not correlate with in vitro findings on the effects of this phosphorylation on SR function. Interventions which increase Ca^{2+} concentration via cAMP-independent mechanisms did not stimulate in vivo phosphorylation of phospholamban in cardiac SR membranes [60] (Garvey, Kranias and Solaro, unpublished). Thus, further studies are required to know better the role of Ca^{2+}/CAM-dependent phosphorylation in the intact myocardium.

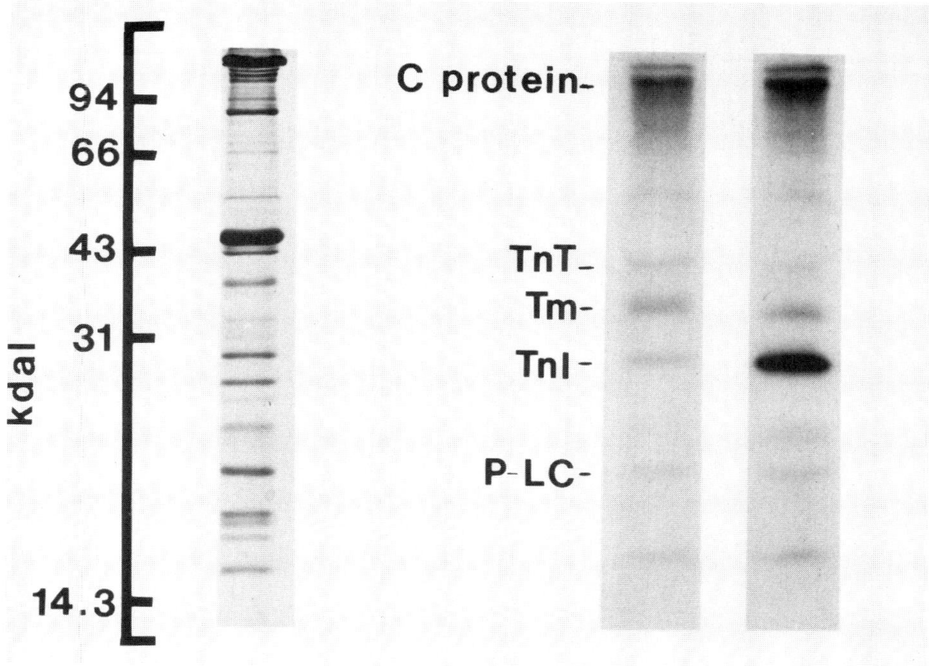

Figure 12-7. Sodium dodecyl sulfate gel electrophoresis (far left lane) and associated autoradiograms showing degree of phosphorylation of myofilaments prepared from hearts freeze-clamped in a control condition or at the peak of the response to perfusion with isoproterenol. See text for details.

Summary and concluding remarks

In vitro, myofilament proteins and phospholamban are phosphorylated by several protein kinases, but results of experiments done so far indicate that regulation of cAMP dependent protein kinase acting through its phosphorylation of TnI, C-protein and phospholamban may be primarily responsible for the mechanical alterations depicted in Fig. 12-1. The scheme shown in Fig. 12-8 provides a summary of a hypothesis for the role of protein phosphorylations in the activating and relaxing effects of catecholamines depicted in Fig. 12-1.

The primary hypothesis illustrated in Fig. 12-8 is that phospholamban phosphorylation is largely responsible for the increased rate of relaxation during β-adrenergic stimulation and the mechanism is an increased rate of Ca^{2+} transport by the Ca^{2+} pump protein. Increased rates of transport allow for a larger amount of $SR-Ca^{2+}$ in the releasable pool and therefore larger amounts of Ca^{2+} for release. A recruitment of Ca^{2+} channels by protein phosphorylation at the surface membrane, alters the inward Ca^{2+} current (Isi) providing an increased 'trigger' and 'loading' component (Fig. 12-2). The deactivating effects of myofilament

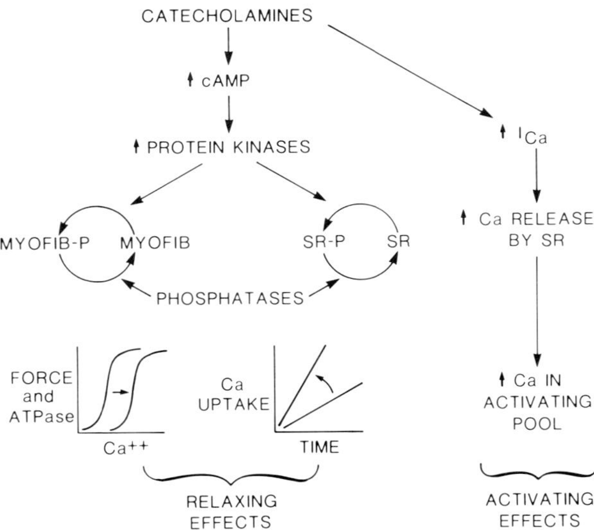

Figure 12-8. Scheme depicting a hypothesis for the mechanism of the activating and relaxing effects of catecholamines on mammalian heart muscle. See text for description.

phosphorylation is proposed to be important in the relaxant effect of catecholamines acting in concert with enhancement of SR-Ca^{2+} uptake. Effects of muscarinic agonists on this system may be due to cAMP formation by adenylate cyclase, but could also be related to effects beyond the receptor involving regulation of protein phosphatase by, as yet, unknown mechanisms. The connection between protein phosphorylation and the effects of frequency on twitch dynamics depicted in Fig. 12-1 is not clear but may involve Ca^{2+} dependent protein kinases.

There is a variety of unanswered questions regarding how protein phosphorylation relates to myocardial contractile state. As yet, there has been no clear evidence for an in situ role of Ca^{2+}/CAM- or Ca^{2+}/phospholipid dependent protein kinase in the regulation of SR or myofilament function. For example, phosphorylation of myosin P-light chains is well known to be regulated by myosin light chain kinase, a Ca^{2+}-CAM-dependent protein kinase, yet levels of light chain phosphorylation appear to remain constant at 0.5 mol/mol over a variety of contractile states varied by alterations certain to alter intracellular Ca^{2+}. This indicates that the Ca^{2+}-dependent kinases are turned on maximally all the time at normal heart rates, and the question remains as to exactly what might regulate the activity of Ca^{2+}-dependent kinases physiologically. A related question that requires further study is the possibility that there are changes in the level of protein phosphorylation during the relaxation/contraction cycle.

At the molecular level, the interrelationships among different phosphorylation sites on phospholamban and among different myofilament proteins remains to be studied. Moreover the specificity and regulation of protein phosphatases for these various sites is not clear. In the case of the SR, the precise mechanism by which phospholamban regulates Ca^{2+}-pumpactivity is unknown as is the stoichiometric correlation of phospholamban to Ca^{2+}-ATPase. In the case of the myofilaments, the functional significance of most of the protein phosphorylations is poorly understood or unknown. Finally, it is clear that relations between the altered contractile dynamics such as those shown in Fig. 12-1, and the dynamics of protein phosphorylation require study utilizing contractile models and approaches that permit more meaningful mechanical measurements. Some of the effects of altered phosphorylation, such as those related to C-protein and TnI, may be too subtle to pick up from gross measurements, such as determination of intraventricular pressure developed in intact hearts.

Acknowledgements

Work described here was supported by N.I.H. Research Grants HL R01-22231, R01-26057 and P01-22619 and by Training Grants 07382 and 07571. We are grateful to Betsy Solaro for typing the manuscript and preparing figures.

References

1. Chapman, R.A.: Control of cardiac contractility at the cellular level. Am. J. Physiol. 245: H535–H552, 1983.
2. Fabiato, A. and Baumgarten, C.M.: Methods for detecting calcium release from the sarcoplasmic reticulum of skinned cardiac cells and the relationships between calculated transsarcolemmal calcium movements and calcium release. In: Physiology and Pathophysiology of the heart. (Sperelakis, N., ed.). pp. 215–254, 1984.
3. Sperelakis, N.: Regulation of calcium slow channels by cyclic nucleotides and phosphorylation. In: Protein Phosphorylation in Heart Muscle. (R.J. Solaro, ed.) CRC Press, Inc. Boca Raton (In Press), 1986.
4. Jones, L.R., Presti, C.F., Presti, F. and Lindemann, J.P.: Protein phosphorylation and the cardiac sarcolemma. In: Protein Phosphorylation in Heart Muscle (R.J. Solaro, ed.) CRC Press Inc. Boca Raton (In Press), 1986.
5. Nishizuka, Y.: Studies and perspectives of protein kinase C. Science. 233: 305–312.
6. Fabiato, A. and Putney, J.W.: Effects of inositol (1, 4, 5)-triphosphate on skinned cardiac cells. Proc. Int. Union. Physiol. Sci. 16: 128, 1986.
7. Tada, M. and Inui, M.: Regulation of calcium transport by the ATPase-phospholamban system. J. Mol. Cell. Cardiol. 15: 565–575, 1983.
8. Kirchberger, M.A. and Antonetz, T.: Phospholamban: dissociation of the 22,000 molecular weight protein of cardiac sarcoplasmic reticulum into 11,000 and 5,500 molecular weight forms. Biochem. Biophys. Res. Comm. 105: 152–156, 1982.
9. LePeuch, C.P., Haiech, J. and Demaille, J.G.: Converted regulation of cardiac sarcoplasmic

150

reticulum calcium transport by cyclic adenosine monophosphate dependent and calcium-calmodulin-dependent phosphorylations. Biochemistry 18: 5150–5157, 1979.

10. Jones, L.R., Maddock, S.W. and Hathaway, D.R.: Membrane localization of myocardial type II cyclic AMP protein kinase activity. Biochim. Biophys. Acta 641: 242–253, 1981.

11. Kirchberger, M.A., Tada, M. and Katz, A.: Adenosine 3′, 5′-monophosphate-dependent protein kinase catalyzed phosphorylation reaction and its relationship to calcium transport in cardiac sarcoplasmic reticulum. J. Biol. Chem., 1974.

12. La Raia, P.J. and Morkin, E.: Adenosine, 3′, 5′-monophosphate-dependent membrane phosphorylation. A possible mechanism for the control of microsomal calcium transport in heart muscle. Circ. Res. 35: 298–306, 1974.

13. Bilezikjian, L.M., Kranias, E.G., Potter, J.D. and Schwartz, A.: Studies on the phosphorylation of canine cardiac sarcoplasmic reticulum by calmodulin-dependent protein kinase. Circ. Res. 49: 1356–1361, 1981.

14. Kirchberger, M.A. and Antonetz, T.: Calmodulin-mediated, regulation of calcium transport and Ca^{2+}-Mg^{2+}-activated ATPase activity in isolated cardiac sarcoplasmic reticulum. J. Biol. Chem. 257: 5685–5691, 1982.

15. Limas, C.J.: Phosphorylation of cardiac sarcoplasmic reticulum by a calcium-activated, phospholipid-dependent protein kinase. Biochem. Biophys. Res. Comm. 96: 1378–1382, 1980.

16. Movsesian, M.A., Nishikawa, M. and Adelstein, R.S.: Phosphorylation of phospholamban by calcium-activated, phospholipid-dependent protein kinase. J. Biol. Chem. 259: 8029–8032, 1982.

17. Kranias, E.G., Schwartz, A. and Jungmann, R.A.: Characterization of cyclic 3′: 5′-AMP-dependent protein kinase in sarcoplasmic reticulum and cytosol of canine myocardium. Biochim. Biophys. Acta 709: 28–37, 1982.

18. Tada, M., Kirchberger, M.A. and Katz, A.M.: Phosphorylation of a 22,000 dalton component of the cardiac sarcoplasmic reticulum by adenosine 3′: 5′-monophosphate dependent protein kinase. J. Biol. Chem. 250: 2460–2467, 1975.

19. Tada, M., Yamada, M. Ohmori, F., Kuzuya, T., Iui, M.- and Abe, H.: Transient state kinetic studies of Ca^{2+}-dependent ATPase and calcium transport by cardiac sarcoplasmic reticulum. Effec of cyclic AMP-dependent protein kinase-catalyzed phosphorylation of phospholamban. J. Biol. Chem. 255: 1985–1992, 1980.

20. Kranias, E.G., Bilezikjian, L.M., Potter, J.D., Piascik, M.T. and Schwartz, A.: The role of calmodulin in regulation of cardiac sarcoplasmic reticulum phosphorylation. Ann. N.Y. Acad. Sci. 356: 279–291, 1980.

21. Kirchberger, M.A. and Wong, D.: Calcium efflux from isolated cardiac sarcoplasmic reticulum. J. Biol. Chem. 253: 6941–6945, 1978.

22. Katz, A., Tada, M. and Kirchberger, M.A.: Control of calcium transport on the myocardium by the cAMP-protein kinase system. In: Advances in Cyclic Nucleotide Research, vol. 5, (G. Drummond, ed.), Raven Press, New York, pp. 453–472. 24a: 6166–6173, 1975.

23. Kranias, E.G., Mandel, F., Wang, T. and Schwartz, A.: Mechanism of the stimulation of calcium ion dependent adenosine triphosphatase of cardiac sarcoplasmic reticulum by adenosine 3′,5′-monophosphate dependent protein kinase. Biochemistry 19: 5434–5439, 1980.

24. Davis, B.A., Schwartz, A., Samaha, F.J. and Kranias, E.G.: Regulation of cardiac sarcoplasmic reticulum calcium transport by calcium-calmodulin-dependent phosphorylation. J. Biol. Chem. 258: 13587–13591, 1983.

25. Plank, B., Pifl, C., Hellman, G., Wyskovsky, W., Hoffman, R. and Suko, J.: Correlation between calmodulin-dependent increase in the rate of calcium transport and calmodulin-dependent phosphorylation of cardiac sarcoplasmic reticulum. Eur. J. Biochem. 136: 215–221, 1983.

26. Kranias, E.G.: Regulation of Ca^{2+} transport by cyclic 3′,5′ AMP-dependent and calcium-calmodulin-dependent phosphorylation of cardiac sarcoplasmic reticulum. Biochim. Biophys. Acta 844: 193–199, 1985.

27. Kranias, E.G.: Regulation of calcium transport by protein phosphatase activity associated with

cardiac sarcoplasmic reticulum. J. Biol. Chem. 260: 11006–11010, 1985.

28. Kranias, E.G. and Blount, A.L.: Regulation of calcium transport in the cardiac sarcoplasmic reticulum by protein kinases and protein phosphatases. In: Advances in Protein Phosphatases II, Leuven Univ. Press, pp. 241–246, 1985.

29. Kranias, E.G., Garvey, J.L, Srivastava, R.D. and Solaro, R.J.: Phosphorylation and functional modifications of sarcoplasmic reticulum and myofibrils in isolated rabbit hearts stimulated with isoprenaline. Biochem. J. 226: 113–121, 1985.

30. Solaro, R.J., Robertson, S.P., Johnson, J.D., Holroyde, M.J. and Potter, J.D.: Troponin-I phosphorylation: A unique regulator of the amounts of calcium required to activate cardiac myofibrils. Cold Spring Harbor Conf. Cell. Prolif. Protein Phosphorylation 8: 901–911, 1981.

31. Chalovich, J.M. and Eisenberg, E.: Inhibition of actomyosin, ATPase activity by troponin-tropomyosin without blocking the binding of myosin to actin. J. Biol. Chem. 2572: 2432–2437, 1982.

32. Stull, J.T., Sanford, C.F., Manning, D.R., Blumenthal, D.K. and High, C.W.: Phosphorylation of Myofibrillar Proteins in Striated Muscle. Cold Spring Harbor Conf. Cell Prolif. Protein Phosphorylation 8: 823–839, 1981.

33. Solaro, R.J.: Protein phosphorylation and the cardiac myofilaments. In: Protein Phosphorylation in Heart Muscle. (R.J. Solaro, ed.) CRC Press, Inc. Boca Raton (In Press), 1986.

34. Malhotra, A., Huang, S. and Bhan, A.: Subunit function of cardiac myosin: effect of removal of LC2 (18,000 molecular weight) on enzymatic properties. Biochemistry 18: 461–467, 1970.

35. Wagner, P.D.: Effect of skeletal muscle myosin light chain 2 on the Ca^{2+} sensitive interaction of myosin and heavy meromyosin with regulated actin. Biochemistry 23: 5950–5956, 1984.

36. Moir, A.G.J. and Perry, S.V.: The sites of phosphorylation of rabbit cardiac troponin-I by adenosine 3',5'-cyclic monophosphate-dependent protein kinase. Biochem. J. 167: 333–343, 1977.

37. Solaro, R.J., Moir, A.J.G. and Perry, S.V.: Phosphorylation of troponin I and the inotropic effect of adrenaline in perfused rabbit heart. Nature 262: 615–616, 1976.

38. Hartzell, H.C. and Glass, D.B.: Phosphorylation of purified cardiac muscle C-protein by purified cAMP-dependent and endogenous Ca^{2+}-calmodulin-dependent protein kinases. J. Biol. Chem. 259: 15587–15596, 1984.

39. Katoh, N., Wise, B.C. and Kuo, J.F.: Phosphorylation of cardiac troponin inhibitory subunit (troponin I) and tropomyosin binding subunit (TnT) by cardiac phospholipid sensitive Ca^{2+}-dependent protein kinase. Biochem. J. 209: 189–195, 1983.

40. Lim, M.S., Sutherland, C. and Walsh, M.P.: Phosphorylation of bovine cardiac C-Protein by kinase C. Biochem. Biophys. Res. Comm. 132: 1187–1195, 1985.

41. Villar-Palasi, C. and Kumon, A.: Purification and properties of dog cardiac troponin-T kinase. J. Biol. Chem. 256: 7409–7415, 1982.

42. Montgomery, K. and Mak, A.S.: In vitro phosphorylation of tropomyosin by a kinase from chicken embryo. J. Biol. Chem. 259: 5555–5560, 1984.

43. Katz, A.M.: Role of the contractile proteins and sarcoplasmic reticulum in the response of the heart to catecholamines, An historical review. Adv. Cyc. Nuc. Res. 11: 303–343, 1979.

44. Stull, J.T.: Phosphorylation of contractile proteins in relation to muscle function. Adv. Cyc. Nuc. Res. 13: 39–93, 1980.

45. Mak, A., Smillie, L.B., Barany, M.: Site of phosphorylation at ser-283. Proc. Nat. Acad. Sci., U.S.A. 75: 3588–3592, 1978.

46. Holroyde, M.J., Howe, E. and Solaro, R.J.: Modification of calcium requirements for activation of cardiac myofibrillar ATPase by cyclic AMP dependent phosphorylation. Biochim. Biophys. Acta 586: 63–69, 1979a.

47. Winegrad, S.: Regulation of cardiac contractile proteins. Circ. Res. 55: 565–574, 1984.

48. Robertson, S.P., Johnson, J.D., Holroyde, M.J., Kranias, E.G., Potter, J.D. and Solaro, R.J.: The effect of troponin-I-phosphorylation on the Ca^{2+}-binding properties of the Ca regulatory site

152

of bovine cardiac troponin. J. Biol. Chem. 257: 260–263, 1982.

49. Hartzell, H.C.: Effects of phosphorylated and unphosphorylated C-protein on cardiac acto-myosin ATPase. J. Mol. Biol. 186: 185–195, 1985.

50. Gevers, W.: The unsolved problem of whether and when light chain phosphorylation is important in the heart. J. Mol. Cell. Cardiol. 16: 587–590, 1984.

51. Persechini, A., Stull, J.T. and Cooke, R.: The effect of myosin phosphorylation on the contractile properties of skinned rabbit skeletal muscle fibers. J. Biol. Chem. 260: 7951–7954, 1986.

52. Kranias, E.G. and Solaro, R.J.: Phosphorylation of troponin I and phospholamban during catecholamine stimulation of rabbit hearts. Nature 298: 182–184, 1982.

53. Lindemann, J.P., Jones, L.R., Hathaway, D., Henry, B. and Watanabe, A.M.: Beta-adrenergic stimulation of phospholamban phosphorylation and Ca^{2+}-ATPase activity in guinea pig ventricles. J. Biol. Chem. 258: 464–471, 1983.

54. England, P.J.: Studies on the phosphorylation of the inhibitory subunit of troponin in perfused rat heart. FEBS Lett. 50: 57–60, 1976.

55. Lindemann, J.P. and Watanabe, A.M.: Muscarinic cholinergic inhibition of beta-adrenergic stimulation of phospholamban phosphorylation and Ca^{2+}-ATPase activity in guinea pig ventricles. J. Biol. Chem. 260: 13122–13129, 1985a.

56. Frearson, N., Solaro, R.J. and Perry, S.V.: Changes in phosphorylation of P light chain of myosin in perfused rabbit heart. Nature 264: 801–802, 1976.

57. Holroyde, M.J., Small, D.A.P., Howe, E. and Solaro, R.J.: Isolation of cardiac myofibrils and myosin light chains with in vivo levels of light chain phosphorylation. Biochim. Biophys. Acta 587: 628–637, 1979b.

58. High, C.W. and Stull, J.T.: Phosphorylation of myosin in perfused rabbit and rat hearts. Amer. J. Physiol. 239: H756–H764, 1980.

59. Westwood, S.A. and Perry, S.V.: The effect of adrenaline on the phosphorylation of the P light chain of myosin and the perfused rabbit heart. Biochem. J. 197: 185–193, 1981.

60. Lindemann, J.P. and Watanabe, A.M.: Phosphorylation of phospholamban in intact myocardium. Role of Ca^{2+}-calmodulin dependent mechanisms. J. Biol. Chem. 260: 4516–4525, 1985a.

General discussion of protein-phosphorylation in EC-coupling

Although some of the presented data show a correspondence between protein-phosphorylation and mechanical properties of the muscle, further studies are required to allow conclusions as to which biochemical steps are related to mechanical events and which are not. Information about phosphorylation of sarcolemmal proteins is still scarce although phosphorylation of a fraction with a molecular weight of 15000 has been observed. Another feature of possible interest is phosphorylation of components of the lipid fraction.

Present evidence suggests that calmodulin dependent kinases that cause phosphorylation of the myosin light-chains are virtually continually active, as was concluded by Dr. Solaro from the observation that lowering of the heart rate caused a dephosphorylation of the light-chains only over a time of 30 minutes.

13. Ventricular pump function and arterial resistance

G. ELZINGA, G.P. TOOROP, G.C. VAN DEN BOS and N. WESTERHOF

Introduction

The function of fluid pumps is characterized by two properties: fluid output and pressure generation. These two variables are not independent from one another but constitute, for a given functional level of the pump, an inverse relationship: the pump function graph.

In the case of the ventricle there are two pressures to consider, ventricular and arterial. Moreover pressures and flow are not constant in this part of the circulatory system but oscillate with the heart beat. Therefore a choice must be made which variable to use to construct the ventricular pump function graph. Some years ago, while we were working on the isolated ejecting cat heart, we chose, on the basis of theoretical and experimental considerations, mean left ventricular pressure and output, as the most appropriate variables in this respect [1, 2]. An example of such a ventricular pump function graph, obtained through changing the arterial load, is shown in Fig. 13-1A.

Recently, however, we found [3] in studies of the anesthetized cat with opened thorax that in the in vivo situation mean aortic and mean left ventricular pressure are proportional ($Plv = a \cdot Pao$). This finding allows us to use mean aortic pressure instead of mean left ventricular pressure for the pump function graph. The use of mean aortic pressure has the advantage that the pump function graph and peripheral resistance, represented by a line through the origin, can be presented in the same plot (Fig. 13-1A). The point of intersection of the pump function graph and the line representing peripheral resistance is the working point, i.e. the pressure and flow present in the steady state situation. From Fig. 13-1A it can be readily seen that the position of the working point on the pump function graph depends on the value of the peripheral resistance, i.e. on the slope of the line through the origin.

The power delivered by the ventricle into the vascular system can almost completely be obtained from the instantaneous product of pressure and flow [4]. In the study describing the proportionality between mean left ventricular and

154

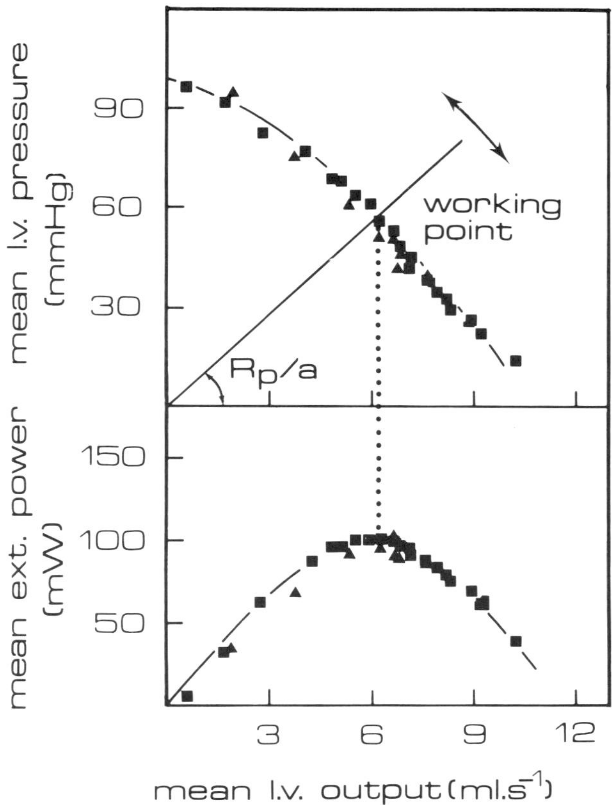

Figure 13-1. A. The relationship between mean output and mean left ventricular pressure, the pump function graph, is obtained by varying the arterial load (steady states, ▲; beat-to-beat, ■). Since mean left ventricular pressure and mean aortic pressure are proportionally related (Pao = a · Plv) it is possible to represent peripheral resistance in this graph by a straight line through the origin. The working point of the ventricle is found at the intersection of this line with the pump function graph. Rp is peripheral resistance. B. Power output of the ventricle depends on the position of the working point on the pump function graph. Power output is zero at the two extremes, while it has an optimum value in between.

mean aortic pressure [3] we found in addition the total external power and the fraction of the power obtained from the product of mean aortic pressure and mean output (steady power), to be proportional as well. This implies that changes in left ventricular external work caused by changes of arterial resistance can be directly derived from the pump function graph. The result is the parabola-shaped function shown in Fig. 13-1B. Power output of the ventricle is thus determined by the value of the peripheral resistance. However the periphery is not the sole determinant, because changes in cardiac function, as occur with changes in inotropic state, end-diastolic volume and heart rate, change the pump function graph [5, 6] and thus the position of the working point at a given value of the peripheral resistance. To illustrate this point we present four of such pump function graphs with the corresponding work output graphs in Fig. 13-2. Changes in pump function were obtained through a change in end-diastolic volume and a change in inotropic state.

Since in the intact body circulatory control affects the heart as a pump as well as the arterial system, the position of the working point in vivo is a result from a complex of mechanisms, all probably tuned to serve the requirements of the body. The question we address here is: What position does the ventricular working point in the intact circulation take relative to the optimum of the power curve under control conditions and in situations where the circulatory system is stressed?

Methods

Anesthetized cat with open thorax

This preparation has been described in detail elsewhere [3]. Therefore a short description will suffice here. Male cats were anesthetized with sodium pentobarbital (40 mg/kg ip) and artificially ventilated. Subsequently a femoral vein and femoral artery were cannulated for infusion of fluid and for measurement of arterial pressure, respectively. Following sternotomy the ascending aorta was dissected free from the surrounding tissues, and a stiff polyethylene catheter was introduced into the left ventricular cavity to measure ventricular pressure. An artificial arterial load, which allowed to increase or decrease aortic pressure on a beat-to-beat basis, was inserted. Blood flow was measured electromagnetically.

Conscious dog

Male mongrel dogs (11.7–20.5 Kg) were selected on their capacity to run 1.56 m · sec^{-1} on a treadmill. Under sterile conditions an aortic flow transducer and a left ventricular pressure transducer (Konigsberg P18) were implanted through a left thoracotomy. An occluding device [7] was placed around the descending branch of the left coronary artery such that blood flow was not impeded. In some dogs a silastic catheter was put into the left atrium. The wires and tubing were passed through an intercostal space and buried under the skin in the neck. The dogs were left to recover for at least one week before the experiments started.

The animals exercised before and four days after occlusion of the coronary artery. They ran 0.67, 0.89, 1.12, 1.34 and 1.56 m · sec^{-1} at a slope of 25% for 5 minutes in random order, with rest periods of 10 minutes between runs. During the experiments aortic flow, left ventricular pressure, maximum rate of rise of left ventricular pressure, heart rate, and cardiac output were continuously recorded

156

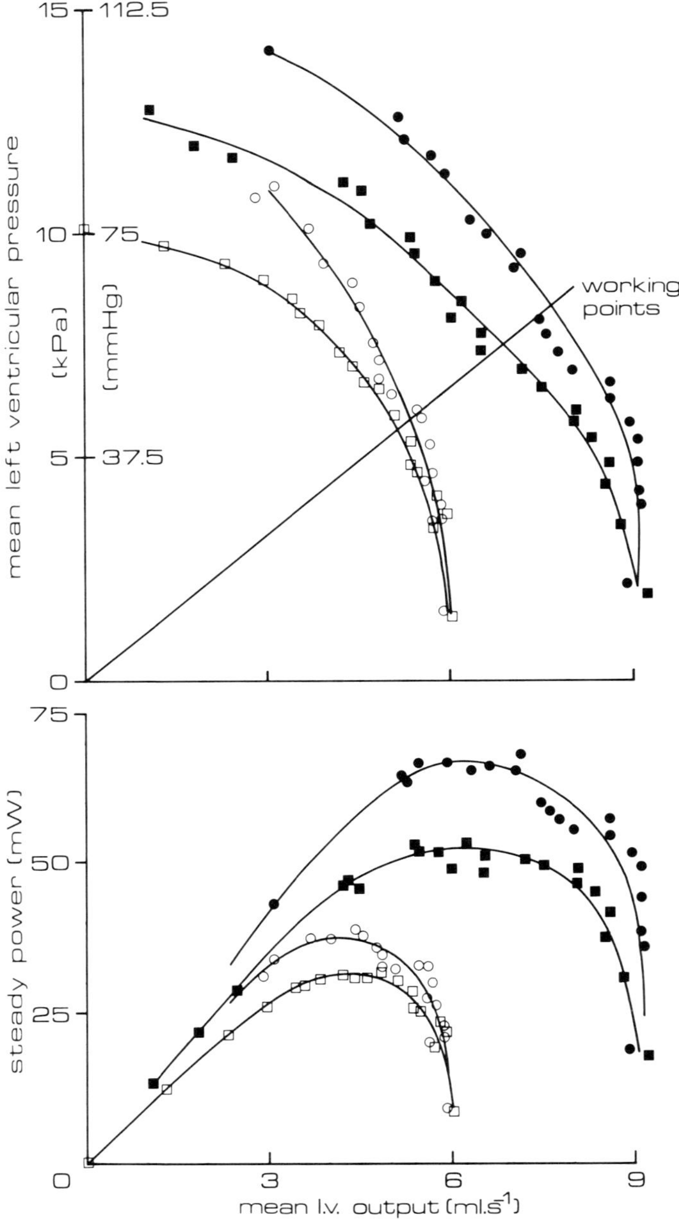

Figure 13-2. Top. The position of the working point is not only affected by the peripheral resistance (cf. Fig. 13-1) but also by the position of the pump function graph. This position changes with changes of the cardiac control mechanisms such as heart rate, filling and inotropic state. Shown here are changes in the position of the pump function graph resulting from two levels in filling (□, ■) and an increase in inotropic state at these two levels, (○, ●). *Bottom.* The power output graphs related to the pump function graphs shown in A.

on paper (Elema EMT 81) and analog tape (HP 3525 A or SE 7000). In dogs in which a left atrial catheter had been implanted mean left atrial pressure was measured at rest with a Statham P23 Db pressure transducer. Mean left ventricular pressure and mean output values were obtained by planimetry in duplicate: two complexes per experimental situation were analyzed (at the same point in a respiratory cycle for all situations). After the dogs had been killed with Na pentobarbital the hearts were removed and cut into 88 pieces as we have described for measurement of coronary blood flow with radioactive microspheres [8]. We decided by macroscopic inspection whether a piece was infarcted or not.

Results and discussion

Anesthetized cats

We found in this preparation under control conditions (n = 18) that the working point was located at optimum power output, which must be the result of mechanisms controlling both arterial resistance and ventricular pump function. Since circulatory control may be affected severely by the anesthesia, we added halothane to the ventilatory gas mixture (n = 6) to see whether this would change the position of the working point relative to optimum power output. This appeared not to be the case, in spite of the changes in pump function and peripheral resistance [3].

Thus a perturbation of the circulation such as caused by halothane did not result in a deviation of the working point from the position of optimum power output. Using other perturbations, such as an increase in heart rate by pacing (n = 8) or infusion of fluid (n = 8) gave similar results: Changes in pump function and arterial resistance were found while the working point was maintained at optimum power output [3, 9]. The results of these experiments strengthen the idea that circulatory control 'tries' to maintain the ventricle to operate at optimum power output. However, it is not very likely that we deal here with the effect of a relatively simple feedback system. A feedback system would therefore imply that power output is sensed by some receptor (in the circulation) and that its value is compared with the optimum value attainable. This is, in the case of power, a rather unlikely possibility. It is much more conceivable to assume that what we found is a result of a combination of circulatory control mechanisms trying to maintain arterial pressure as well as blood flow to the tissues.

Since maintenance of arterial pressure is a very stringent requirement the circulation has to deal with and since the body also requires a certain flow, it seems fair to take the point of view that the power to be delivered by the ventricle is set by the body. In principle, this amount of work can be delivered by the ventricle in many ways (cf. Fig. 13-2). What then, is the reason that the ventricle does this at the optimum of the power output curve?

At first sight it seems even more logical to think that the ventricle would 'rather' operate at optimum efficiency (i.e. the ratio of the external work done and the energy liberated) than at optimum power output. This idea has been supported also by arguments. For instance, recently it has been postulated on basis of considerations which regard the ventricle to behave as a time varying compliance [10], that it is unlikely that in the intact animal the working point of the ventricle is found at optimum power output, but that it is probably located more closely to the optimum efficiency. (One of the major arguments is that ejection fraction would be 0.5 for the optimum power output point, which is lower than normally observed.)

However, some years ago [6] we showed that the point of optimum efficiency on the pump function graph is found well to the right (higher output, lower pressure) of the point of optimum power output. In those experiments, which were done on isolated ejecting cat hearts, we were unable to find the point of optimum efficiency during a steady state because pressure became so low that coronary perfusion became insufficient.

The fact that the theoretical prediction based on the time varying elastance model [10] leads to a result which differs from the experimental findings follows from the assumptions made for the calculations. If, for instance, it is assumed that the steepest elastance line (Emax) is not straight but convex to the pressure axis as was shown experimentally [11] the optimum power output would have been found at a higher ejection fraction.

In addition, one has to realize that the notion that the ventricle tends to operate at optimum efficiency does not mean that when a certain amount of work is required from the heart by the circulation (cf. above) this could be done at the lowest cost at the point of optimum efficiency.

Assuming that the tendency to maintain the position of the working point at optimum power output is a result of a complex, integrated circulatory control mechanism, we set out to find experimental conditions where the ventricle no longer would operate at this specific point. Such conditions could teach us more about the nature of the overall control and the limits thereof. In the open thorax cat we found that infusion of norepinephrine (n = 8) caused a consistent deviation of the working point from optimum power output [9].

In addition to this finding a study appeared recently on anesthetized dogs [12] showing that when a sufficient number of 50 μm microspheres are injected into the coronary arterial system to cause the ventricle to fail, the working point is no longer found at optimum power output. In preliminary experiments on the open thorax cat we confirmed these results when an infarct was made through occlusion of the anterior descending branch of the left coronary artery (Fig. 13-3).

From these findings the conclusion may be drawn that when the circulation is more severely perturbed the working point is no longer maintained at optimum power output.

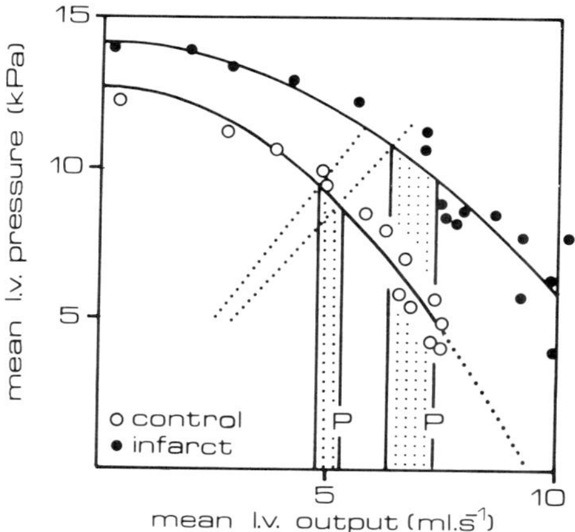

Figure 13.3. Left ventricular pump function graphs before and after infarction obtained in the open thorax cat. The working points are indicated by the dotted lines. The vertical lines indicated by a P represent the power optima. The deviation of the working point from the point of optimum power increases with infarction. The finding that the intercept on the pressure axis increases can be explained by the activation of circulatory control mechanisms following the infarct.

Conscious dogs

Circulatory control mechanisms and the importance thereof can be studied most appropriately in conscious animals. More than 20 years ago Wilcken [13] showed for the conscious dog at rest that the working point is located at optimum power output. These investigators could conclude this because they were able to occlude the aorta and to open an arterio-venous shunt on a beat-to-beat basis. Both interventions resulted in a decrease of ventricular power output.

Assuming, on the basis of this study, that in the normal conscious dog at rest the working point is again found at optimum power output we studied how infarction would affect the position of the working point. The results for the dog at rest (n = 6) are shown in Fig. 13-4A. It can be seen that no change in position of the working point was found 4 days after infarction (infarct size 18.7% of left ventricular mass). However, this does not imply that the position of the optimum power output point may not have changed. On the contrary, the infarct must have decreased the pressure generating capacity. Moreover we found in these dogs a significant increase in left atrial filling pressure with infarction (from 4.4 to 12.1 mm Hg). On the basis of these two effects it is likely that due to infarction the pump function graph rotated such that the intercept on the pressure axis became lower and that on the output axis higher than during control (Fig. 13-4B). This would mean that the working point would then no longer be at optimum power output. A similar change of the pump function graph due to infarction, as hypothesized here, can be seen in Fig. 13-3, although the effect of infarction in the

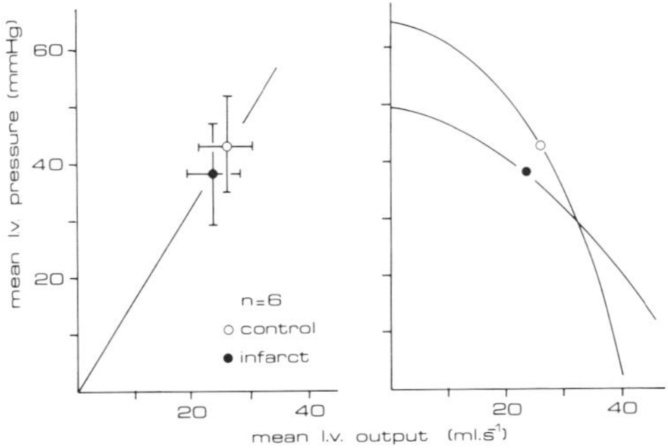

Figure 13-4. Left. In conscious dogs at rest the working point is not affected by a ventricular infarct. *Right.* However, this does not mean that the position at optimum power output is necessarily maintained. It is more likely that an infarct causes the pump function graph to rotate such that the intercept on the pressure axis decreases and that on the output axis increases.

open thorax cat appears to be masked by other changes in circulatory control, probably related to the occlusion of the coronary artery.

We did not only study the position of the working point in the dogs at rest but also during different levels of treadmill exercise. When dogs exercise on the treadmill heart rate increases considerably, stroke volume does not change very much or increases slightly, left ventricular end-diastolic volume remains approximately the same, and the rate of rise of left ventricular pressure increases considerably [14]. An increase in contractility causes the pump function graph to rotate around the intercept on the output axis (cf. Fig. 13-2), while an increase in heart rate causes a parallel shift [6]. From these two changes, the area in the pressure output plane toward where the working point would have to go in order to remain at optimum power output (Fig. 13-5B, hatched area) can be determined.

However, we found for the six dogs that during exercise the working point moved to higher outputs and pressures along a line which had an intercept on the pressure axis (Fig. 13-5A). This implies that they moved outside the hatched area, which leads us to conclude that during exercise the ventricle does no longer operate at the point of optimum power output.

The working points of dogs with a myocardial infarct were found on the same pressure output line as found prior to coronary occlusion (Fig. 13-5A). This leads to the conclusion that the deviation between optimum power output and working point most likely present for the infarcted dog at rest, increased even further during exercise.

Taking all experimental results presented here together it may be concluded that under basal conditions the left ventricle operates at optimum power output and that small perturbations of the circulation cannot force the working point away from that optimum. However, when the system is more severely perturbed

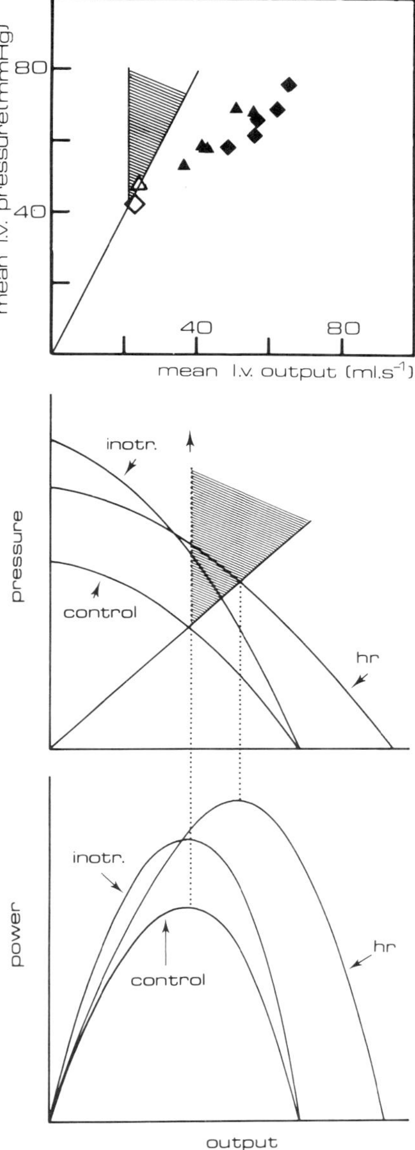

Figure 13-5. Top. During exercise the working point of the dog left ventricle: control (▲, ◆) and infarct (△, ◇) moves outward along a line which has an intercept on the pressure axis. The hatched area indicates where the workpoint would go if optimum work output would be maintained (cf. Figure 13-5B). The open symbols represent the situation at rest. *Bottom* two panels. An increase in heart rate (hr) shifts the control pump function graph outwards in a parallel fashion. An increase in inotropic state (inotr.) causes the pump function graph to rotate around an intercept on the abscissa. Each pump function graph corresponds with a power output graph (panel C). The hatched areas in panels B and A correspond to the area where the working point should go to maintain optimum power output when heart rate and inotropic state change simultaneously.

through ventricular infarction or by infusion of nor-epinephrine, the working point is no longer maintained at that specific position.

During exercise the working point moves away from the point of optimum power output along a straight line. If there would have been the tendency to keep the working point at optimum power output under these conditions, the working point would have moved, into the hatched area (Fig. 13-5B). Since this was not the case it may be that exercise changes the circulatory control such that the required increase in output is a stronger determinant of the working point than the optimum of the power output curve.

Summary and conclusions

Pump function of the ventricle can be characterized by an inverse relationship between mean pressure and cardiac output, obtained by changing the arterial load. The proportional relationship between mean arterial pressure and output, representing the peripheral resistance, intersects the pump function graph at the working point, i.e. the point constituted by the pressure and output generated in the steady state. The position of the working point relative to the power (pressure times flow) output curve is determined by ventricular pump function and arterial resistance and appears to be of importance in circulatory control.

Experiments on anesthetized cats with an open thorax and on intact conscious dogs showed the working point to be located at the optimum of the power output curve. This position is no longer maintained when pump function is impaired by a myocardial infarction, suggesting inadequacies in circulatory control under this condition. During exercise the working point probably also deviates from the point of optimum power output. In this case, however, other control mechanisms or controlled variables come into play, rather than inadequacies in circulatory control.

References

1. Elzinga, G. and Westerhof, N.: Pressure and flow generated by the left ventricle against different impedances. Circ. Res., 32: 178–186, 1973.
2. Elzinga, G. and Westerhof, N: How to quantify pump function of the feline left heart; changes with heart rate and its bearing on the energy balance. Cardiovasc. Res., 14: 81–92, 1979.
3. Horn, G.J. van den, Westerhof, N. and Elzinga, G.: Optimum power generation by the left ventricle; a study in the anesthetized open thorax cat. Circ. Res., 56: 252–261, 1985.
4. McDonald, D.A.: Blood flow in arteries. Arnold, London, 1974.
5. Elzinga, G. and Westerhof, N.: The effect of an increase in inotropic state and end-diastolic volume on the pumping ability of the feline left heart. Circ. Res., 42: 620–628, 1978.
6. Elzinga, G. and Westerhof, N.: Pump function of the feline left heart; changes with heart rate and its bearing on the energy balance. Cardiovasc. Res., 14: 303–308, 1980.
7. Jagenau, A.H.M., Schaper, W.K.A. and Reus, W.: A simple pneumatic cuff for occlusion of

small arteries in dogs, pigs and sheep. Pflugers Arch., 310: 185–188, 1969.
8. Kiewit de Jonge, M.: Circulatory effects of myocardial infarction at rest and during exercise. Ph.D. Dissertation. Free University of Amsterdam, 1980.
9. Horn, G.J. van den, Westerhof, N. and Elzinga, G.: The feline left ventricle does not always operate at optimum power output. Am. J. Physiol., 250: H961–H967, 1986.
10. Burkhoff, D. and Sagawa, K.: Ventricular efficiency predicted by an analytical method. Am. J. Physiol. R1021–R1027, 1986.
11. Maughan, W.L., Sunagawa, K., Burkhoff, D. and Sagawa, K: Effect of arterial impedance changes on end-systolic pressure-volume relationship. Circ. Res., 54: 595–602, 1984.
12. Myhre, E.S.P., Johansen, A., Bjornstad, J. and Piene, H.: The effects of contractility and preload on matching between canine left ventricle and afterload. Circulation 73: 161–171, 1986.
13. Wilcken, D.E.L., Charlier, A.A., Hoffman, J.I.E. and Guz, A.: Effects of alterations in aortic impedance on the performance of the ventricles. Circ. Res., 14: 283–293, 1964.

14. Ventricular wall motion

JIM W. COVELL and LEWIS K. WALDMAN

Introduction

Before discussing Dr. Elzinga's work, I thought it might be appropriate to take a moment to ease the transition from the first chapters on the mechanics of the isolated myocardium to ventricular mechanics and describe briefly the relationship between forces and deformation in the wall of the ventricle. To translate the elegant studies on isolated muscle discussed in the previous chapters to the intact heart, one must find a way to measure force and deformation in the complex thick wall of the ventricle. Most investigators have used membrane theory to calculate wall-forces and have measured deformation in the wall with some type of uniaxial measurement. As I will attempt to show you in recent data from our laboratory, motion in the ventricular wall is probably much too complex to allow either of these two analyses.

Wall-strain measurements

The data I will show you is similar to the work of Fenton and Klassen [1] from this country and from Dieudonne [2] in France. The information shown, was obtained from collaborative work performed at San Diego with Dr. Lewis Waldman and Dr. Yuang-Cheng Fung [3]. In our studies, we have implanted three columns of beads in the anterior free wall of the left ventricle. We then select any four non-coplanar beads to form an arbitrary tetrahedron of the ventricular wall. Each of these tetrahedra are approximately 0.1 ml in volume. By measuring the sides of this tetrahedron, using high speed bi-plane cineradiography, one can calculate strains in any cardiac reference system.

Figure 14-1 shows data calculated using this technique during two cardiac contractions. In this case, there is substantial circumferential strain (E_{11}) and little longitudinal strain (E_{22}), substantial wall thickening (E_{33}) and substantial transverse shear (E_{23}; shown in Fig. 14-2). Such large radial shears, as are documented

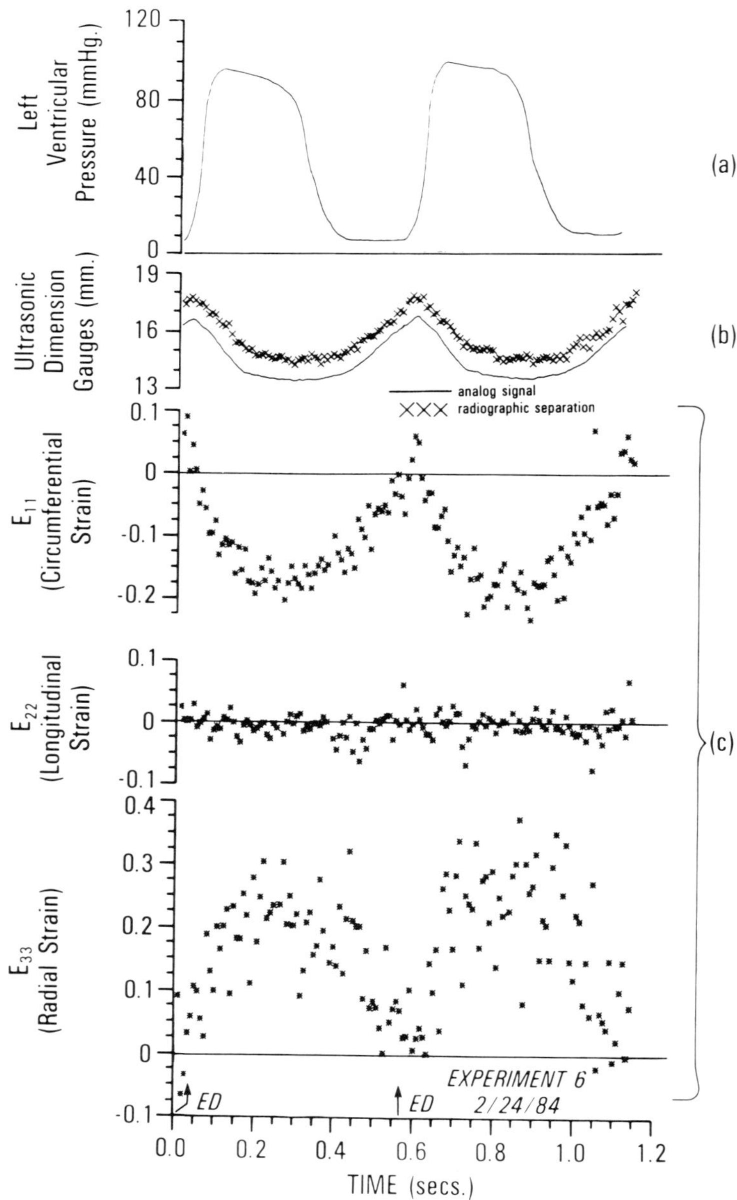

Figure 14-1. Shows pressure development and simultaneously calculated strain in circumferential, longitudinal and radial direction of the left ventricle.

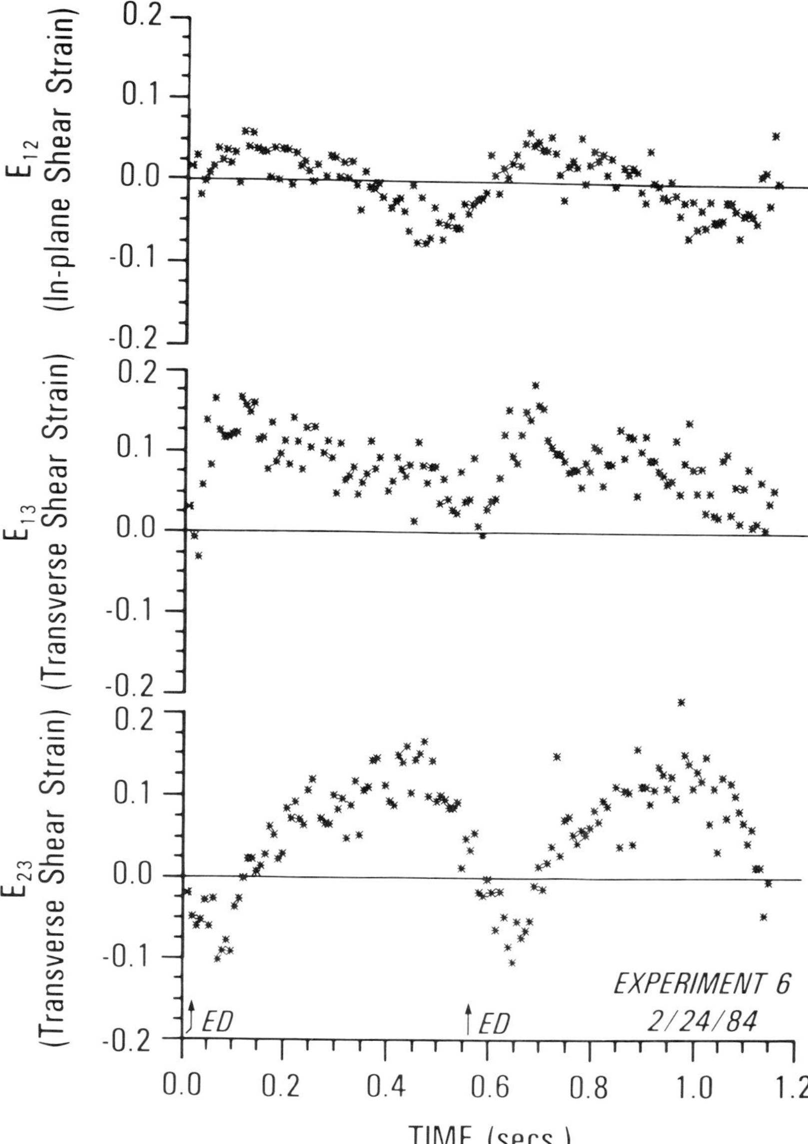

Figure 14-2. Illustrates inplane – and transverse shear streams during the same heartbeats as in Figs. 14-3 (see text).

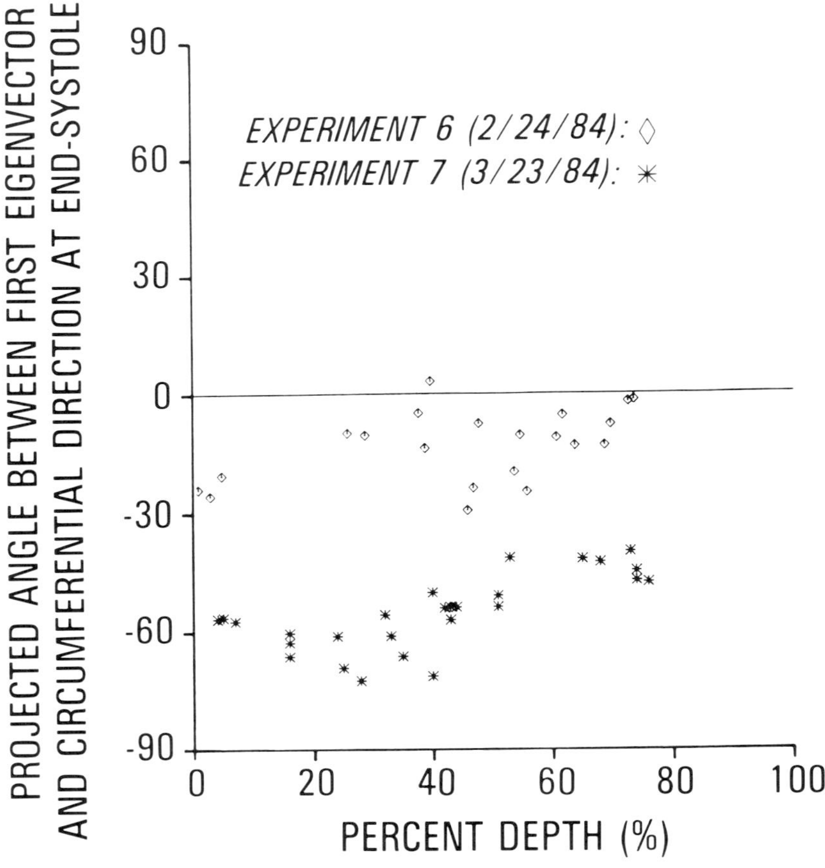

Figure 14-3. Shows the direction of the first principle stream as a function of depth (see text).

in the subendocardial tetrahedron and occur across the wall, invalidate the use of membrane theory in determining forces. The latter theory assumes that there are no transverse shearing forces. With this technique we can also measure principle strains. Principle strains are three orthogonal strains which, with their directions, account for all deformation within this arbitrary tetrahedron.

In Fig. 14-3 the direction of the first principle (greatest shortening) strain at end-systole in two representative experiments is plotted against the depth of the center of the tetrahedron. The direction of end-systolic principle strain, is quite constant. Fiber direction across the wall at this site changes approximately 140 degrees. These results indicate that there is substantial deformation away from the fiber direction, particularly at deeper layers of the wall; thus all deformation is not in line with the fibers implying that there must be substantial rearrangement or shape change of myofibers during contraction.

I have selected these two findings from our current work to emphasize that it is difficult to directly extrapolate the myocyte mechanics, that we heard so eloquently described in the previous part of the symposium, directly to the intact heart. Perhaps the approach to pump function, discussed by Dr. Elzinga or that elaborated in some detail by Dr. Sagawa is a more practical way to deal with ventricular function.

In reference to Dr. Elzinga's studies, perhaps the most difficult conceptual problem is that they imply that ventricular power is somehow sensed and controlled by the circulatory systems. I would like to ask Dr. Elzinga, how he proposes that ventricular power is sensed and how matching of the heart and the arterial system is carried out?

References

1. Fenton, T.R., Cherry, J.M., Klassen, G.H. and Outerbridge, J.S.: Transmural myocardial deformation in the canine left ventricular wall. Am. J. Physiol. 235: H523–H530, 1978.
2. Dieudonne, J.M.: Gradients de direction et de deformation principaux dans la paroi ventriculaire gauche normale. J. Physiol. (Paris) 61: 305–330, 1969.
3. Waldman, L.K., Fung, Y.C. and Covell, J.W.: Transmural myocardial deformation in the canine left ventricle. Circ. Res. 57: 152–163, 1985.

General discussion of pumpfunction properties

Some features of the pump function analysis were clarified. Infarction shifts the curve to the right because increased diastolic filling increases output at lower pressures. However, the curve rotates counter-clockwise since the capacity to develop pressure at low cardiac outputs is diminished for the given preload. It was acknowledged that changes of efficiency are difficult to interpret when contractility and preload change simultaneously.

There was discussion of several aspects of the control system. Although the normal working point coincides with peak external power, it seems unlikely that there are 'power receptors' and there is no reason to reject the conventional concept that the system is regulated by mechanisms which maintain oxygen flow and systemic arterial pressure. The short-term response to a transient perturbation (e.g. heart rate) involves a change in peripheral resistance and a shift to a different pump function curve; therefore, a new working point. It is not yet clear whether this is neurally mediated; systematic denervation experiments are in progress. (In denervated animals cardiac output is maintained and the pump function curve is generally unchanged even though heart rate falls.) Long-term responses are more complex (e.g. the development of the ventricles from birth to maturation). Early results indicate that even though the geometry of each ventricle changes considerably, the working points tend to correspond to near-optimal efficiency.

15. Mechanics of the ventricular septum

ELDON R. SMITH and JOHN V. TYBERG

Introduction

Traditionally, the ventricular septum has been viewed as part of the left ventricle (Fig. 15-1), both from an anatomic [1] and functional viewpoint. Support for this concept is widespread and is illustrated in the echocardiographic study shown in Fig. 15-2. Thus, the septum is the same thickness as the left ventricular free wall and (at both end-diastole and end-systole) is concave to the left ventricle with a radius of curvature which is not noticeably different from that of the free wall. The M-mode echocardiogram in Fig. 15-1 demonstrates the normal motion pattern of the ventricular septum; during systole the septum thickens and moves toward the center of the LV cavity.

The fact that the septum is not always oriented in this manner has been noted under pathological conditions. Kieffer and co-workers [2] reported the findings from 5 patients who died from severe pulmonary hypertension; in these patients the septum was displaced to the left so that it was actually convex to the LV cavity. The advent of echocardiography has allowed the ready recognition of this phenomenon during life as is illustrated in Fig. 15-3. The two-dimensional image at end-diastole reveals that the septum is inverted and convex to the LV cavity with a resultant large right ventricular cavity. During systole the LV cavity becomes more rounded although the septum remains flattened. The M-mode echocardiogram from the same patient shows the motion of the septum. At end-diastole the septum is displaced far to the left (with a resultant large RV cavity) and then moves sharply rightward (paradoxically) during systole.

Although this represents an extreme case of abnormal septal shape and motion, abnormalities of variable degrees are noted in a wide variety of clinical conditions. Patients with right ventricular volume overload [3–7], right ventricular pressure overload [8], pericardial disease [9–10] and many of those in the post cardiac surgery state [11–14] all have findings similar to those noted in Fig. 15-2. Patients with left bundle branch block [15–16], ventricular pacing and those with left ventricular volume loads have different, although nonetheless abnormal,

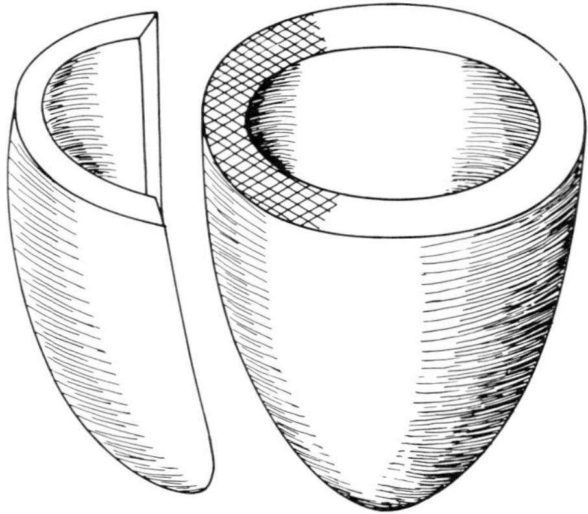

Figure 15-1. A schematic illustrating the traditional view of the ventricles with the right ventricle 'wrapping around' approximately one-third of the circumference of the thicker left ventricle. The cross hatching indicates the zone of the ventricular septum.

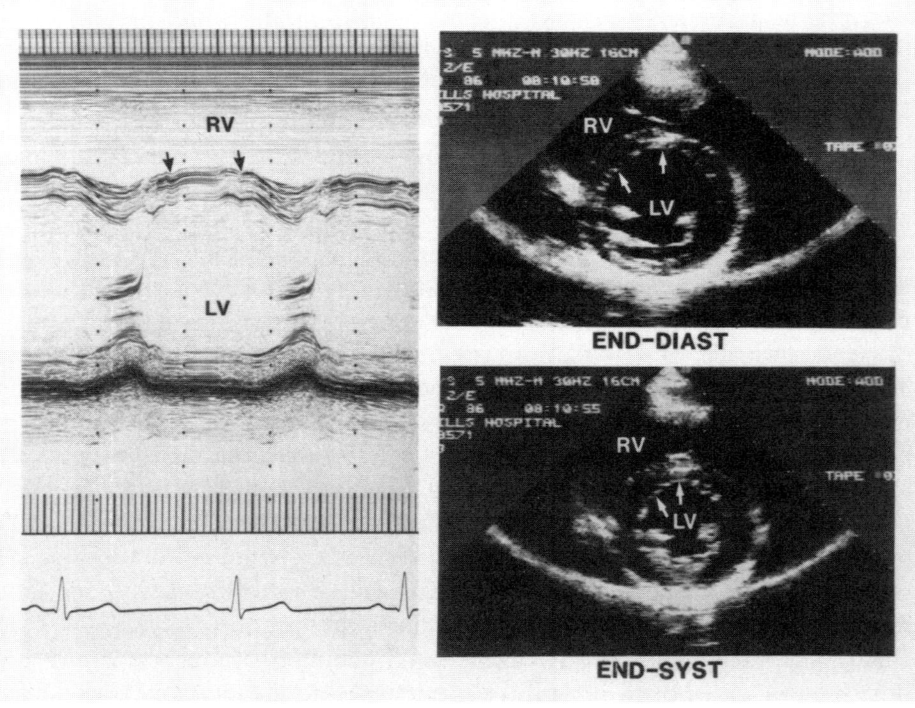

Figure 15-2. M-mode (left panel) and two-dimensional (right panel) echocardiographic images from a normal subject. The two-dimensional images (short axis) demonstrate the circular shape of the left ventricle (LV) both at end-diastole (top) and end-systole (bottom). The septum is indicated by the white arrows on the two-dimensional images and the black arrows on the M-mode tracing. RV = right ventricle.

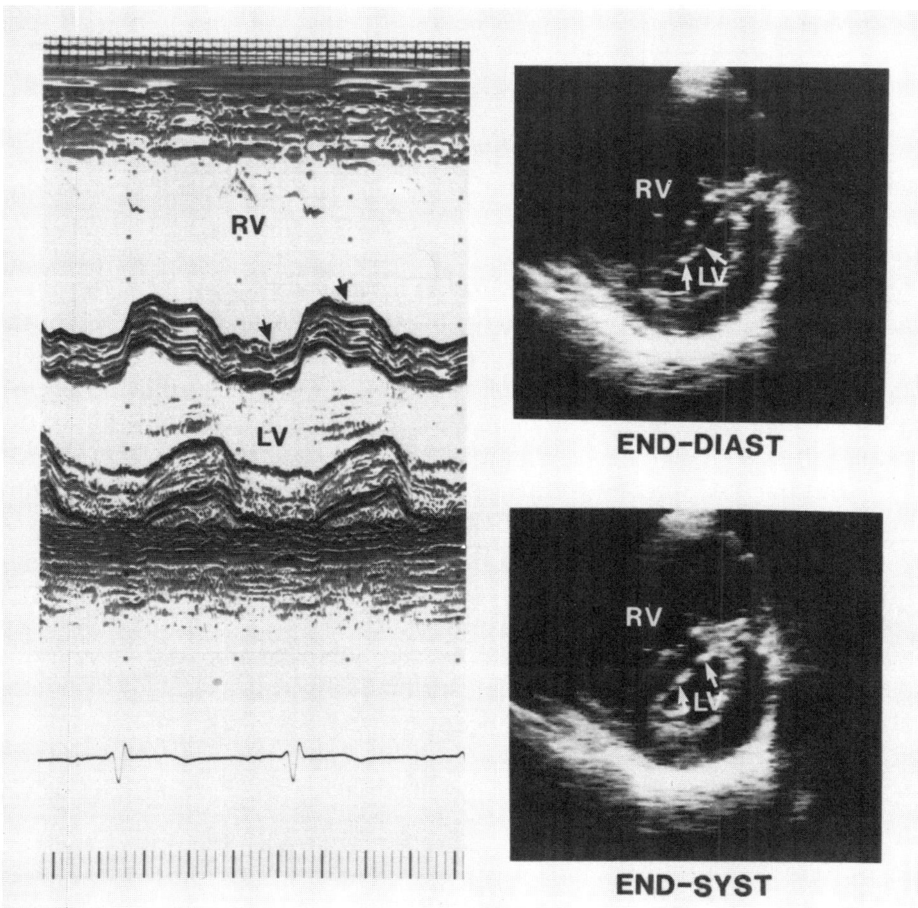

Figure 15-3. M-mode and two-dimensional echocardiographic images from a patient with primary pulmonary hypertension. Description is as for Fig. 15-2. Note that at end-diastole the septum is inverted and actually concave to the right ventricle (RV). At end-systole, the septum is still displaced leftward compared to normal. Note also the marked paradoxic movement of the septum demonstrated on the M-mode tracing.

septal movement patterns. Although a number of theories have been advanced to explain these abnormalities, until recently the subject has continued to be controversial with no single hypothesis being widely accepted.

In this presentation the basic and clinical studies which have led to improving our understanding of septal mechanics will be reviewed and an attempt made to place this new information in the context of our current understanding of cardiac structure and function.

Diastolic mechanics

Right ventricular volume overload

As early as 1914, Henderson and Prince [17] noted that filling of one ventricle impacted on the performance of the other and speculated that their observations could be explained by displacement of the septum during diastole. Much later, Bemis and co-workers [18] utilized a contracting dog heart model (in which the right and left ventricles could be loaded independently) to study the same problem. They noted that increasing right ventricular volume resulted in proportional increases in left ventricular end-diastolic pressure without detectable changes in the estimated left ventricular volume. They concluded that this altered pressure-volume relationship in the LV was the result of a leftward shift of the septum with resultant alteration in LV geometry. Similar findings were reported by Elzinga and co-workers [19] using an isolated cat heart preparation. Santamore et al. [20] used isolated rabbit hearts and also demonstrated that LV diastolic pressure was altered when RV volume was manipulated. In addition, they demonstrated that right ventricular diastolic pressure could be increased by increasing LV volume. These changes were believed to be due to a shift in the diastolic position of the ventricular septum and, although there was a demonstrable influence of the pericardium [19], qualitatively similar changes were also observed after the pericardium had been removed.

Popp and his colleagues [3] were the first to note that patients with right ventricular volume overload, as occurs with atrial septal defect, had not only a large RV during diastole but also had paradoxic (rightward) systolic motion of the septum. Later, using an animal model, Kerber et al. [21] demonstrated that acutely opening a shunt from the left to the right atrium resulted in paradoxic motion in most experiments. Pearlman and his associates [4], as well as Laurenceau and Dumesnil [6] found a correlation between the position of the septum relative to the two ventricles at end-diastole and the occurrence of abnormal septal motion during systole. Thus, the more leftward the septum within the heart at end-diastole, the more likely was the systolic motion to be abnormal. Using two-dimensional echocardiography, Weyman et al. [7] observed that patients with atrial septal defect had a leftward displaced (flattened) septum at end-diastole which moved rightward or paradoxically during systole as the LV reassumed its circular shape.

In an effort to define the hemodynamic correlates of septal position and movement, we developed an open-chest dog model in which we could study the effects of RV volume load by means of a reversible shunt from the pulmonary artery to the right atrium [22]. This same preparation also allowed us to study RV pressure overload (pulmonary artery constriction) and simulated left bundle branch block (RV pacing). Pressures in the RV and LV were measured with catheter tip transducers and cardiac dimensions were obtained with ultrasonic crystals; a double-faced crystal was inserted into the ventricular septum and single crystals were mounted on the RV and LV free walls. This allowed accurate assessment of RV septal-to-free wall and LV septal-to-free wall diameters throughout the cardiac cycle. Crystals were also positioned to measure the anterior-posterior diameter of the LV. Septal shape was continuously monitored by two-dimensional echocardiography while an M-mode tracing was derived to assess septal motion.

When the shunt was acutely opened there was an immediate increase in RV diastolic pressure, a progressive increase in RV septal-to-free wall diameter and a reciprocal decrease in LV septal to free wall diameter. The two dimensional echo images revealed that the septum became displaced toward the LV so that it appeared flattened at end-diastole (LV minor axis at the level of the papillary muscles). The M-mode tracings revealed that septal motion during systole was indeed a function of the end-diastolic position; if the septum became displaced enough toward the LV at end-diastole systolic motion became paradoxic. Intermediate degrees of displacement resulted in intermediate changes in septal motion. The fundamental observation in this study, however, was that there was a tight linear relationship between septal position at end-diastole (as reflected by the septal-to-free wall diameters) and the instantaneous transseptal pressure gradient. Normally LV pressure exceeds RV pressure throughout the cardiac cycle. Thus, the transseptal gradient (LV-RV) at end-diastole is normally positive by several mm Hg and the septum is concave to the LV. With reduction (or reversal) of this gradient, the septum became displaced leftward – this displacement was not an all-or-none phenomenon, but rather was progressive and proportional to the magnitude of the alteration in transseptal gradient.

Right ventricular pressure overload

Right ventricular systolic hypertension usually results in elevated diastolic pressure. Thus, it is not surprising that RV pressure overload produces similar changes in septal position and motion to that observed in volume overload states. Stool et al. [23] produced progressive RV hypertension in conscious dogs by constriction of the pulmonary artery and observed a progressive increase in RV diastolic pressure and a decrease in LV septal-to-free wall diameter at end-diastole – a finding which was speculated to be due to a septal shift. Other workers have noted similar findings during experimental acute [8, 22, 24–26] or chronic [24, 27–28] RV hypertension. In our open-chest model, we also assessed the effect of acute pulmonary artery constriction on septal position and motion [22]. Figure 15-4 shows the tight linear relation between transseptal pressure difference and the septal-to-free wall diameters of both the RV and LV in response to pulmonary artery constriction in a representative experiment. As end-diastolic transseptal gradient declined and then reversed in response to the pulmonary

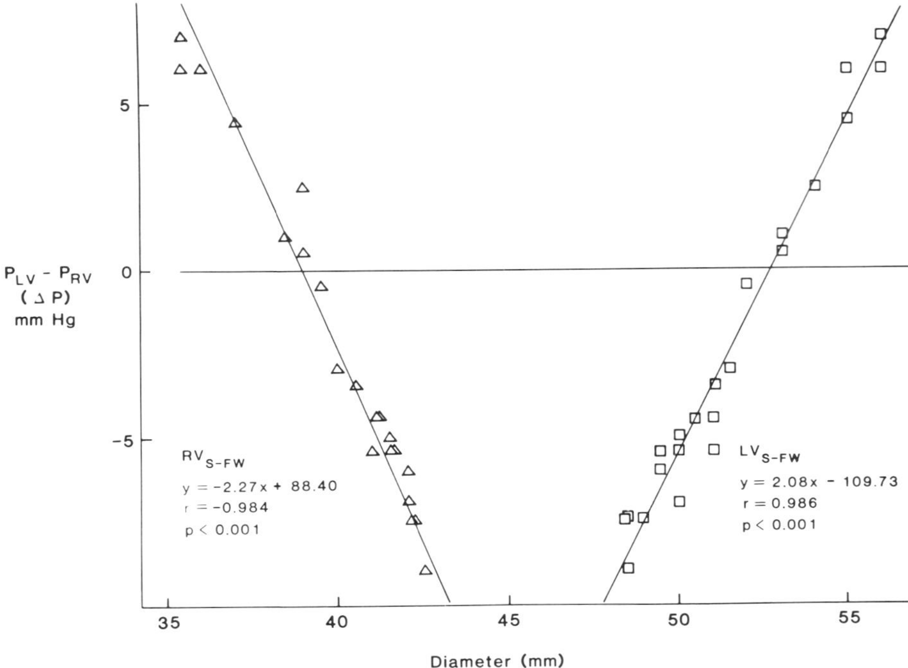

Figure 15-4. End-diastolic RV (triangles) and LV (squares) septal-to-free wall diameters (horizontal axis) plotted against end-diastolic transseptal pressure gradient (vertical axis) for 22 consecutive beats following the onset of PA constriction. The lines represent results of the least squares linear regression. (Reproduced with the permission of the American Heart Association.) [22]

artery constriction, there was a progressive increase in the RV septal-to-free wall diameter and a reciprocal decrease in the corresponding LV diameter. There was no difference in the LV anteroposterior diameter or in total cardiac diameter. The echocardiographic images confirmed that this reflected a leftward septal shift at end-diastole and the derived M-mode tracings showed that as the septum shifted there was first a progressive decrease in normal leftward systolic septal motion, then akinesis and eventually frankly paradoxic systolic movement.

The earlier observations in man by Tanaka and co-workers [8] are compatible with these conclusions. They noted leftward septal bulging at end-diastole by echocardiography in 4 patients with pulmonary hypertension and correlated this leftward bulging with a reversed transseptal pressure gradient (in the 2 in whom invasive studies were performed). This is well illustrated in Fig. 15-3. It is interesting to note that in this situation, the LV cavity assumes the slit-like appearance of the normal RV. Figure 15-5 is a schematic which illustrates the profound alteration in cardiac geometry which can occur with reversed transseptal pressure gradient at end-diastole; the septum actually becomes inverted so that the RV assumes a circular shape. In this situation, the LV becomes the

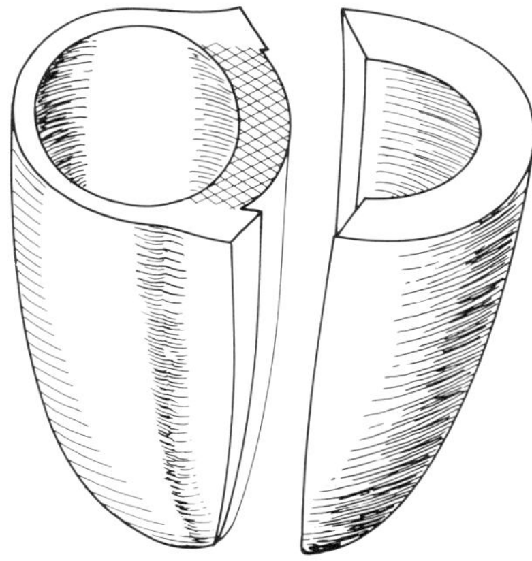

Figure 15-5. Schematic of the ventricles to illustrate the relationship of the septum to the right ventricle when the end-diastolic transseptal gradient is reversed. Note the circular shape to the right ventricle.

crescent shaped cavity similar to that of the normal RV. Based on these observations, it is not surprising that the ventricles of the human fetus have been noted to have a similar shape [29].

Left bundle branch block

Figure 15-6 shows the M-mode echocardiogram from a patient with complete left bundle branch block. The septal motion is abnormal with a leftward motion soon after the onset of electrical systole followed by a rightward movement during the rest of systole. There is another leftward motion in early diastole. Earlier investigators postulated that this motion pattern reflected the abnormal activation sequence of the septum in left bundle branch block [15–16]. However, Little et al. [30] used RV pacing to simulate left bundle branch block and noted that the abnormal motion pattern was readily explained by abnormalities in transseptal gradient. Thus, with left bundle branch block, there is delayed activation of the LV so that pressure begins to rise in the RV before that in the LV. This causes a brief period of transseptal pressure reversal resulting in the early systolic (or late diastolic) leftward septal motion. The normal transseptal gradient is re-established when LV contraction occurs resulting in the septum moving back to the right. The late (early diastolic) leftward motion reflects another period of reduced or reversed transseptal pressure gradient probably secondary to the fact that RV systole terminates before that in the LV so that RV filling begins earlier.

These findings were confirmed by data from our laboratory in the open-chest dog model [22]. In this preparation, therefore, RV volume load (by opening a shunt) RV pressure load (pulmonary artery constriction) and left bundle branch

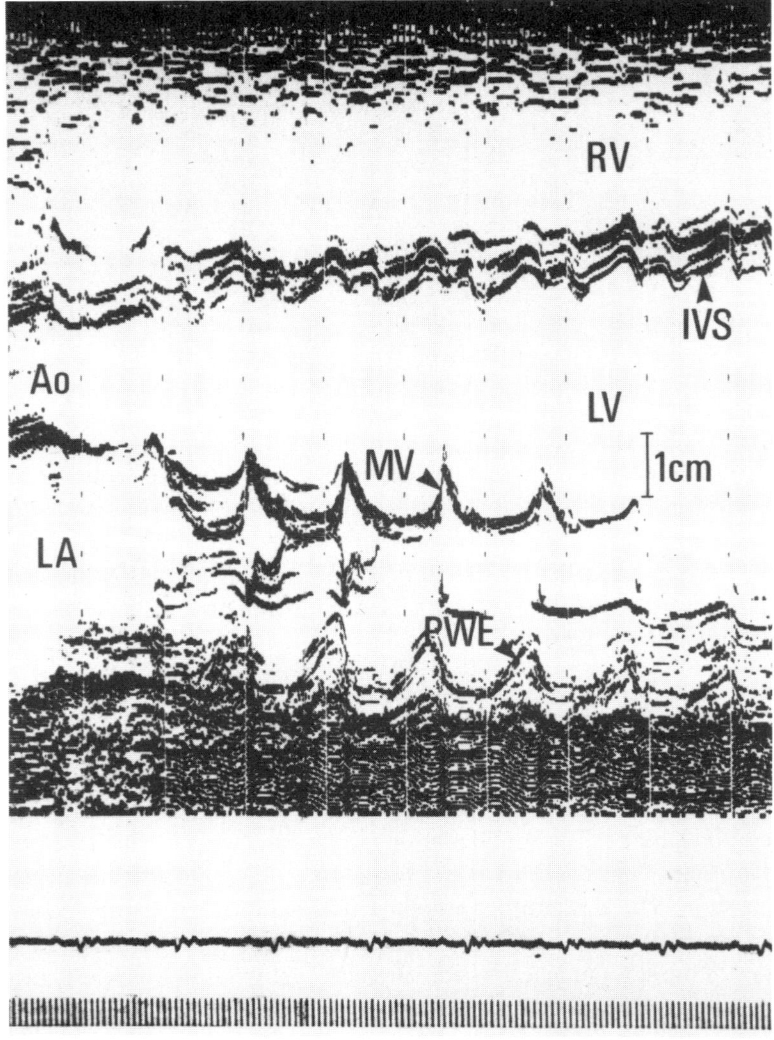

Figure 15-6. M-mode echocardiogram from a patient with left bundle branch block. See text for description of ventricular septal motion pattern. Ao = aorta; LA = left atrium; MV = mitral valve; IVS = interventricular septum; PWE = posterior wall endocardium.

block (RV pacing) all caused abnormalities of transseptal pressure gradient at end-diastole with resultant abnormal positioning of the septum. The subsequent systolic motion was readily explained on the basis of the end diastolic septal position.

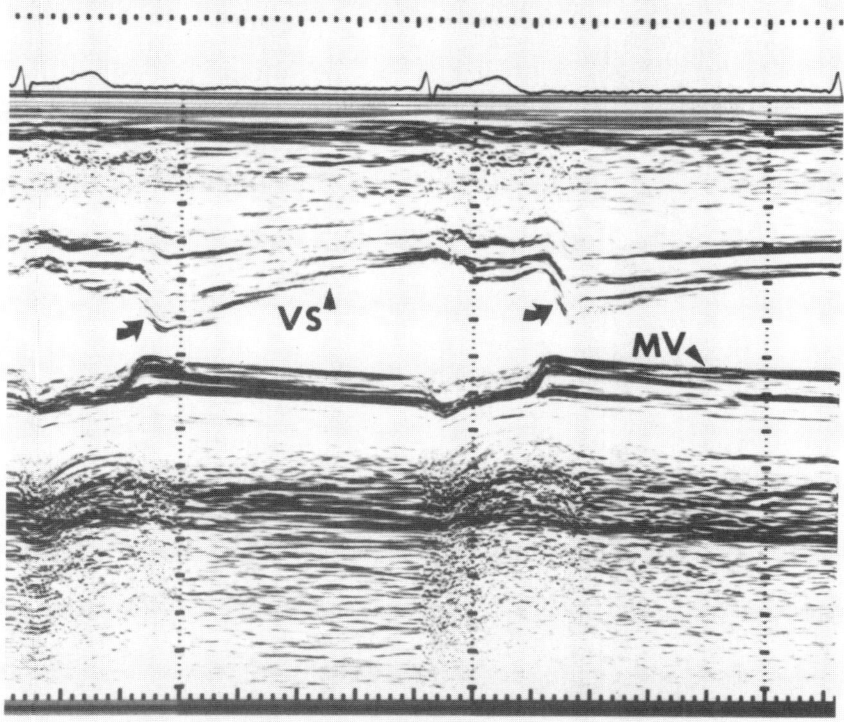

Figure 15-7. M-mode echocardiogram from a patient with mitral stenosis illustrating the marked leftward (paradoxic) diastolic septal movement (curved arrows). MV = mitral valve; VS = ventricular septum.

Mitral stenosis

It has been reconized for some time that patients with mitral stenosis have an abnormal leftward (paradoxic) motion of the ventricular septum during early diastole (Fig. 15-7).

This occurs at a time when the septum normally moves rightward as the LV fills during the rapid filling phase. Thus, there is an abnormal shape to the LV septum during the early phase of diastolic filling as viewed on two-dimensional echocardiographic images. Weyman and co-workers [31] noted that the degree of this distortion correlated with the severity of the mitral stenosis. Thompson et al. [32] in our laboratory have recently demonstrated that the abnormal diastolic movement represents an abnormal transseptal gradient during early diastole. Since left ventricular filling is impeded by the stenotic mitral valve, right ventricular filling occurs more rapidly, causing right ventricular pressure to equal or exceed that in the LV; this results in a brisk leftward septal motion. As the gradient normalizes the septum is displaced back toward the RV cavity. By analysing transseptal pressure-septal position coordinates at frequent time intervals throughout diastole in a group of patients with mitral stenosis, we have demonsrated that the septal position at any time during diastole is determined by the instantaneous transseptal gradient. However, only the position at end-diastole (reflecting the transseptal gradient at that instant) influences the systolic septal motion.

Normal physiology

Echocardiography frequently allows recognition of displacement of the septum toward the LV during normal inspiration [33]. This would be expected if the increased RV filling occurring during inspiration resulted in a decrease in the normal transseptal gradient. Ieri and Zipoli [34] reported marked leftward diastolic displacement of the septum followed by paradoxic systolic motion in a patient during forced inspiration. This patient did have pulmonary disease which may have caused abnormal RV hemodynamics although this was not evident clinically. Brinker and co-workers [35] assessed the degree of leftward septal displacement occurring in normal subjects secondary to a Mueller manoeuvre. The septal displacement (as reflected by a change in the septal radius of curvature) was most marked during diastole and was observed [36] to be a function of the transseptal pressure gradient. Studies in our laboratory in patients undergoing diagnostic cardiac catheterization revealed similar findings [37]. Moreover, a Mueller manoeuvre of 40–60 mm Hg negative pressure caused sufficient reduction in the end-diastolic transseptal gradient with associated leftward septal shift to result in paradoxic systolic septal motion for a few cardiac cycles. Although Mueller manoeuvres as performed in this study represent unusually large inspiratory efforts, the results clearly demonstrate the responsiveness of diastolic septal position to even minor changes in transseptal pressure gradient.

Left ventricular volume load

An empiric observation in patients with a volume load on the LV has been excessive systolic motion of the ventricular septum, a sign now widely used clinically in echocardiography (Fig. 15-8). Experimentally, Molaug et al. [38] assessed the effect of opening a shunt between the subclavian artery and the left atrium on septal position. This intervention resulted in an increase in the end-diastolic transseptal gradient, an increase in the LV septal-to-free wall diameter and a decrease in the reciprocal RV dimension – all observations in keeping with a rightward shift of the septum at end-diastole. We made similar observations in patients undergoing cardiac catheterization [37]. Isometric hand grip exercise increased LV diastolic pressure and the transseptal gradient at end-diastole. This

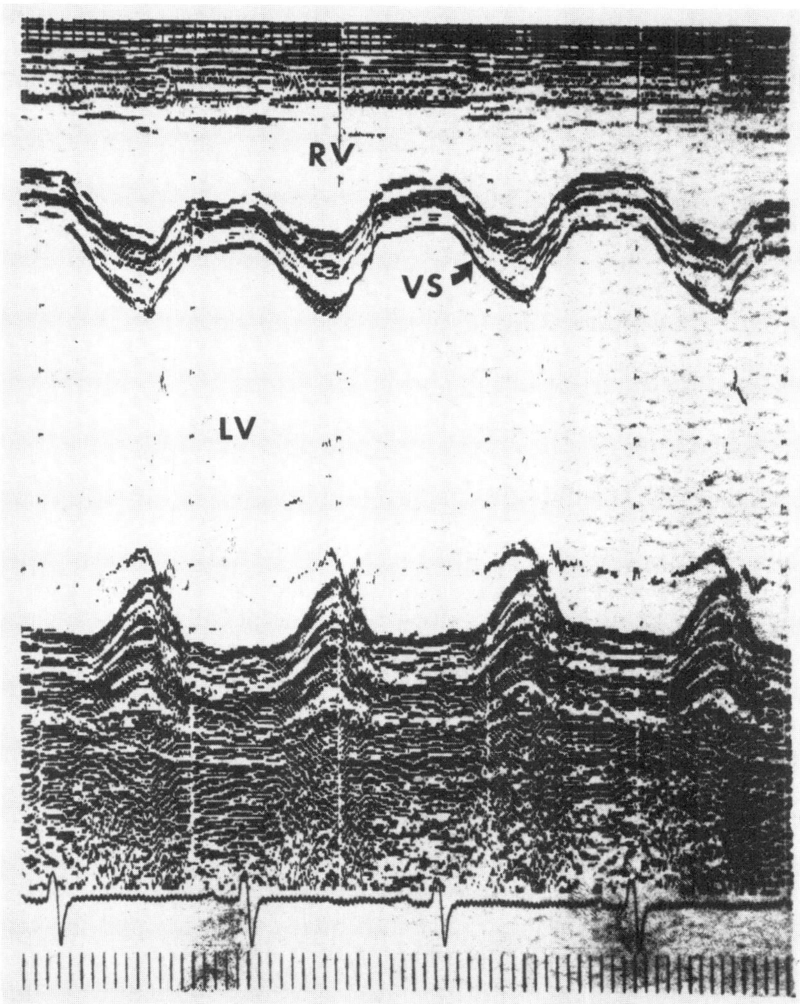

Figure 15-8. M-mode echocardiogram from a patient with a volume load on the left ventricle. Note the marked (leftward) excursion of the ventricular septum (VS) during systole.

resulted in an increase in LV diameter and in leftward systolic septal motion.

Based on the results of these many studies, it seems clear that during diastole the septum is a very compliant membrane between the two ventricles with its position responsive to even minor alterations in transseptal pressure gradient. Abnormalities of transseptal gradient explain the abnormal diastolic motion in patients with mitral stenosis and is responsible for the abnormal position of the septum at end-diastole in a number of clinical conditions. When the septum is shifted to the left at end-diastole secondary to a decreased transseptal gradient, the subsequent systolic motion will be abnormal – either reduced, akinetic or frankly paradoxic depending on the magnitude of the diastolic septal shift. If the septum is displaced rightward at end-diastole, secondary to an increased transseptal gradient, the subsequent systolic motion will be exaggerated in the normal direction.

Systolic mechanics

There are two important considerations in dealing with mechanics of the septum during systole. The first relates to the effect of abnormal transseptal gradient during systole on septal position and movement. The second relates to the effect of the systolic motion pattern on ventricular performance.

Effects of abnormal systolic transseptal gradient

Normally the pressure in the LV exceeds that in the RV during systole by approximately 100 mm Hg. As previously mentioned, the septum normally maintains a concave orientation to the LV during systole with the septal radius of curvature equal to that of the free wall. However, in the presence of RV hypertension, a number of investigators have noted that the septum remains displaced (flattened) leftward at end-systole [8, 23–24, 27–28]. In a study using chronically instrumented dogs we recently reported similar findings and confirmed that the end-systolic septal displacement also reflected altered transseptal gradient [39]. Figure 15-9 shows RV septal-to-free wall diameters at end-diastole and at end-systole (measured by sonomicrometry) plotted against transseptal gradient from 18 consecutive cardiac cycles during inflation of a pulmonary artery occluder. There was a tight linear relationship between transseptal gradient and both end-diastolic and end-systolic RV diameter. However, the slopes of these relationships were significantly different; during systole a much greater change in transseptal gradient was required to effect a given change in RV dimension than that during diastole. This is in keeping with the greater stiffness of the myocardium during systole. There were reciprocal changes of similar magnitude in the LV septal-to-free wall diameter.

Similar displacement of the septum at end-systole has been noted in patients with RV hypertension. Note in Fig. 15-2 that the end-systolic shape of the LV is more circular than at end-diastole but that the septal curvature is still quite different from that of the LV free wall. Such observations may prove to be very useful clinically. Ryan et al. [40] were able to separate volume from pressure overload states by two-dimensional echocardiography by assessing the shape of the septum during diastole and systole. In RV volume overload without pulmonary hypertension, the septum is displaced leftward (flattened) during diastole but the LV reassumes its circular shape during systole. In RV pressure overload,

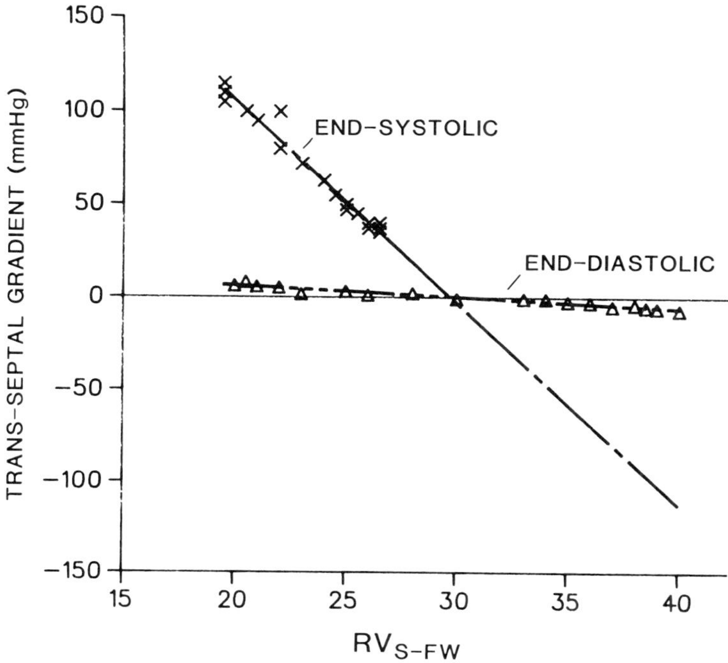

Figure 15-9. End-diastolic (triangles) and end-systolic (crosses) right ventricular septal-to-free wall diameters (horizontal axis) plotted against transseptal (LV-RV) pressure gradient (vertical axis) for 18 consecutive beats following the onset of pulmonary artery constriction in a conscious dog model. The slopes of these relationships were significantly different reflecting the greater stiffness of the contracted myocardium.

the septum is displaced leftward during both diastole and systole. Shimada and co-workers [41], using a similar approach were able to identify those patients with atrial septal defect who were complicated by pulmonary hypertension. Thus, such observations allow rapid non-invasive assessment of RV hemodynamics – during both diastole and systole – at least in comparison to those in the LV.

Effect of abnormal septal mechanics on ventricular performance

Displacement of the septum to the left secondary to a reduced transseptal gradient results in a change in the pressure-volume relationship of the LV – that is, the change in configuration of the LV cavity causes an apparent decrease in LV compliance. This has been demonstrated in isolated hearts [17–20], as well as in intact animals. Similarly, a volume load to the LV shifts the septum rightward and may alter the pressure-volume characteristics of the right ventricle [38]. In both situations, the loading conditions of the contralateral ventricle can be altered and ventricular performance affected.

Perhaps of greater importance, however, is the implication of the altered systolic septal motion to respective ventricular function. During experimental RV volume overload, Molaug and co-workers [42], noted that RV stroke volume increased more than could be explained by RV free wall segment length changes. Rather, the major fraction of the increased stroke volume was due to a marked increase in RV septal-to-free wall axis shortening – an observation consistent with there having been a marked leftward septal displacement at end-diastole with consequent paradoxic systolic motion. Interestingly, in their model systolic performance of the LV was not adversely affected. In a model of LV volume overload, these same investigators [38] noted an increase in the transseptal gradient, an increase in LV septal-to-free wall diameter and an increase in LV stroke volume. The increased stroke volume resulted largely from the increased systolic shortening of the LV septum-to-free wall axis.

Thus, septal displacement at end-diastole secondary to an altered transseptal gradient may impact in a major way on systolic performance of the ventricles. An altered end-systolic transseptal gradient may also modulate the systolic septal motion making the final contribution of septal contraction to either ventricle the result of a rather complex set of variables.

Implications

Appreciation of the influence of transseptal gradient on both diastolic and systolic position and motion makes it clear that the ventricular septum cannot simply be considered part of the LV. Thus, it seems necessary to consider the ventricles as a three component system, the LV free wall, the RV free wall and the ventricular septum (Fig. 15-10). Although the septum is normally concave to the LV during diastole (panel A), in a number of clinical states it becomes concave to the RV (panel B).

This more complete understanding of septal mechanics also has important implications to currently utilized methods for the assessment of ventricular function. It is apparent that systolic septal motion may not only reflect contractile function of the myocardium. Indeed, normally contractile septal muscle might be assocated with hyperkinesis, hypokinesis, akinesis or dyskinesis depending on the transseptal gradients throughout the cardiac cycle. Methods of assessment of LV function which rely to greater or lesser degrees on septal motion may, therefore, provide misleading information. This includes echocardiography, as well as contrast and nuclide angiography (left anterior oblique projections). This is most important to the increasingly common practice of analysing regional myocardial function by these techniques to make decisions on viability of segmental myocardium. Clearly, septal motion should not be included in such studies unless the presence of a normal transseptal gradient is documented throughout the cardiac cycle.

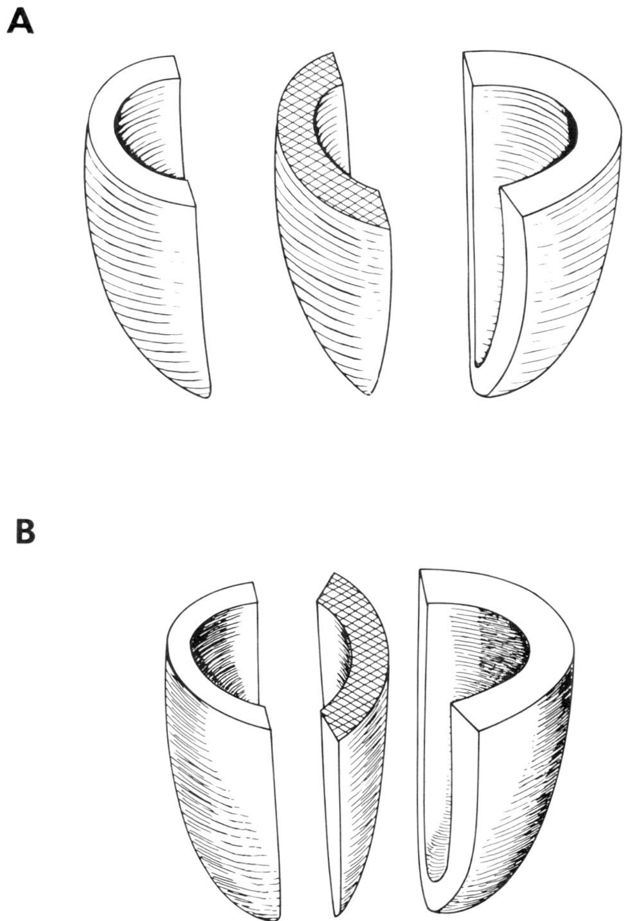

Figure 15-10. Schematic of the ventricles to illustrate the three component system. Panel A represents the orientation of the septum (cross hatched) given a normal transseptal gradient at end-diastole. Panel B illustrates the orientation of the septum when the end-diastolic transseptal gradient is reversed. Adapted from Kieffer et al. [2].

Conclusions

An impressive body of experimental and clinical data is now available to provide new insight into the mechanics of the ventricular septum. Given normal hemodynamics, the septum is structurally and funtionally part of the LV. Abnormalities of transseptal gradient during diastole result in displacement of the septum and subsequent abnormal systolic motion patterns. During diastole, the septum is very compliant membrane between the ventricles with its position responsive to even small changes in transseptal gradient. During systole, septal position is also responsive to the instantaneous transseptal gradient although the contracted myocardium is considerably stiffer. Abnormalities of systolic motion secondary to abnormal end-diastolic transseptal position can have a major impact on the systolic performance of the ventricles.

Acknowledgements

Work reported here was supported by grants from the Alberta Heart and Stroke Foundation.

References

1. Armour, J.A. and Randall, W.C.: Structural basis for cardiac function. Am. J. Physiol. 218: 1517–1523, 1970.
2. Kieffer, R.W., Hutchins, G.M., Moore, G.W. and Bulkley, B.H.: Reversed septal curvature. Association with primary pulmonary hypertension and Shone Syndrome. Am. J. Med. 66: 831–835, 1979.
3. Popp, R.L., Wolfe, S.B., Hirata, T. and Feigenbaum, H.: Estimation of right and left ventricular size by ultrasound. A study of the echoes from the interventricular septum. Am. J. Cardiol. 24: 523–530, 1969.
4. Pearlman, A.S., Clark, C.E., Henry, W.L., Morganroth, J., Itscoitz, S.B. and Epstein, S.E.: Determinants of ventricular septal motion. Influence of relative right and left ventricular size. Circulation 54: 83–91, 1976.
5. Meyer, R.A., Schwartz, D.C., Benzing, G. III and Kaplan, S.: Ventricular septum in right ventricular volume overload. An echocardiographic study. Am. J. Cardiol. 30: 349–353, 1972.
6. Laurenceau, J.L. and Dumesnil, J.G.: Right and left ventricular dimensions as determinants of ventricular septal motion. Chest 69: 388–393, 1976.
7. Weyman, A.E., Wann, S., Feigenbaum, H. and Dillon, J.C.: Mechanism of abnormal septal motion in patients with righ ventricular volume overload. Circulation 54: 179–186, 1976.
8. Tanaka, H., Tei, C., Nakao, S., Tahara, M., Sakurai, S., Kashima, T. and Kanehisa, T.: Diastolic bulging of the interventricular septum toward the left ventricle. An echocardiographic manifestation of negative interventricular pressure gradient between left and right ventricles during diastole. Circulation 62: 558–563, 1980.
9. Candell-Riera, J., Garcia del Castillo, H., Permanyer-Miralda, G. and Soler-Soler, J.: Echocardiographic features of the interventricular septum in chronic constrictive pericarditis. Circulation 57: 1154–1158, 1978.
10. Payvandi, M.N. and Kerber, R.E.: Echocardiography in congenital and acquired absence of the pericardium. An echocardiographic mimic of right ventricular volume overload. Circulation 53: 86–92, 1976.
11. Schuler, G., Peterson, K.L., Johnson, A.D., Francis, G., Ashburn, W., Dennish, G., Daily, P.O. and Ross, J. Jr.: Serial noninvasive assessment of left ventricular hypertrophy and function after surgical correction of aortic regurgitation. Am. J. Cardiol. 44: 585–594, 1979.
12. Waggoner, A.D., Shah, A.A., Schuessler, J.S., Crawford, E.S., Nelson, J.G., Miller, R.R. and Quinones, M.A.: Effect of cardiac surgery on ventricular septal motion: assessment by intra-

operative echocadiography and cross-sectional two-dimensional echocardiography. Am. Heart J. 104: 1271–1278, 1982.

13. Schabelman, S.E., Jackson, J.G., Schulz, E.E. and Jutzy, R.V.: Pericardial closure and para-doxic septal motion after surgery. South Med. J. 74: 1353–1356, 1981.

14. Kerber, R.E. and Litchfield, R.: Postoperative abnormalities of interventricular septal motion: Two-dimensional and M-mode echocardiographic correlations. Am. Heart. J. 104: 263–268, 1982.

15. McDonald, I.G.: Echocardiographic demonstration of abnormal motion of the interventricular septum in left bundle branch block. Circulation 48: 272–280, 1973.

16. Gomes, J.A.C., Damato, A.N., Akhtar, M., Dhatt, M.S., Calon, A.H., Reddy, C.P. and Moran, H.E.: Ventricular septal motion and left ventricular dimensions during abnormal ven-tricular activation. Am. J. Cardiol. 39: 641–650, 1977.

17. Henderson, Y. and Prince, A.L.: The relative systolic discharges of the right and left ventricles and their bearing on pulmonary congestion and depletion. Heart 5: 217–226, 1914.

18. Bemis, C.E., Serur, J.R., Borkenhagen, D., Sonnenblick, E.H. and Urschel, C.W.: Influence of right ventricular filling pressure on left ventricular pressure and dimension. Circ. Res. 34: 498–504, 1974.

19. Elzinga, G., Van Grondelle, R., Westerhof, N. and Van Den Bos, G.C.: Ventricular inter-ference. Am. J. Physiol. 226: 941–947, 1974.

20. Santamore, W.P., Lynch, P.R., Meier, G., Jeckman, J. and Bove, A.A.: Myocardial interaction between the ventricles. J. Appl. Physiol. 41: 362–368, 1976.

21. Kerber, R.E., Dippel, W.F. and Abboud, F.M.: Abnormal motion of the interventricular septum in right ventricular volume overload. Circulation 48: 86–96, 1973.

22. Kingma, I., Tyberg, J.V. and Smith, E.R.: Effects of diastolic transseptal pressure gradient on ventricular septal position and motion. Circulation 68: 1304–1314, 1983.

23. Stool, E.W., Mullins, C.B., Leshin, S.J. and Mitchell, J.H.: Dimensional changes of the left ventricle during acute pulmonary arterial hypertension in dogs. Am. J. Cardiol. 33: 868–875, 1974.

24. Badke, F.R.: Left ventricular dimensions and function during right ventricular pressure over-load. Am. J. Physiol. 11: H611–H618, 1982.

25. Slutsky, R.A., Peck, W.W. and Mancini, G.B.J.: The effect of pulmonic and aortic constriction on regional left ventricular thickening dynamics, geometry and the radius of septal curvature. Analysis by gated computed transmission tomography. Invest. Radiol. 19: 374–379, 1984.

26. Molaug, M., Stokland, O., Ilebekk, A., Lekven, J. and Kiil, F.: Myocardial function of the interventricular septum. Effects of right and left ventricular pressure loading before and after pericardiotomy in dogs. Circ. Res. 49: 52–61, 1981.

27. Visner, M.S., Arentzen, C.E., O'Connor, M.J., Larson, E.V. and Anderson, R.W.: Alterations in left ventricular three-dimensional dynamic geometry and systolic function during acute right ventricular hypertension in the conscious dog. Circulation 67: 353–365, 1983.

28. Olsen, C.O., Tyson, G.S., Maier, G.W., Spratt, J.A., Davis, J.W. and Rankin, J.S.: Dynamic ventricular interaction in the conscious dog. Circ. Res. 52: 85–104, 1983.

29. Azancot, A., Caudell, T.P., Allen, H.D., Horowitz, S., Sahn, D.J., Stoll, C., Thies, C., Valdes-Cruz, L.M. and Goldberg, S.J.: Analysis of ventricular shape by echocardiography in normal fetuses, newborns, and infants. Circulation 68: 1201–1211, 1983.

30. Little, W.C., Reeves, R.C., Arciniegas, J., Katholi, R.E. and Rogers, E.W.: Mechanism of abnormal interventricular septal motion during delayed left ventricular activation. Circulation 65: 1486–1491, 1983.

31. Weyman, A.E., Heger, J.J., Kronik, G., Wann, L.S., Dillon, J.C. and Feigenbaum, H.: Mechanism of paradoxical early diastolic septal motion in patients with mitral stenosis. A cross-sectional echocardiographic study. Am. J. Cardiol. 40: 691–699, 1977.

32. Thompson, C.R., Kingma, I., MacDonald, R.P., Belenkie, I., Tyberg, J.V. and Smith, E.R.:

Transseptal pressure gradient determines diastolic ventricular septal motion in patients with mitral stenosis. Circulation 72 (Suppl III): III–410, 1985.

33. Meyer, R.A.: Pediatric Echocardiography. Philadelphia, Lea and Febiger, 1977.

34. Ieri, A. and Zipoli, A.: Abnormal diastolic motion of interventricular septum during inspiratory phase. Echocardiographic study. Br. Heart J. 43: 702–704, 1980.

35. Brinker, J.A., Weiss, J.L., Lappe, D.L., Rabson, J.L., Summer, W.R., Permutt, S. and Weisfeldt, M.L.: Leftward septal displacement during right ventricular loading in man. Circulation 61: 626–633, 1980.

36. Guzman, P.A., Maughan, W.L., Yin, F.C.P., Eaton, L.W., Brinker, J.A., Weisfeldt, M.L. and Weiss, J.L.: Transseptal pressure gradient with leftward septal displacement during the Mueller manoeuvre in man. Br. Heart H. 46: 657–662, 1981.

37. Kingma, I., Smiseth, O.A., Belenkie, I., MacDonald, R.P.R., Knudtson, M.L., Tyberg, J.V. and Smith, E.R.: Ventricular septal dynamics in response to altered transseptal pressure in man. J. Am. Coll. Cardiol. 5: 511, 1985 (Abstract).

38. Molaug, M., Geiran, O. and Kiil, F.: Dynamics of the interventricular septum and free ventricular walls during selective left ventricular volume loading in dogs. Acta. Physiol. Scand. 119: 81–89, 1983.

39. Smith, E.R., Kingma, I., Smiseth, O.A., MacDonald, R.P.R., Groves, G., Pawlak, C., Kondo, C. and Tyberg, J.V.: Ventricular septal responses to acute constriction of the pulmonary artery in conscious dogs. Am. Rev. Respir. Dis. 131: A57, 1985 (Abstract).

40. Ryan, T., Petrovic, O., Dillon, J.C., Feigenbaum, H., Conley, M.J. and Armstrong, W.F.: An echocardiographic index for separation of right ventricular volume and pressure overload. J. Am. Coll. Cardiol. 5: 918–924, 1985.

41. Shimada, R., Takeshita, A. and Nakamura, M.: Noninvasive assessment of right ventricular systolic pressure in atrial septal defect: Analysis of the end-systolic configuration of the ventricular septum by two-dimensional echocardiography. Am. J. Cardiol. 53: 1117–1123, 1984.

42. Molaug, M., Geiran, O., Stokland, O., Thorvaldson, J. and Ilebekk, A.: Dynamics of the interventricular septum and free ventricular walls during blood volume expansion and selective right ventricular volume loading in dogs. Acta. Physiol. Scand. 116: 245–256, 1982.

16. Mechanics of the interventricular septum

A. ILEBEKK

Introduction

Dr. Eldon Smith has just pointed out that the interventricular septum is a compliant membrane during diastole. Although stiffer during systole, the shape and position of the septum is also determined by the instantaneous transseptal pressure gradient. I'll try to show that contractions of septal muscle fibers influence cardiac pump-function depending on the end-diastolic position of the septum and illustrate this by presenting examples from selective right- and left ventricular volume loading. The experiments I'll refer to were performed at the Institute for Experimental Medical Research, University of Oslo, Norway. The results have been published by Dr. Molaug and co-workers. We used mongrel dogs, anesthetized with sodium pentobarbital. The chest was opened and segment lengths were recorded in the right and left ventricular free walls and the interventricular septum. Pairs of piezoelectric crystals were sewn into midwall positions, and segment lengths were recorded by an ultrasonic technique.

The tracings of Fig. 16-1 show an example of a segment length obtained from the interventricular septum (lower line) [1]. The cyclic variations of the segment length in the septum paralleled those in the left ventricular free wall (the line above). Furthermore, the segment length in the septum responded in a typical way to local ischemia. Figure 16-2 shows that segment lengths recorded in the longitudinal and the transverse direction of the septum behaved equally during variations in cardiac filling [2]. Accordingly, we usually recorded only one segment length in the septum.

Figure 16-3 shows function curves of stroke volume and end-diastolic segment lengths in the free wall of the right ventricle, the septum, and the free wall of the left ventricle during variations in cardiac filling in one dog [3]. When the Frank-Starling mechanism was activated by uniform cardiac dilation, the systolic shortening of the segment lengths increased in all three locations. In the next few figures we will see how data deviate from these function curves during selective left- and right ventricular volume loading.

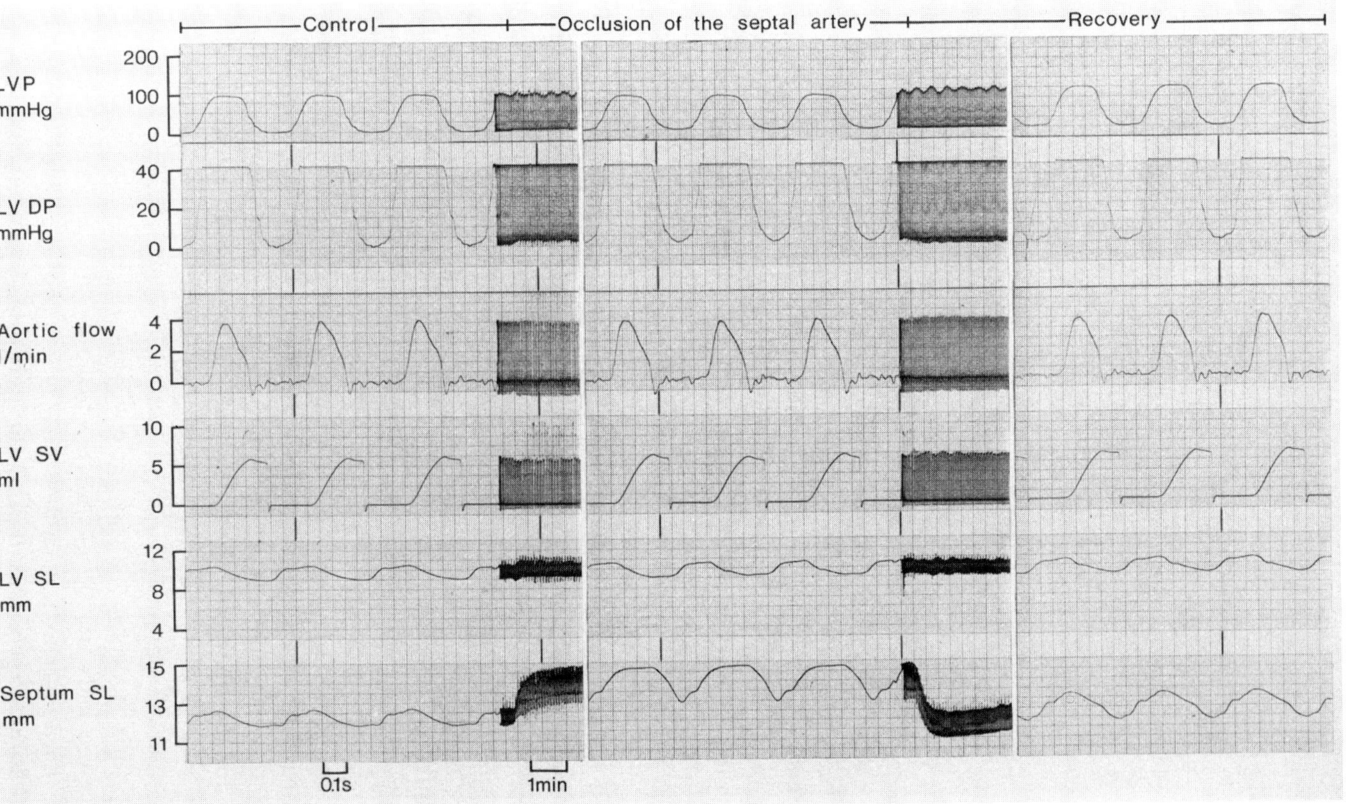

Figure 16-1. Tracings from dog weighing 15 kg. The two lower lines demonstrate parallel cyclic changes in the septal- and LV-free wall segment length (SL) in the control setting, and typical changes in the septal-SL by localized ischemia. Reproduced by permission from Molaug M et al. [1].

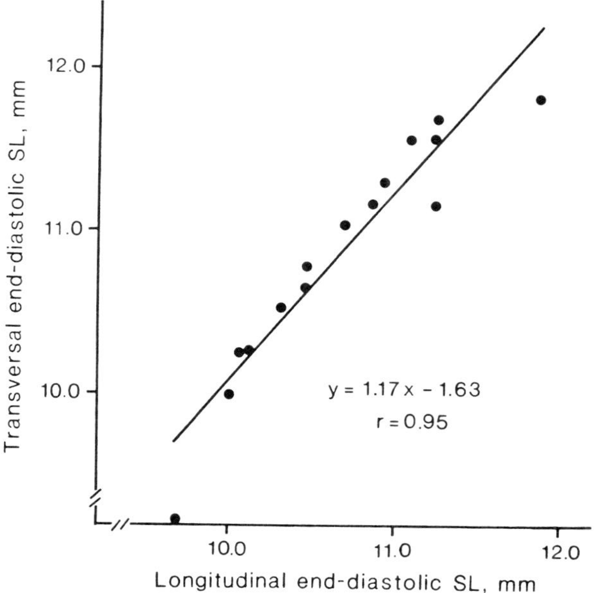

Figure 16-2. Similar changes in end-diastolic segment lengths (SL) in the transverse and longitudinal direction of the septum were obtained during variations in cardiac filling. Reproduced by permission from Molaug M et al. [2].

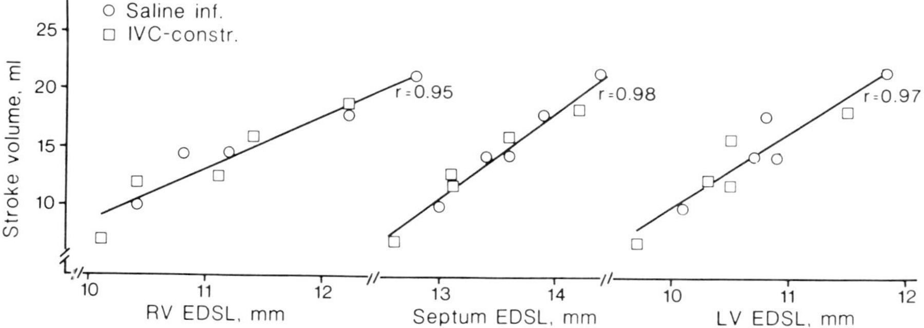

Figure 16-3. Relations between stroke volume and end-diastolic segment lengths (EDSL) in the right ventricle (RV), the septum, and the left ventricle (LV) during variations in cardiac filling IVC = inferior vena cava. Reproduced by permission from Molaug M et al. [3].

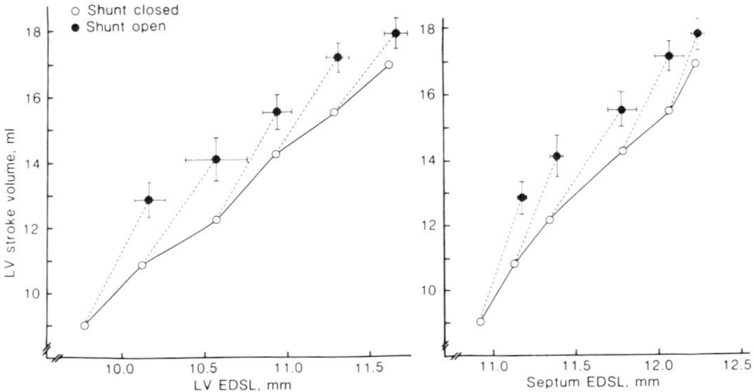

Figure 16-4. Relations between LV-stroke volume and EDSL in the LV-free wall and the septum. By opening a shunt between the left subclavian artery and the left atrium, left ventricular pump function was improved (filled symbols). Reproduced by permission from Molaug M et al. [4].

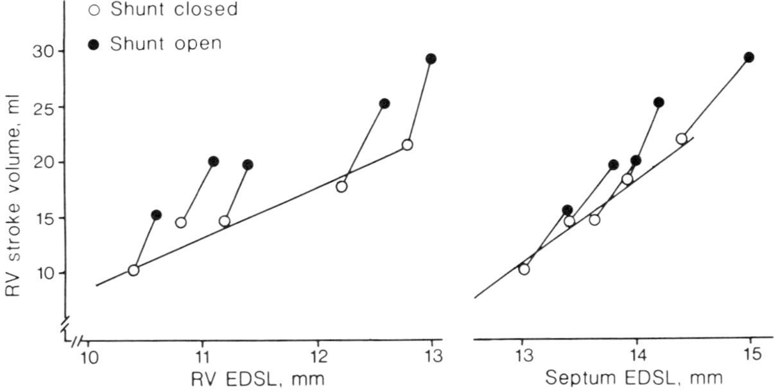

Figure 16-5. Relations between right ventricular stroke volme and end-diastolic segment lengths (EDSL) in the RV free wall and in the septum. By opening a shunt between the pulmonary artery and the superior vena cava, rightventricular pump function was improved (filled symbols). Reproduced by permission from Molaug M et al. [3].

First, the effects of selective left ventricular volume loading are shown (Fig. 16-4) [4]. This loading was achieved by opening a shunt between the left subclavian artery and the left atrium. When the shunt was opened at different degrees of blood volume expansion, a new cardiac function curve was established. Left ventricular stroke volume became greater than expected from the increments in segment lengths in the left ventricular free wall and the septum.

Right ventricular output, decreased by about 15%, despite an almost unchanged end-diastolic segment length. This signifies a decline of right ventriculr function from the normal function curve. The results can be explained by the

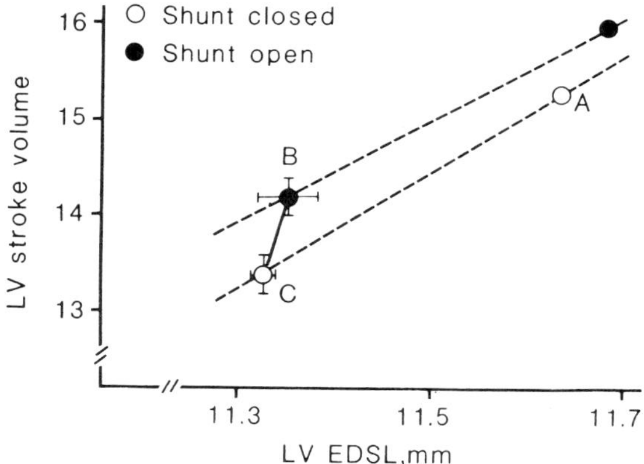

Figure 15-6. Function curves (stippled lines) between LV stroke volume and LV-EDSL before (open symbols) and during selective RV-volume loading (filled symbols). By opening the pulmonary artery-superior vena cava shunt, left ventricular stroke volume and EDSL in the free wall of the left ventricle both declined (A–B), but stroke volume fell less than expected according to comparison at similar LV EDSL with the shunt open and closed (B and C). Drawn from data published by Molaug M et al. with permission [3].

rightward displacement of the septum, improving left- an diminishing right ventricular pump function.

Some of the effects of selective right ventricular volume loading are shown in Fig. 16-5 [3]. This loading was achieved by opening a shunt between the pulmonary artery and the superior vena cava. In Fig. 16-5 the open symbols constitute the basal function curve of right ventricular stroke volume and end-diastolic segment lengths in the right ventricular free wall and in the septum. Deviations from the function curves appeared when the shunt was opened, probably because of a leftward displacement of the septum as a consequence of a reduced left-to-right diastolic pressure gradient.

The effect of right ventricular volume loading on left ventricular function is shown in Fig. 16-6 [3]. This figure shows that left ventricular stroke volume is larger than expected from the function curve and the concomitant decrease in end-diastolic segment length of the free wall of the left ventricle when the shunt is opened. The alteration in the left ventricular function curve indicates improved left ventricular function when the right ventricle is selectively volume-loaded by opening a shunt between the pulmonary artery and the superior vena cava.

In conclusion. A selective right ventricular volume loading reduces the left-to-right diastolic pressure difference and changes the geometric configuration of the left ventricle. This leads to a passive stretching of the septal muscle fibers, which in turn induces an increased active systolic shortening. This apparently counteracts any negative effects on left ventricular stroke volume by the changes in configuration. Thereby the pump function of both the right and left ventricle is improved.

References

1. Molaug, M., Geiran, O. and Kiil, F.: Compensatory cardiac mechanisms evoked by septal ischemia in dogs. Am. J. Cardiol. 51: 201–206, 1983.
2. Molaug, M., Stokland, O., Ilebekk, A., Lekven, J. and Kiil, F.: Myocardial function of the interventricular septum. Effects of right and left ventricular pressure loading before and after pericardiotomy in dogs. Circ. Res. 49: 52–61, 1981.
3. Molaug, M., Geiran, O., Stokland, O., Thorvaldson, J. and Ilebekk, A.: Dynamics of the interventricular septum and free ventricular walls during blood volume expansion and selective right ventricular volume loading in dogs. Acta. Physiol. Scand. 116: 245–256, 1982.
4. Molaug, M., Geiran, O. and Kiil, F.: Dynamics of the interventricular septum and free ventricular walls during selective left ventricular volume loading in dogs. Acta. Physiol. Scand. 119: 81–91, 1983.

General discussion of septal mechanics

The desirability of describing the motion of the ventricular septum by measuring the change in radius of curvature was discussed. While measurement of the radius of curvature can be helpful in interpreting changes in absolute ventricular diameters, Dr. Smith and his colleagues ascertained the relative motion of the septum by 2-D echocardiography and by expressing the motion of the septum in relation to the combined width of the two ventricles.

17. On the interaction between the pericardium and the heart

JOHN V. TYBERG and ELDON R. SMITH

Introduction

This review focuses on the concept of pericardial 'pressure', an issue which is critical to understanding the physiology of the pericardium. The quotation marks anticipate our final conclusion – that pericardial constraint cannot be measured by measuring pressure (as defined strictly) and that some of the confusion and misunderstanding of the physiologic role of the pericardium is really a semantic issue. We will survey the observations which contradict the current consensus position – that pericardial pressure is near zero and cannot change acutely [1] and suggest a perspective which agrees more closely with experimental and clinical observations.

Load-mediated shifts in the LV diastolic P-V relationship

This series of studies began several years ago in search of an explanation for an observation that was completely unexpected. At that time it was generally believed that the left ventricular (LV) diastolic pressure-volume relationship was a constant, simple curvilinear one. However, several observations made a decade ago indicated that, in patients with a degree of congestive heart failure, the LV diastolic pressure volume relation could be shifted upward [2, 3] or downward [3, 4] in a generally parallel fashion (see Fig. 17-1). (This observation is to be distinguished from those made somewhat earlier by Dwyer et al. [5] and confirmed by others [6, 7] which showed an upward shift lasting for several seconds following a period of tachycardia in the presence of ischemia. More recently the latter phenomenon was conclusively shown to be due to a transient change in the distensibility of the ventricular myocardium [8].) The hypothesis that we advanced in 1978 to explain the mechanism of load mediated shift in the LV diastolic pressure-volume relationship [9] is represented in Fig. 17-2. If pericardial 'pressure' is elevated in the presence of congestive heart failure, the administration of

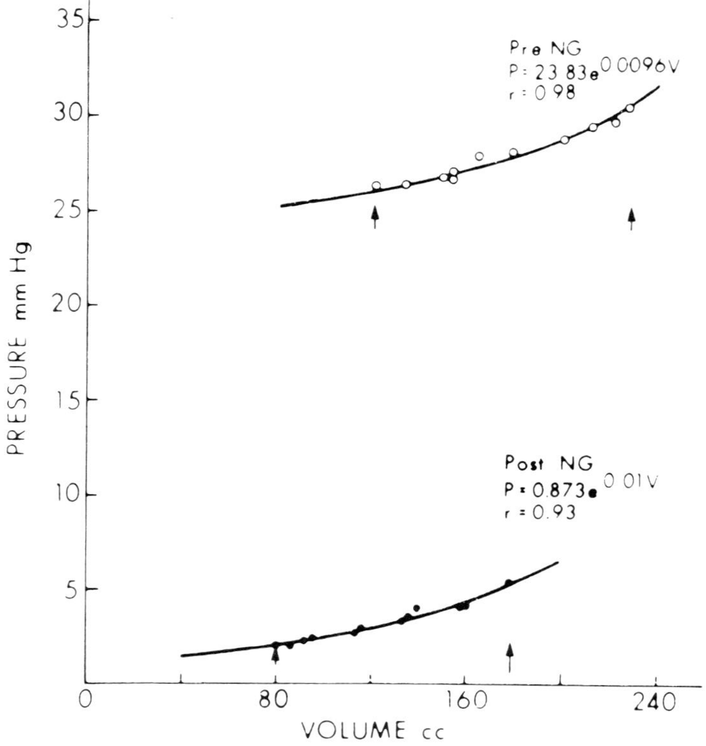

Figure 17-1. An example of a large load-mediated shift in the left ventricular diastolic pressure-volume relationship. At the top in the diastolic portion of a pressure-volume loop in a patient with congestive heart failure (note that the end diastolic pressure is approximately 30 mm Hg). At the bottom of the figure is the diastolic pressure-volume relationship shortly after the administration of sublingual nitroglycerin. Note that, in spite of the large fall in end diastolic pressure, end diastolic volume decreases by less than 10%. From Ludbrook et al. [4] with permission of the American Heart Association.

a vasodilator such as nitroprusside or nitroglycerin might produce peripheral venous pooling which would make the heart smaller and lower pericardial 'pressure'. If the reduction in pericardial pressure is almost as great as the reduction in LV diastolic pressure, the fall in preload (i.e., LV end diastolic transmural pressure) might be relatively small. This would tend to explain the surprisingly modest reduction in end diastolic volume (Fig. 17-1) and may explain in part why cardiac output is so well maintained even when vasodilator therapy lowers LV filling pressure dramatically [10].

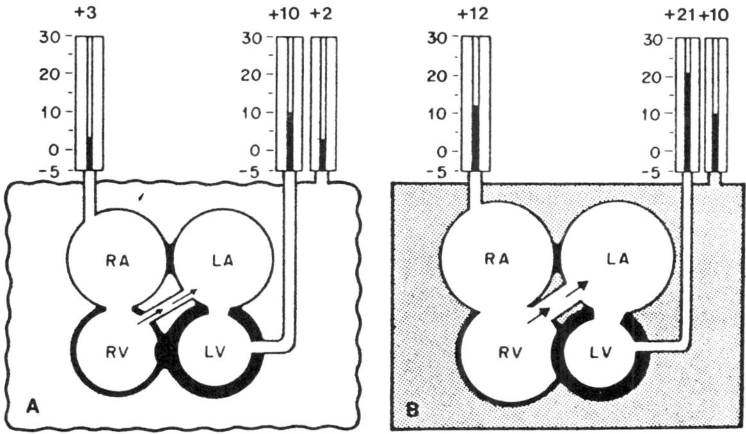

Figure 17-2. A schematic representation of our hypothesis to explain the phenomenon illustrated by Fig. 17-1. In the right hand panel the situation of acute congestive heart failure is represented. Because the heart is enlarged pericardial pressure is increased. The left hand panel represents the situation after nitroglycerin administration. Peripheral systemic pooling allows the heart to become smaller which lowers pericardial pressure. The modest reduction in LV volume is consistent with the fall in LV transmural pressure (i.e. LV end diastolic pressure – pericardial pressure) but less than would have been predicted using LV end diastolic pressure alone as a measure of preload. [N.B. The careful reader will note that the water manometer pictured would not measure the true effect of the pericardial constraint unless considerable pericardial fluid was present. This device is used in the diagram for the sake of simplicity, only]. Modified from Shabetai [23] with permission.

Measuring pericardial pressure

Of course, the correctness of this hypothesis depended on demonstrating that pericardial pressure was greater than was generally believed. We [11] compared two techniques for measuring pericardial pressure, a conventional open catheter and a liquid-containing balloon used earlier by Holt et al. [12]. Although previous measurements had been made carefully, the results were inconclusive because there was no rationale to determine what was the true, effective pericardial pressure. We made the following assumption illustrated in Fig. 17-3. At end diastole, when viscous and inertial terms can be neglected, a static equilibrium exists at the endocardial surface of the free wall of the left ventricle. The intracavitary pressure is exactly opposed by the sum of the transmural pressure, which the ventricular wall itself is able to sustain at that volume, and the effective 'pressure' exerted by the pericardium. The same assumption is represented differently in Fig. 17-4. In this LV pressure-diameter diagram, pericardial 'pressure' ('calculated pericardial pressure') is equal to the difference between the LV end diastolic intracavitary pressures recorded with the pericardium present and with it absent, respectively. The pressure measured by the pericardial balloon

198

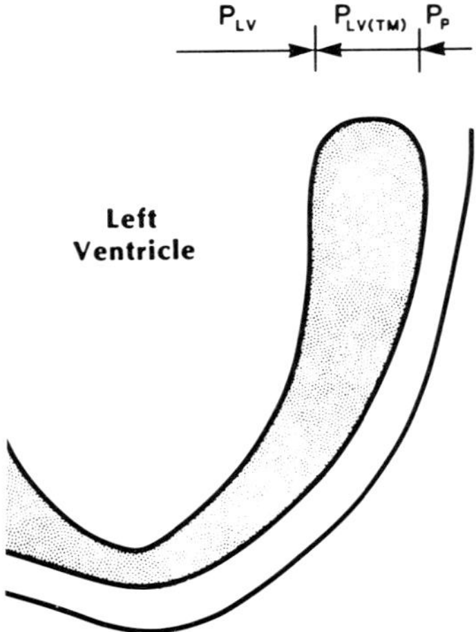

Figure 17-3. At end diastole, a static equilibrium exists at the endocardial surface of the left ventricular free wall. Intracavitary LV pressure (P_{LV} is exactly opposed by the sum of the transmural pressure the ventricular wall can sustain at this volume ($P_{LV(TM)}$ plus the force per unit area (i.e., the effective pericardial 'pressure') applied by the pericardium (Pp). This is the fundamental assumption for the series of investigations we have carried out.

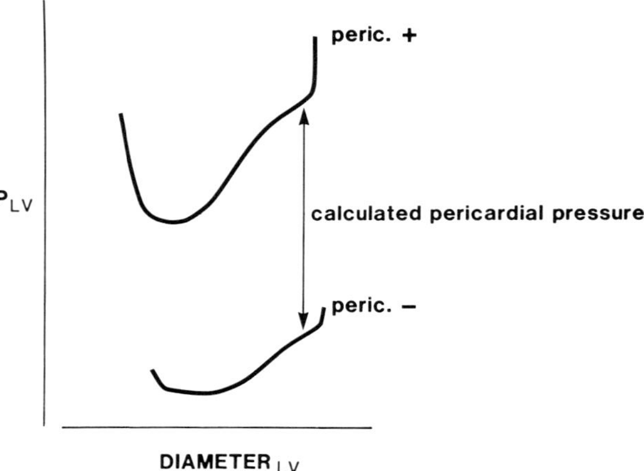

Figure 17-4. A schematic representation of the rationale used to determine effective pericardial 'pressure'. At end diastole it is assumed that there is no motion of the left ventricle so inertial and viscous forces can be ignored. Thus, when the pericardium is intact [upper pressure-diameter (volume) loop], the intracavitary pressure must be equal to the sum of the transmural pressure that the ventricular wall is capable of sustaining at that volume and the effective 'pressure' that the pericardium exerts. The bottom loop indicates the directly measured transmural pressure, since this was recorded when the chest was open and the lungs held back. The difference between LV end diastolic pressure ('calculated pericardial pressure') must be the effective pericardial 'pressure'. This value was used as a gold standard against which to compare the balloon- and the open-catheter-measured pericardial pressures. From Smiseth et al. [11] with permission of the American Heart Association.

proved to be equal to the calculated pressure regardless of the volume of liquid in the pericardium; on the contrary, the pressure measured by the open catheter was zero when the pericardium was empty and was less than the calculated value until at least 30 ml had been added to the pericardium. Perhaps the contrast between the methods was shown even more clearly when we cut several small slits in the pericardium (see Fig. 17-5). Although calculated pressure decreased somewhat because of the experimental manipulation, the decrease was exactly matched by the fall in balloon pressure. However, pericardial pressure measured with the open catheter quickly fell to zero as the fluid escaped. Thus, according to the criterion developed from the rationale diagrammed in Fig. 17-3, the balloon correctly measured effective pericardial pressure regardless of the volume of fluid in the pericardium whereas the open catheter measurement is subject to serious inaccuracy unless the pericardium is tightly sealed and a modest effusion is present.

'Pericardial surface pressure'

Agostini and Mead [13, 14] developed the concept of surface pressure in their earlier, similar studies of pleural mechanics. They suggested that surface pressure is equal to the sum of liquid pressure plus 'deformational force', which for the pericardial situation is perhaps better termed compressive radial contact stress. Although this formulation is unsatisfactory to some because contact stress is vectorial and pressure is not (Pascal's Law), we will nonetheless apply this concept to our observations. We speculate that when the heart is dilated by expansion of the vascular blood volume and the sealed pericardium is still empty, radial contact stress increases and entirely accounts for the rise in surface pressure since liquid pressure remains negligible. When fluid is infused into the pericardium pericardial liquid pressure rises quickly from zero and approaches the value of surface pressure. Since the relationship between liquid pressure and contact stress is an additive, complementary one, we believe that contact stress would have fallen to zero had we measured it. This is intuitively correct as the heart is suspended increasingly freely by the expanding volume of liquid until finally all contact between the heart and the pericardial surface is lost.

Pericardiocentesis

We have shown that pericardial pressure (as measured by the balloon) is approximately equal to right ventricular diastolic or mean right atrial pressure under many conditions in dogs [15] or in patients [16]. However, previous investigators [17, 18] showed that mean right atrial pressure failed to correspond to pericardial pressure as measured through a catheter. Upon draining a pericardial effusion,

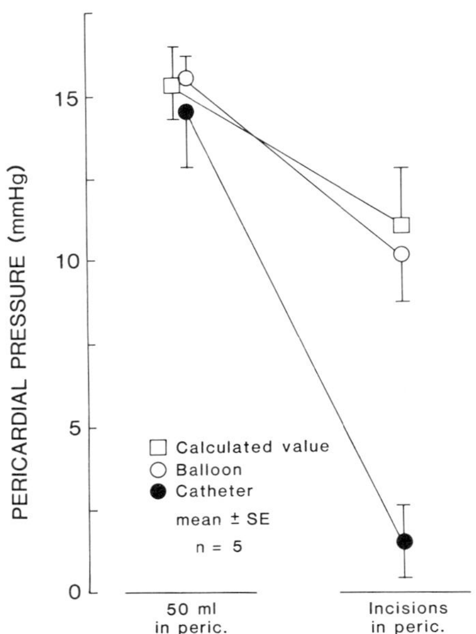

Figure 17-5. The pericardium effectively resists left ventricular filling even when several small incisions have been cut in it. Under these conditions an open catheter cannot measure the pericardial effect. On the left side the calculated pericardial pressure (see Fig. 17-4), the pressure measured with the pericardial balloon and the pressure measured with the open catheter are all equal since 50 ml of liquid had been infused into the pericardium. On the right side is shown the effect of making several small incisions in the pericardium. The pressure measured with the pericardial balloon remained equal to the calculated pressure but the fundamental inadequacy of the open-catheter measurement is obvious. From Smiseth et al. [11] with permission of the American Heart Association.

they showed that mean right atrial pressure plateaus while pericardial pressure as measured through the drainage catheter continued to fall toward zero. They [17, 18] also observed that cardiac output increased only until pericardial (catheter) pressure fell below right atrial pressure. We [19] repeated part of their observations in patients and constructed a parallel experiment in dogs (see Fig. 17-6). In this experiment (Fig. 17-6, bottom panel) although pericardial pressure measured with the open catheter fell toward zero as is observed in patients, pericardial pressure measured with the balloon remained high and exactly equal to right ventricular diastolic pressure.

These observations lead to the hypothesis diagrammed in Fig. 17-7. Characteristically, in the presence of a large pericardial effusion, pressures in all four chambers of the heart are equal during diastole and equal to pericardial pressure. As the fluid is drained, LV end diastolic pressure decreases somewhat but RV diastolic (and right atrial) and pericardial pressure fall more and remain equal. Thus, during this interval LV transmural end diastolic pressure increases which stretches the ventricle and increases cardiac output by the Frank-Starling mecha-

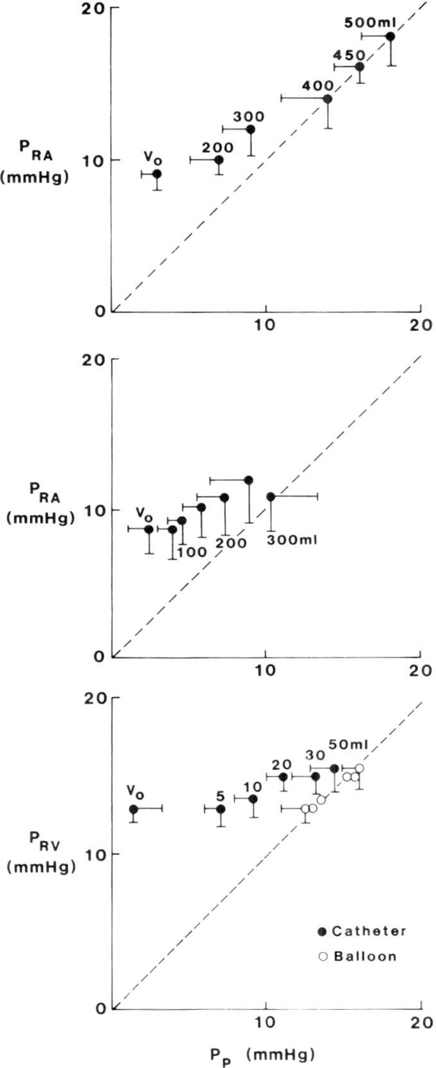

Figure 17-6. The relation of right ventricular filling pressure to pericardial pressure during pericardio-centesis. In the top panel data from Grose et al. [18] are plotted. As the pericardium was progressively drained (numbers refer to ml in excess of minimal volume), right atrial and pericardial pressure measured through the drainage catheter were initially equal and declined together. However, after an average of 100 ml had been removed, pericardial pressure continued to decrease while right atrial pressure tended to stabilize. The middle panel shows the confirming result of our smaller clinical study. The bottom panel shows the results of the study in dogs. When pressure was measured with an open catheter, results qualitatively identical to the clinical observations were seen. However, when the pressure measured with the pericardial balloon was plotted, the identity between right ventricular filling pressure and pericardial (balloon) pressure was maintained. This again suggests that an open catheter measures the effect of the pericardium only when considerable volume is contained. From Smiseth et al. [19] with permission of the publisher.

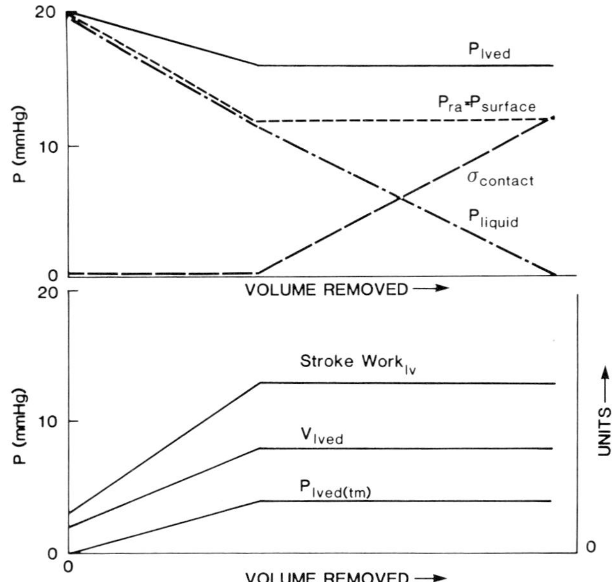

Figure 17-7. A hypothesis to explain the correspondence of the plateau in cardiac output [17, 18] with the divergence between the right atrial pressure and the pericardial pressure measured with an open catheter (see Fig. 17-6). At the beginning before any fluid is withdrawn, diastolic intracardiac and pericardial pressures are equal, LV end diastolic volume is small and cardiac output is low. As some fluid is removed right atrial and pericardial pressures remain equal but decrease faster than LV end diastolic pressure. This increase in LV transmural pressure increases end diastolic volume and thereby cardiac output (via the Frank-Starling mechanism). However, at the point that right atrial pressure and pericardial pressure diverge, transmural LV end diastolic pressure increases no further [if right atrial pressure is equal to the effective pericardial pressure as measured by the balloon (Psurface)]. Therefore, LV end diastolic volume remains constant as does cardiac output. Note that if the pericardial pressure measured with the catheter had been the true measure of pericardial constraint, LV end diastolic transmural pressure, end diastolic volume and cardiac output all should have continued to increase. This hypothesis requires experimental verification. (σcontact represents radial contact stress which may be proportional to the difference between the pericardial pressures measured with the balloon and the open catheter).

nism. As more fluid is withdrawn, right atrial pressure plateaus but pericardial (catheter) pressure continues to fall. If pericardial pressure (as measured by the catheter) accurately represents the effective pressure on the outside of the left ventricle, preload (i.e. transmural diastolic pressure) should continue to increase and one might expect a continued increase in cardiac output. Thus, the fact that cardiac output and right atrial pressure apparently plateau at the same point suggests that right atrial pressure (which, as we have shown, is usually approximately equal to pericardial pressure recorded with the balloon [15, 16]) is a better measure of effective pericardial pressure than the pressure measured by the open catheter. These speculations regarding the plateau in cardiac output (stroke work) require experimental verification.

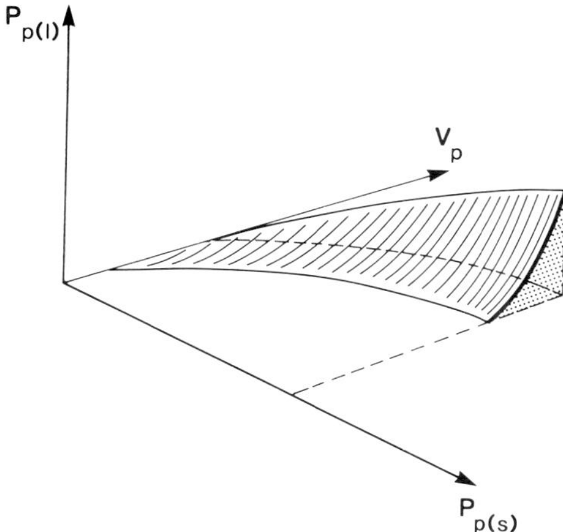

Figure 17-8. Hypothetical relationships among the pericardial pressure measured with an open catheter [Pp (1), pericardial liquid pressure], the pressure measured with a balloon [Pp (s), pericardial 'surface pressure'], and the volume of the pericardium. When the heart is dilated acutely and the pericardium is empty, balloon pressure increases with a negligible increase in the pressure measured with an open catheter (note solid line on the bottom of the curved surface). Regardless of the size of the heart, as fluid is infused the catheter-measured pressure increases until it equals the balloon-measured pressure (to be visualized as a vertical progression up the curved surface). Further infusion would result in equal increases in both pressures and an increase in total pericardial volume (see solid lines on top of the surface which has a slope of 45° in the pressure-pressure plane). These relationships require experimental verification.

Regional pericardial surface pressure

Recently, in an attempt to demonstrate the possibility that balloon-measured pericardial pressure could be different at different locations on the epicardial surface, we examined the effects of acute constrictions of the aorta and of the main pulmonary artery [20]. Such differences have also recently been found by others [21]. In these experiments the pericardium was only loosely approximated after instrumentation and an open catheter would, presumably, have recorded zero pressure. Aortic constriction raised the pericardial pressures recorded by balloons placed over the right and left ventricular free walls but the pressure measured over the left ventricle increased more. The results with pulmonary artery constriction were even more dramatic. As peak systolic right ventricular pressure was rapidly increased to 70–80 mm Hg, pericardial pressure over the right ventricle increased sharply but the pressure measured by the left ventricular balloon actually decreased. This demonstrates that balloon-measured pressures can be importantly different, at least with these relatively extreme, acute interventions, although the physiological importance of these observations remains to be explored.

Pericardial P-V relationships

Various experimental observations suggest that the relationship between the pericardial pressure measured with a balloon and pericardial volume may be more simple and regular than one might suppose (see Fig. 17-8). The study described above shows that in a pericardium that contains no liquid, an open catheter will record negligible pressure, even when expansion of the heart causes pressure measured with a balloon to rise [11].

When the heart is dilated and the pericardial pressure measured by a balloon is high, the pressure measured by the catheter infusion of liquid into the sealed pericardium causes increase until it becomes equal to the balloon pressure [11]. Presumably, if the infusion were continued, both catheter- and balloon-measured pressures would increase further and remain equal as suggested by the pericardiocentesis experience. Thus, it may be that all possible combinations of catheter pressure, balloon pressure and pericardial volume can be represented by a curved surface as illustrated in Fig. 17-8. Experiments are underway to test this hypothesis [22].

Conclusions

The pressure measured using the pericardial balloon seems to provide the best estimate of the pericardial constraint at any volume of pericardial liquid or even if the pericardium is completely empty.

Pericardial pressure as measured with an open catheter accurately measures the constraining effect exerted by the pericardium on the external surface of the heart only if a considerable amount of liquid is present (in our dogs, >30 ml).

When less that 30 ml of liquid is present or when the pericardium is unsealed the pericardium still restricts left ventricular diastolic filling by exerting a radially directed contact stress. It may be possible to measure this stress directly, depending on the development of appropriate methodology. When there is a small amount of liquid present, this stress may be proportional to the difference between the pressure measured with a balloon and the pressure measured with an open catheter.

Acknowledgements

This work was supported by grants from the Alberta Heart and Stroke Foundation and the Alberta Heritage Foundation for Medical Research of which Dr. Tyberg is a Medical Scientist.

References

1. Spodick, D.H.: The normal and diseased pericardium: Current concepts of pericardial physiology, diagnosis and treatment. J. Am. Coll. Cardiol. 1: 240–51, 1983.
2. Flessas, A.P., Connelly, G.P., Hands, S., Tilney, C.R., Kloster, C.K., Rimmer, P.H. Jr, Keefe, J.F., Klein, D.M. and Ryan, T.J.: Effects of isometric exercise on the end diastolic pressure, volumes, and function of the left ventricle in man. Circulation 53: 839–847, 1976.
3. Alderman, E.L. and Glantz, S.A.: Acute hemodynamic interventions shift the diastolic pressure-volume curve in man. Circulation 54: 662–671, 1976.
4. Ludbrook, P.A., Byrne, J.D., Kurnick, M.S. and McKnight, R.C.: Influence of reduction of preload and afterload by nitroglycerin on left ventricular diastolic pressure-volume relations and relaxation in man. Circulation 56: 937–943, 1977.
5. Dwyer, E.M., Jr.: Left ventricular pressure-volume alterations and regional disorders of contraction during myocardial ischemia induced by atrial pacing. Circulation 42: 1111–1122, 1970.
6. McLaurin, L.P., Rolett, E. and Grossman, W.: Impaired left ventricular relaxation during pacing-induced ischemia. Am. J. Cardiol. 32: 751–757, 1973.
7. Barry, W.H., Brooker, J.Z., Alderman, E.L. and Harrison, D.C.: Changes in diastolic stiffness and tone of the left ventricle during angina pectoris. Circulation 49: 255–263, 1974.
8. Serizawa, T., Carabello, B.A. and Grossman, W.: Effect of pacing-induced ischemia on left ventricular diastolic pressure-volume relations in dogs with coronary stenoses. Circ. Res. 46: 430–439, 1980.
9. Tyberg, J.V., Misbach, G.A., Glantz, S.A., Moores, W.Y. and Parmley, W.W.: A mechanism for shifts in the diastolic, left ventricular pressure-volume curve: The role of the pericardium. Eur. J. Cardiol. 7 (Suppl.): 163–175, 1978.
10. Tyberg, J.V., Misbach, G.A., Parmley, W.W. and Glantz, S.A.: Effects of the pericardium on ventricular performance. In Cardiac Dynamics, Ed. Baan J, Yellin EL, Arntzenius AC. Martinus Nijhoff, The Hague, Boston, 1980, pp 159–168.
11. Smiseth, O.A., Frais, M.A., Kingma, I., Smith, E.R. and Tyberg, J.V.: Assessment of pericardial constraint in dogs. Circulation 71: 158–164, 1985.
12. Holt, J.P., Rhode, E.A. and Kines, H: Pericardial and ventricular pressure. Circ. Res. 8: 1171–1181, 1960.
13. Agostoni, E.: Mechanics of the pleural space. eds. Fishman AP, Macklem, P.T., Mead, J. and Geiger, S.R.: In Handbook of Physiology. Section 3, The Respiratory System. Washington, D.C. American Physiological Society, Bethesda, 1986, Vol. III, pp. 531–559.
14. Agostoni, E.: Mechanics of the pleural space. Physiol Rev 52: 57–128, 1972.
15. Smiseth, O.A., Refsum, H. and Tyberg, J.V.: Pericardial pressure assessed by right atrial pressure: A basis for calculation of left ventricular transmural pressure. Am Heart J 108: 603–605, 1984.
16. Tyberg, J.V., Taichman, G.C., Smith, E.R., Douglas, N.W.S., Smiseth, O.A. and Keon, W.J.: The relation between pericardial pressure and right atrial pressure: An intraoperative study. Circulation 73: 428–432, 1986.
17. Reddy, P.S., Curtiss, E.I., O'Toole, J.D. and Shaver, J.A.: Cardiac tamponade: Hemodynamic observations in man. Circulation 58: 265–272, 1978.
18. Grose, R., Greenberg, M., Steingart, R. and Cohen, M.V.: Left ventricular volume and function during relief of cardiac tamponade in man. Circulation 66: 149–155, 1982.
19. Smiseth, O.A., Frais, M.A., Kingma, I., White, A.V.M., Knudtson, M.L., Cohen, J.M., Manyari, D.E., Smith, E.R. and Tyberg, J.V.: Assessment of pericardial constraint: The relation between right ventricular filling pressure and pericardial pressure measured after pericardiocentesis. J. Am. Coll. Cardiol. 7: 307–314, 1986.
20. Smiseth O.A., Scott-Douglas, N.W., Smith, E.R. and Tyberg, J.V.: Non-uniformity of pericardial surface pressure in dogs. Circulation (In press).

21. Hoit, B., Lew, W. and LeWinter, M.: Regional variation in pericardial contact pressure. J. Am. Coll. Cardiol. 7: 205A, 1986 (Abstract).
22. Scott-Douglas, N.W, Thompson, C., Bergman, D., Hamilton, D., Dani, R., Smith, E. and Tyberg, J.V.: Effects of heart size on the pericardial (liquid) pressure-volume relation. Clin. Invest. Med. 9 (Suppl B): 13–44, 1986. (Abstract).
23. Shabetai, R.: The Pericardium. Grune and Stratton, New York, 1981, p 63.

18. The mechanical effects of the pericardium on the left ventricle

EDWARD L. YELLIN

Introduction

Before discussing John Tyberg's presentation on measuring pericardial constraint, I would like to first describe work from my laboratory on right and left ventricular filling patterns during cardiac tamponade – the ultimate in pericardial constraint.

The growing use of high-tech, non-invasive methods to study ventricular filling (e.g. radionuclide ventriculography and ultrasonography) and the concomitant ambiguities and potential errors in these methods make it particularly important to also study filling dynamics using highly invasive but highly accurate methods in the animal laboratory. Intracardiac electromagnetic flowmetry and micromanometer pressure measurement is the approach used in our lab.

Methods

Large mongrel dogs (25 kg) were given fentanyl (10 mcg/kg) and vecuronium (2 mg), artificially ventilated and placed on cardiopulmonary bypass. An electromagnetic flow probe (Carolina Medical Electronics) was implanted above the mitral valve (5 dogs) or the tricuspid valve (5 dogs). Micromanometers (Millar) were placed in all four cardiac chambers. A large bore catheter was introduced into the pericardial space for infusion of warm saline and positioned at the left ventricular posterior wall. The pericardium was sutured closed using dacron strips to reinforce the suture line and to minimize the overlap of pericardial tissue.

Oscillographic records were taken at slow speed on a pen recorder (Gould 2600) and at high speed, high gain, on a photographic recorder (Electronics for Medicine DR-12). The records were manually digitized with a sonic digitizer (Science Accessories) coupled to a microcomputer (IBM-XT).

208

Results and discussion

Figure 18-1 illustrates a typical response to an infusion of 120 ml of warmed saline into the pericardial space. As expected, tricuspid flow decreased (as did mitral flow, not shown), right and left ventricular diastolic pressures increased and systolic pressures decreased. The changes in phasic filling patterns of both ventricles are shown in the next two figures.

The changes in right ventricular filling patterns after cardiac tamponade are shown in Fig. 18-2. The rate of rise of tricuspid flow, the peak flow rate, and the atrial booster function are all depressed, leading to a severe decrease in filling volume, and, of course, to right and left side output. (The quality of the right heart pressure tracings after tamponade was poor and only the control pressures are shown.)

Figure 18-3 illustrates a typical response to tamponade of the left heart. It is similar to the right side response: flow acceleration, peak flow rate, and atrial pump function are all depressed leading to a decrease in filling volume and in stroke volume. Note particularly that after tamponade there is a large increase in the absolute values of the pressures in the left atrium and ventricle during diastole. But because the increase in left atrial pressure was not as much as the increase in left ventricular diastolic pressure, the normal atrioventricular pressure gradient was not maintained and transmitral flow decreased. On occasion, we also found the ST segment elevation seen in Fig. 18-3 due, presumably, to a reduction in coronary flow at large radial stresses. Blood volume expansion tended to restore atrial pressures and to increase filling volumes, but during severe tamponade cardiac output remained well below control. Similarly, attempts to decrease heart volume and improve filling with infusions of dopamine were only partially successful.

In summary, severe cardiac tamponade leads to severe pericardial constraint thereby influencing the factors that determine filling: rate of left ventricular relaxation, left ventricular diastolic pressure, and left atrial diastolic pressure. We are all aware of the importance of maintaining a low left ventricular diastolic pressure; it keeps the left atrial pressure low, preventing pulmonary congestion, and it allows the ventricle to operate on the more compliant part of its pressure-volume relation – again, to keep the left atrial pressure low. It is clear from the force balance described by John Tyberg that a low intrapericardial pressure is required to maintain a low left ventricular diastolic pressure. The method of measuring that pressure, as well as the concepts underlying the method, was the main subject of John Tyberg's presentation.

Offering a critical evaluation of John Tyberg's outstanding work on pericardial contraint is somewhat like piping oil to Alberta and makes me uncomfortable. Furthermore, I have had little personal involvement in the measurement of intrapericardial pressure, and frankly, I am not comfortable dealing with concepts, assumptions, data, and conclusions, that are not a part of my own labora-

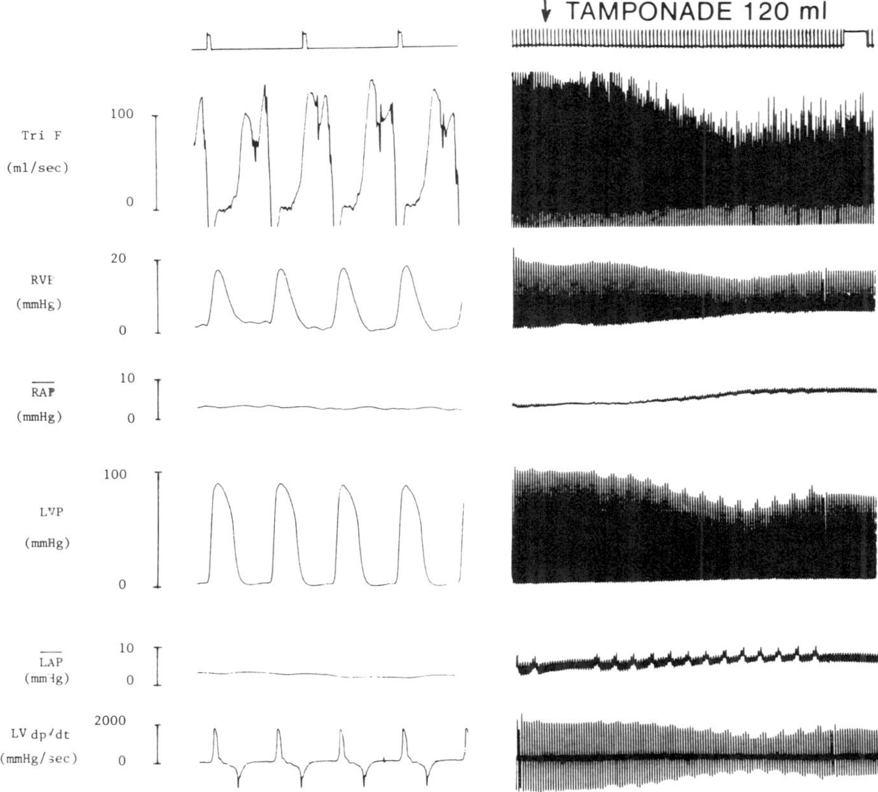

Figure 18-1. Oscillographic demonstration of the effects of severe cardiac tamponade on right heart filling. Heart rate = 90/min. Tri F = tricuspid flow; RVP = right ventricular pressure; RAP = mean right atrial pressure; LVP = left ventricular pressure; LAP = mean left atrial pressure; LVdP/dt = derivative of LVP. Time marks are one/sec.

tory experience. Nevertheless, I am more uncomfortable with John's analysis of pericardial contraint based on the concepts of liquid (or hydrostatic) pressure, and surface (or contact) pressure. I am therefore using this opportunity to provoke discussion of this most important subject.

I agree with John that the radial stress acting on the epicardial surface of the heart is the sum of a liquid pressure and any local deformational stress, due to a contact pressure. I also agree that there is so little fluid in the normal pericardial space that using a multihole, fluid-filled catheter to measure pressure is fraught with danger. Finally, I accept the data comparing the multihole catheter measurements with the flat balloon and I conclude that at the very large cardiac volumes and the small amount of pericardial effusion of Smiseth's experiment (see Fig. 17-5 and ref. [11]) the flat balloon is indeed superior to the catheter. My concern is with extending these conclusions to the measurement of local differences in

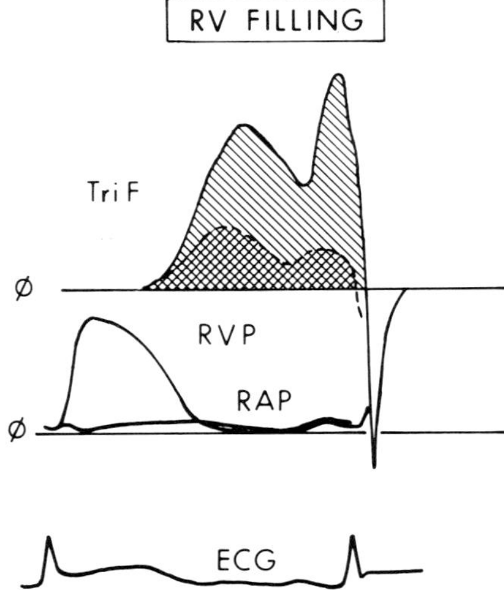

Figure 18-2. High speed oscillographic record illustrating the effects of tamponade on right ventricular filling dynamics. The lightly shaded area of tricuspid flow is control and the dark area is post tamponade. (The post tamponade pressures are not shown.) The large increase in flow due to the atrial contraction is typical of tricuspid flow and shows large variations with respiration. This record was taken at the height of increased venous return.

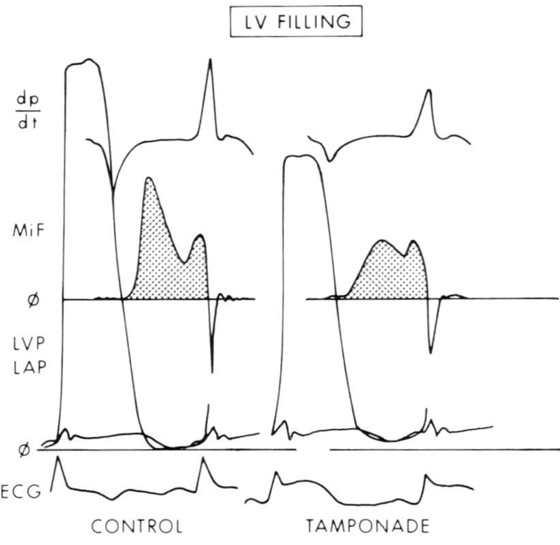

Figure 18-3. High speed oscillographic records illustrating the effects of tamponade on left ventricular filling patterns. The mitral flow patterns (MiF) are shaded for clarity.

intrapericardial pressure by the use of the balloon.

The knee joint analogy advanced by John to justify the significance of contact stress is misleading. The solid structures of the knee undergo such small deformations that they do not transmit the stress to the surrounding fluid. The pericardium, on the other hand, is highly deformable and able to transmit stresses to the fluid medium. Furthermore, it is not likely that the surface of the heart will produce large local deformations. Until we follow Jim Covell's suggestion that lubrication theory may have the answer to the study and measurement of intrapericardial constraint, I am concerned that even with the flat balloon, we may be looking at artifacts introduced by the balloon. This is particularly true with the intact beating heart; perhaps the dynamic effects of cardiac motion within the pericardial sac are amplified by the balloon and produce what appear to be local differences in surface pressure. I think further studies are in order and we should proceed with caution in measuring pericardial pressure, particularly in the normal situation where there is very little fluid in the intrapericardial space.

General discussion on pericardial mechanics

The quantitative description of the mechanical interaction between the heart and the pericardium is still very incomplete and present attempts to provide a conceptual framework for experimental observations may prove to be incorrect. It is useful to emphasize the observations about which agreement seems possible: first, fluid pressure is an adequate measure of the mechanical effect of the pericardium when an excess of liquid is present and, second, the pressure within a Holt-type balloon correctly measures (assuming the rationale described above) the mechanical effect of the pericardium when it is empty as well as when a variable amount of liquid is present. When the pericardium contains an intermediate amount of liquid (e.g., 5 ml in Smiseth's experimental animals) the situation is less clear. Then the mechanical effect of the pericardium cannot be measured with an open catheter. Agostoni suggested that under these conditions there are 'deformational forces' in addition to fluid pressure. While the nature of the forces is not yet understood, they may be clarified with the development of small transducers that measure radial stress directly and are unresponsive to changes in pressure in the fluid medium. While a rigorous physical analysis of the problem is not yet available there may be some agreement with a further simple statement. The pericardium develops an inwardly-directed radial stress which, when the pericardium contains an excess of liquid, is equal to pericardial pressure. The left ventricle also develops an outwardly directed radial stress of the same magnitude. When the pericardium is empty of fluid, the opposing stresses developed in the pericardium and the LV are still equal and opposite but it may be impossible to measure true pressure between the surfaces. At this time the pressure elsewhere in the pericardial cavity may be less than the value of the opposing stresses between the heart and pericardium.

19. Role of a changing venous capacitance in cardiovascular homeostasis

CLIVE V. GREENWAY

Introduction

This chapter summarizes studies on the role of the splanchnic venous system in overall cardiovascular homeostasis, with emphasis on work carried out in the author's laboratory. Several recent reviews present more complete and balanced accounts of this field [1, 2, 3, 4].

Hepatic sympathetic venoconstriction

Stimulation of the sympathetic nerves to the liver causes up to a 50% reduction in hepatic blood volume [5]. This response is illustrated in Fig. 19-1 and has been confirmed many times in cats and dogs [6, 7, 8, 9]. In cats there is little change in hepatic blood flow and, since intrahepatic pressure increases, this response must be an active contraction of the capacitance vessels [10]. Activation of these hepatic nerves seems to be the major mechanism which can produce a large venous response in the liver. Norepinephrine and epinephrine infusions can produce hepatic venoconstriction, [11] but endogenous levels of these catecholamines do not normally increase sufficiently to constrict the hepatic venous bed [12]. Angiotensin can produce hepatic venoconstriction [11] and in cats, the hepatic venoconstriction seen after administration of nifedipine appears to be mediated by endogenous angiotensin [13]. Beta-adrenergic agonists such as isoproterenol can also cause venoconstriction in cats mediated by an indirect but as yet unknown mechanism [14]. However, the importance of these humoral mechanisms is not yet clear and activation of the hepatic nerves appears to be the major physiological mechanism for hepatic venoconstriction.

This sympathetic response is unusual in that it is mediated through innervated adrenoceptors of the alpha-2 subtype in cats [15]. The response is produced by alpha methylnorepinephrine but not by phenylephrine and is blocked by yohimbine but not by prazosin. These data do not support the hypothesis that only

214

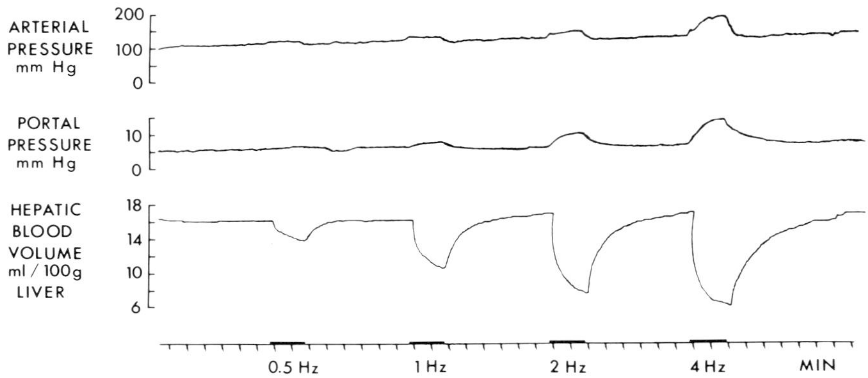

Figure 19-1. Responses to stimulation of the hepatic nerves in a representative cat anesthetized with pentobarbital. (Reproduced with permission from ref. 41).

alpha-1 adrenoceptors are innervated, but do support the concept that while innervated alpha-1 adrenoceptors predominate on the arterial side, innervated alpha-2 adrenoceptors predominate on the venous side of the circulation [16]. Thus alpha-2 adrenoceptors may play an important role in postural and other venous mechanisms.

Role of splanchnic bed as blood volume reserve

In 1974 we suggested that the splanchnic bed represented a major, if not the only, venous reservoir in the body [17]. Subsequent work has supported this conclusion. Recent studies [18], and reviews [2, 3, 4], have suggested that the venous system in skeletal muscle may be less responsive to sympathetic nerve stimulation than originally suggested by Mellander in 1960 [19]. Blood volume changes in muscle may be passive consequences of changes in flow and venous pressure. Also the lungs may be a smaller reservoir than we estimated ten years ago [20, 21]. Table 1 updates our previous estimates of the distribution of the blood volume and of the proportions which can be mobilised by maximal stimulation of the sympathetic nerves. The extensive publications on which this revised table is based are cited in a review to be published shortly [2]. Thus the splanchnic bed, including the liver, is an important venous reservoir which can be mobilized by the central nervous system.

Mechanism of hepatic venoconstriction

Blood volume within an organ is partly determined by the product of transmural pressure and vascular compliance. This is the stressed volume. Compliance appears to be relatively constant over the physiological range and volume/ pressure relationships in the liver are linear [22, 10]. However, capacitance, or total organ blood volume at a particular pressure, exceeds the stressed volume and extrapolation of this linear volume/pressure relationship results in an apparent volume intercept at zero pressure. This is the unstressed volume [23, 2, 3, 4, 24, 25]. One difficulty in studies on the venous system is measurement of transmural pressure within the capacitance vessels. Accurate measurement of this pressure is essential to separate passive changes in blood volume secondary to transmural pressure changes, from active changes in blood volume due to contraction or relaxation of the vessel walls.

Measurement of this pressure is easier in the hepatic venous bed than in any other organ because the hepatic venular pressure is closely similar to portal pressure. The major sites of resistance in the liver are the hepatic arterioles and the post-sinusoidal hepatic veins. Pressure within the capacitance vessels of the liver is close to, and usually not significantly different from portal pressure. It can be measured either by a catheter in the portal vein or by one within a hepatic vein proximal to the resistance site [2, 26, 10, 27, 28]. Since intrahepatic pressure increases while hepatic blood volume decreases during hepatic nerve stimulation (Fig. 19-1) or infusion of norepinephrine, these changes in blood volume must result from an active contraction of intrahepatic vessels.

The decrease in hepatic blood volume produced by hepatic nerve stimulation

Table 19-1. Regional distribution of blood volume and mobilization by sympathetic nerve stimulation (reproduced from ref. 16).

Organ	Blood volume		% Total blood volume mobilized by symp.
	% Body weight	% Total blood volume	
Splanchnic bed	9.5	33	21
Liver[1]	2.5	12	6
Spleen	1	14	12
Intestine	6	7	3
Skeletal muscle[2]	45	17	5
Adipose tissue[2]	14	9	3
Skin[3]	3	2	1
Lungs	1.5	10	1
Heart chambers	5		
Kidneys	0.5	1	
Rest	26.5	23	
100	100	31	

[1] Parenchymal tissue excluding residual blood and bile.
[2] Mobilization may be entirely passive secondary to flow change.
[3] Involved in temperature regulation.

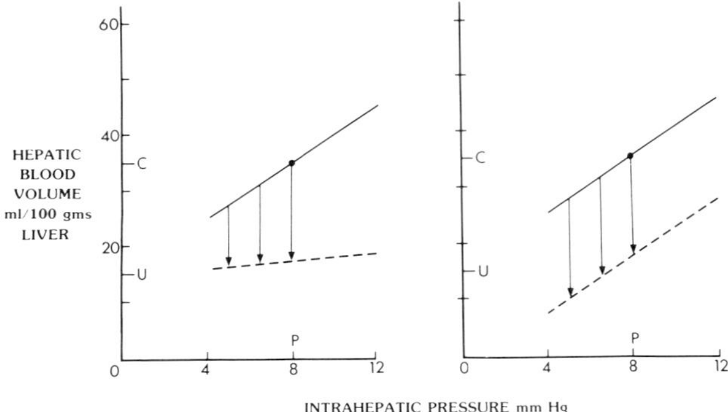

Figure 19-2. The pressure-volume relationship in the hepatic venous bed (solid line). Hepatic blood volume or capacitance (C) at a normal portal pressure is made up of the unstressed volume (U) plus the stressed volume. The slope of the relationship (solid line) is the compliance. The transmural pressure (P) is determined by the stressed volume and the compliance. Venoconstriction shown by the arrows could result from a change in compliance with no change in unstressed volume (dotted line left panel), a change in unstressed volume with no change in compliance (dotted line right panel), or a combination of changes in both compliance and unstressed volume. (Reproduced from ref. [23]).

or infusion of norepinephrine could be due to a decrease in venous compliance or to a decrease in unstressed volume. These possibilities are illustrated in Fig. 2 and were discussed recently [27, 10]. If venoconstriction occurred by a decrease in compliance (left panel in Fig. 19-2), the distention of the capacitance vessels caused by the intravascular transmural pressure would be reduced. The stressed volume, the product of compliance and pressure, would be less at each pressure. However the effect of hepatic nerve stimulation would decrease as transmural pressure decreased and the active response would be smallest in those situations where it would be most beneficial for survival, for example, when pressure decreased after hemorrhage. In contrast, contraction of the hepatic venous system might occur by a parallel downward shift in the volume/pressure relationship (right panel in Fig. 19-2). In this case, the volume of blood mobilized by the hepatic nerves would be independent of pressure and, after a hemorrhage, the active response and the passive response to reduction in intravascular pressure would be additive. This mechanism would have the greatest survival value. We can express this parallel shift in the curve as a change in unstressed volume – the apparent blood volume which the liver contains when intravascular pressure is extrapolated to zero.

Figure 19-3 shows measurements of volume/pressure relationships in the livers of anesthetized cats before, during and after infusions of norepinephrine [10]. In the left panel, intrahepatic pressure was varied by changing blood flow, while in the right panel it was varied by changing inferior vena caval pressure. Both sets of curves are very similar and norepinephrine clearly produced a change in unstressed volume with no significant change in vascular compliance. If these data

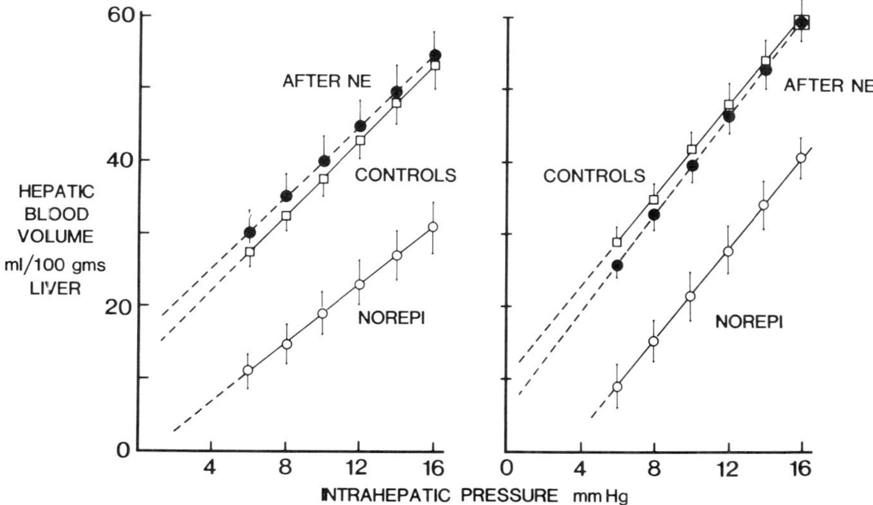

Figure 19-3. Relationships between hepatic blood volume and intrahepatic pressure before (CONTROLS), during (NOREPI) and after infusion of norepinephrine (AFTER NE), determined by varying portal flow (left panel) or by varying outflow pressure (right panel). Values are means ± S.E. n = 9 cats. (Reproduced with permission from ref. [10]).

can be extrapolated to other stimuli, other vascular beds and other species, then venoconstriction is brought about by CONVERSION OF UNSTRESSED VOLUME TO STRESSED VOLUME [23]. In the control situation, the hepatic blood volume is about 50% stressed volume and 50% unstressed volume and the unstressed volume represents a blood volume reserve which can be mobilised by the hepatic nerves or norepinephrine infusions.

The unstressed volume which is mobilized from the splanchnic bed is converted to stressed volume which will then be distributed elsewhere in the circulation in accordance with the pressures and vascular compliances in the different parts. Prediction of the resulting changes is complex but can be approximated using a computer program of the type described previously [27] and recently updated to incorporate the concepts described here [23].

Thus we can form a working hypothesis on the function of the venous system, illustrated in Fig. 19-4. Venoconstriction converts unstressed volume to stressed volume, this increases the pressure-gradient for venous return and increases cardiac preload. This may or may not change cardiac output depending on interaction with the other factors which control cardiac output [30, 23]. At rest total stressed volume is approximately 40% of total blood volume (see below). This is the 'effective blood volume' which determines vascular pressures and flows. The unstressed volume is 60% of the total of which about half is required to fill pipes and chambers while the remaining half forms a blood volume reserve

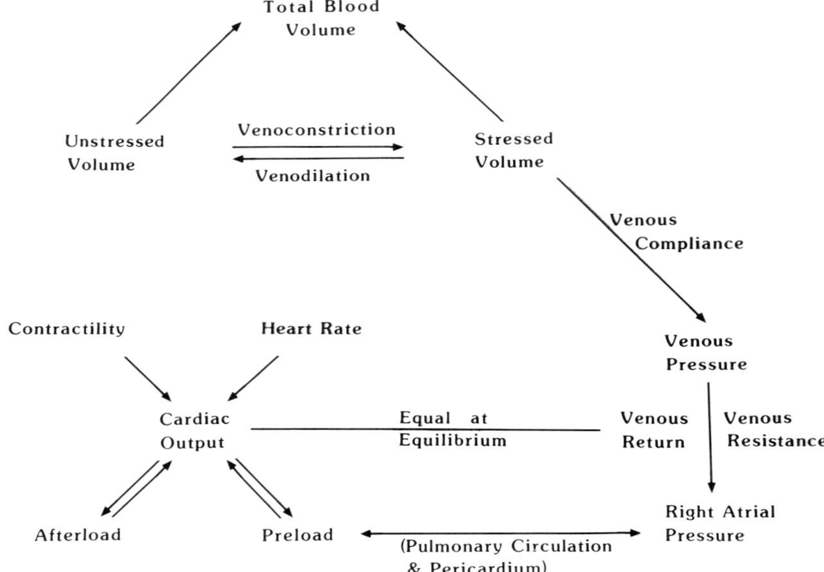

Figure 19-4. Simplified summary diagram of the relationships between blood volume and cardiac output. (Reproduced from ref. [23]).

which can be mobilized and converted to stressed volume by the CNS or by drugs [23, 2].

Other approaches to the venous system

These studies in the liver fit together quite well with other types of studies on the venous sytem reviewed recently by Rothe [3, 4]. In the preparation used by Shoukas and Sagawa and their colleagues [31, 32, 24, 25] cardiac output is held constant by a pump while venous return flows into an extracorporeal reservoir. In this preparation, changes in reservoir volume reflect the changes in the animal's blood volume required to hold the cardiac output at a predetermined level. If cardiac output is held constant, venoconstriction appears as a displacement of blood volume from the animal into the reservoir. By raising venous outflow pressure and noting the decrease in reservoir volume, an estimate of whole body vascular compliance can be obtained. The studies cited indicated that in this preparation, stressed volume was some 30% of the total blood volume. This is probably an underestimate since the rise in venous outflow pressure is not fully transmitted to the splanchnic bed [22, 2, 10, 5] and compliance is therefore underestimated. In this preparation, the venoconstriction induced in dogs by reduction in arterial baroreceptor activity diverted blood to the reservoir with only a small change in total vascular compliance. Thus, the baroreceptor reflex moved unstressed volume from the animal to the reservoir.

If the reservoir had not been present, the unstressed volume mobilised by the venoconstriction would have been converted to stressed volume in the animal raising pressure in the venous system. Other workers, following the classical work of Guyton and his colleagues, have examined this effect by measuring mean circulatory pressure – the instantaneous equilibrium pressure in the circulation when cardiac output is suddenly stopped. Mean circulatory pressure equals stressed volume divided by whole body vascular compliance, and it increases when stressed volume increases [3, 4].

Although these and other approaches have yielded a large body of interesting data [33, 34, 35, 36, 3, 4, 37], precise measurement of volume/pressure relationships have not yet been made. The data appear compatible with the hypotheses presented here but were often interpreted in other ways by the authors. The basic concept of the relation between stressed and unstressed volumes needs further validation in other organs, in other species and under a variety of different conditions.

Reflex control of vascular capacitance

The reflex systems which activate and control the sympathetic innervation of the capacitance vessels need to be clarified. In anesthetized cats, we have made several unsuccessful attempts to demonstrate reflex control of the hepatic venous bed [1]. In anesthetized dogs, a variety of studies (reviewed by Dr. Carl Rothe [3]) have demonstrated reflex control of the venous system. Afferent mechanisms include the arterial baroreceptors, chemoreceptors and cardiopulmonary receptors. The overall role of the venous system in cardiovascular reflexes is controversial [3, 38]. There is a large body of circumstantial evidence in favour or reflex control of the venous system, and of the splanchnic and hepatic beds in particular [2], but definitive experiments are difficult to carry out. Many studies neglected measurements of pressure in the capacitance vessels and measurements of the effects of reflexes on volume/pressure relationships in individual organs have not yet been made. Baroreceptor and cardiopulmonary receptor reflexes appear to be inhibitory to sympathetic tone on the capacitance vessels but the central mechanisms responsible for this tone are unknown. It is not clear whether the central nervous system can produce selective venous responses independently from resistance responses. I believe the evidence is overwhelming that reflex mechanisms control the venous system and that this plays an important role in control of cardiac output, but much work remains to be done to clarify and quantitate these mechanisms in animals and especially in humans.

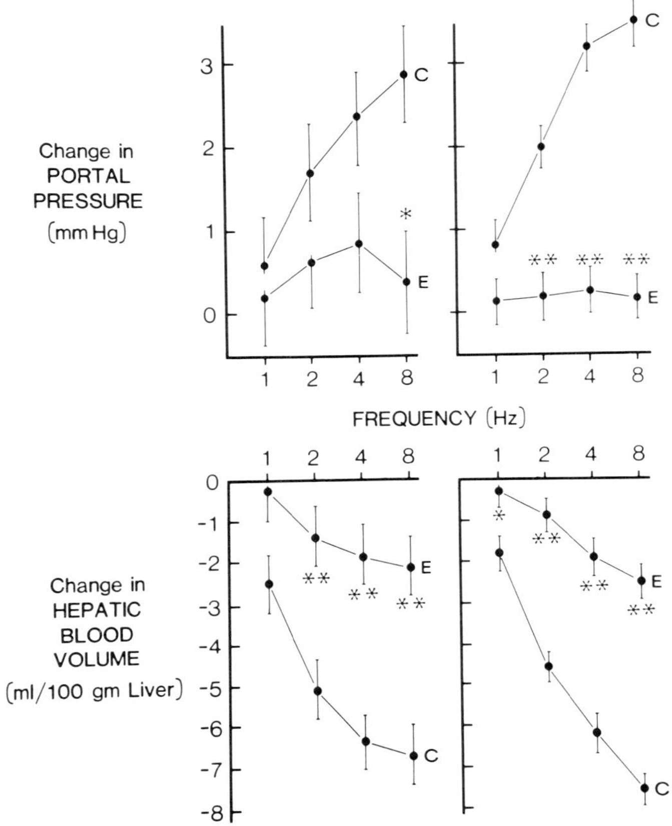

Figure 19-5. Changes in portal pressure and hepatic blood volume during hepatic nerve stimulation before (C) and 150 min after injection of endotoxin (E) in cats pretreated with indomethacin (left panel n = 4) and before (C) and 150 min after slow infusion of endotoxin (E) without indomethacin pretreatment (right panel n = 4). *P<0.05 **P<0.01 comparison of before and after endotoxin. (Reproduced from ref. [39]).

Effects of drugs on venous system and cardiac output

There are a number of pharmacological studies which suggest the importance of venous responses in control of cardiac output. 1. After endotoxin in anesthetized cats the hepatic venous responses to sympathetic nerve stimulation are rapidly and severely impaired. This is illustrated in Fig. 19-5. Responses to infused norepinephrine and angiotensin were also impaired. This type of impairment may play a role in the development of circulatory shock [39]. It seems possible that in this situation, unstressed volume increases leading to reduced stressed volume, preload and cardiac output even though total blood volume is unchanged. However volume/pressure relationships in the venous system during shock have not yet been studied. 2. Many drugs which cause postural hypotension during clinical use also impair the hepatic venous responses to sympathetic nerve stimulation. An example which we studied recently is bromocryptine [40]. We suggested that one mechanism which can cause postural (orthostatic) hypotension is failure of the splanchnic venous reserve to compensate for venous pooling in the lower limbs, but a definitive test of this hypothesis has not yet proved possible. 3. A variety of studies, reviewed in 1981 [29], led to the hypothesis that venoconstriction is an essential component of the actions of drugs which increase cardiac output. At that time, the volume/pressure relationships in the liver had not been clarified and this work assumed that venoconstriction involved a change in compliance which was calculated incorrectly as total organ blood volume divided by intrahepatic pressure [41, 27, 42]. Nevertheless the data still support our hypothesis. Cardiac stimulation alone produces only a modest increase in cardiac output accompanied by a marked decrease in preload and an increase in afterload [43, 44]. The potential increase in cardiac output is limited by the decrease in preload. Conversely, splanchnic nerve stimulation which produces splanchnic venoconstriction does not increase cardiac output in anesthetized cats, in spite of an increased preload because of the concomitant opposing increase in afterload [30]. Maximal sustained increases in cardiac output occur when cardiac stimulation is accompanied by venoconstriction and by arteriolar dilatation thus maintaining preload and preventing elevation of afterload [29]. This is exemplified by epinephrine and isoproterenol [33, 41, 29, 42]. In a recent study, abolition of the indirect venoconstrictor action of nifedipine by removal of the kidneys also abolished the increase in cardiac output in anesthetized cats [13].

Vasodilator drugs used in treatment of heart failure can be classified into those with a predominant effect of increasing cardiac output, those with a balanced effect on cardiac output and pulmonary congestion, and those with a predominant effect of reducing pulmonary congestion. These differences can be explained on the basis of a venoconstrictor action, no action on the venous system, and a venodilator action for the three groups respectively [29, 2]. This is illustrated with examples in Table 19-2.

Thus there is evidence from pharmacological studies that venoconstriction is a prerequisite for large sustained increases in cardiac output. If this is true, then venoconstriction should also occur in muscular exercise and some circumstantial evidence suggests that this occurs [3]. However, with the exception of norepinephrine [10], the effects of drugs and of physiological procedures such as exercise on the volume/pressure relationships, on stressed and unstressed volumes, and on venous compliance have not yet been analysed.

Summary and conclusions

Stimulation of the hepatic sympathetic nerves reduces hepatic blood volume by up to 50%. Since intrahepatic pressure increases, this is an active contraction of the capacitance vessels and it is mediated by innervated alpha-2 adrenoceptors in cats. This response illustrates the role of the liver, which together with intestine and spleen, constitute the major blood volume reserve from which up to 20% of the total blood volume can be mobilised. The mechanism of this hepatic venoconstriction involves conversion of unstressed volume to stressed volume with no significant change in hepatic vascular compliance. Conversion of unstressed to stressed volume increases the pressure gradient for venous return and cardiac preload. This may or may not increase cardiac output depending on interactions with afterload, contractility and heart rate. Reflex control of the venous system appears to be important but measurements of the effects of reflexes on volume/pressure relationships have not yet been made in the splanchnic bed. Based on pharmacological studies, three hypotheses were presented: that loss of splanchnic venous responsiveness is important in development of endotoxin shock, that interference with splanchnic venoconstriction may be one cause of postural hypotension, and that venoconstriction is an essential prerequisite for large sustained increases in cardiac output. In conclusion, knowledge of the role of venous capacitance in cardiovascular homeostasis has been steadily increasing in recent years. Some hard data and many questions and ideas have been raised for discussion. Many of these questions are hard to answer until experiments can be

Table 19-2. Effects of arteriolar vasodilator drugs on the hepatic venous system, in relation to the observed clinical effects on cardiac output and pulmonary congestion during treatment of heart failure.

	Cardiac output	Pulmonary congestion
Group 1: Venoconstrictors		
a) Direct		
Epinephrine	Marked	Little
Dopamine	increase	change
b) Indirect		
Isoproterenol		
Hydralazine		
Group 2: No effect on veins		
Nitroprusside[1]	Modest	Modest
Diazoxide	increase	decrease
Prazosin		
Group 3: Venodilators		
Nitroglycerin	Little	Marked
Isosorbide	change	decrease

[1] Nitroprusside relaxes venous smooth muscle but tissue uptake is so great that concentrations reaching the capacitance vessels are probably insufficient to cause relaxation except at high doses [8, 9].

done in animals and man without anesthesia and with minimal surgical intervention, but new techniques, particularly blood pool imaging, are on the horizon. I look forward to many exciting new discoveries in this field over the next few years.

Acknowledgements

Work from my laboratory described in this chapter would not have been possible without the enthusiastic efforts of my graduate students and technicians or without the support of the Medical Research Council of Canada, the Manitoba Heart Foundation and the Canadian Liver Foundation. I am also very grateful for many vigorous and exciting discussions with colleagues, especially Drs. Carl Rothe and Wayne Lautt.

References

1. Greenway, C.V.: The role of the splanchnic venous system in overall cardiovascular homeostasis. Fed. Proc. 42: 1678–1684, 1983.
2. Greenway, C.V. and Lautt, W.W.: The hepatic vascular bed. In: Handbook of Physiology, Gastroenterology Section, Motility and Circulation, ed. by J.D. Wood. American Physiological Society, Washington (in press).
3. Rothe, C.F.: Reflex control of veins and vascular capacitance. Physiol. Rev. 63: 1281–1342, 1983.
4. Rothe, C.F.: Venous system: physiology of the capacitance vessels. In: Handbook of Physiology Section II Cardiovascular System, Vol. III Peripheral Circulation and Organ Blood Flow, edited by J.T. Shepherd and F.M. Abboud, American Physiological Society, Washington. Chapter 13 pp 397–452, 1983.
5. Greenway, C.V., Stark, R.D. and Lautt, W.W.: Capacitance responses and fluid exchange in the cat liver during stimulation of the hepatic nerves. Circ. Res. 25: 277–284, 1969.
6. Bennett, T.D., MacAnespie, C.L. and Rothe, C.F.: Active hepatic capacitance responses to neural and humoral stimuli in dogs. Am. J. Physiol. 242: H1000–H1009, 1982.
7. Brooksby, G.A. and Donald, D.E.: Dynamic changes in splanchnic blood flow and blood volume in dogs during activation of sympathetic nerves. Circ. Res. 29: 227–238, 1971.
8. Greenway, C.V. and Oshiro, G.: Comparison of the effects of hepatic nerve stimulation on arterial flow, distribution of arterial and portal flows and blood content in the livers of anaesthetized cats and dogs. J. Physiol. (London) 227: 487–501, 1972.
9. Karim, F. and Hainsworth, R.: Responses of abdominal vascular capacitance to stimulation of splanchnic nerves. Am. J. Physiol. 231: 434–440, 1976.
10. Greenway, C.V., Seaman, K. and Innes, I.R.: Norepinephrine on venous compliance and unstressed volume in the cat liver. Am. J. Physiol. 248: H468–476, 1985.
11. Greenway, C.V. and Lautt, W.W.: Effects of infusions of catecholamines, angiotensin, vasopressin and histamine on hepatic blood volume in the anaesthetized cat. Br. J. Pharmacol. 44: 177–184, 1972.
12. Greenway, C.V., Dettman, R., Burczynski, F. and Sitar, D.S.: Effects of circulating catecholamines on hepatic blood volume in anesthetized cats. Am. J. Physiol. 250: H992–H997, 1986.
13. Segstro, R., Seaman, K.L., Innes, I.R. and Greenway, C.V.: Effects of nifedipine on hepatic blood volume in cats: indirect venoconstriction and absence of inhibition of postsynaptic alpha-2

adrenoreceptor responses. Can. J. Physiol. Pharmacol. 64: 615–620, 1986.

14. Seaman, K. and Greenway, C.V.: Hepatic venoconstrictor effects of isoproterenol and nifedipine in anesthetized cats. Can. J. Physiol. Pharmacol. 62: 665–672, 1984.

15. Segstro, R. and Greenway, C.V.: Alpha adrenoceptor subtype mediating sympathetic mobilization of blood from the hepatic venous system in anesthetized cats. J. Pharmacol. Exp. Ther. 236: 224–229, 1986.

16. Ruffolo, R.R.: Distribution and function of peripheral alpha adrenoceptors in the cardiovascular system. Pharmacol. Biochem. Behav. 22: 827–833, 1985.

17. Greenway, C.V. and Lister, G.E.: Capacitance effects and blood reservoir function in the splanchnic vascular bed during non-hypotensive haemorrhage and blood volume expansion in anaesthetized cats. J. Physiol. (London) 237: 279–294, 1974.

18. Hainsworth, R., Karim, F., McGregor, K.H. and Wood, L.M.: Hind-limb vascular-capacitance responses in anaesthetized dogs. J. Physiol. (London) 337: 417–428, 1983.

19. Mellander, S.: Comparative studies on the adrenergic neuro-hormonal control of resistance and capacitance vessels in the cat. Acta. Physiol. Scand. 50: Suppl. 176, pp 1–86, 1960.

20. Thorvaldson, J., Ilebekk, A., Leraand, S. and Kiil, F.: Determinants of pulmonary blood volume. Effects of acute changes in pulmonary vascular pressures and flow. Acta Physiol. Scand. 121: 45–56, 1984.

21. Thorvaldson, J., Stokland, O., Molaug, M. and Ilebekk, A.: Cardiopulmonary blood volume during acute blood pressure elevations in dog. Acta Physiol. Scand. 122: 137–144, 1984.

22. Bennett, T.D. and Rothe, C.F.: Hepatic capacitance responses to changes in flow and hepatic venous pressure in dogs. Am. J. Physiol. 240: H18–H28, 1981.

23. Greenway, C.V. and Lautt, W.W.: Blood volume, the venous system, preload and cardiac output. Can. J. Physiol. Pharmacol. 64: 383–387, 1986.

24. Shoukas, A.A. and Sagawa, K.: Total systemic vascular compliance measured as incremental volume-pressure ratio. Circ. Res. 28: 277–289, 1971.

25. Shoukas, A.A. and Sagawa, K.: Control of total systemic vascular capacity by the carotid sinus baroreceptor reflex. Circ. Res. 33: 22–33, 1973.

26. Greenway, C.V. and Oshiro, G.: Effects of histamine on hepatic volume (outflow block) in anaesthetized dogs. Br. J. Pharmacol. 47: 282–290, 1973.

27. Lautt, W.W., Greenway, C.V., Legare, D.J. and Weisman, H.: Localization of intrahepatic portal vascular resistance. Am. J. Physiol. 251: G375–G381, 1986.

28. Lautt, W.W., Greenway, C.V. and Legare, D.J.: Effect of hepatic nerves, norepinephrine, angiotensin and elevated central venous pressure on postsinusoidal resistance sites and intrahepatic pressures in cats. Microvasc. Res. 33: 50–61, 1987.

29. Greenway, C.V.: Mechanisms and quantitative assessment of drug effects on cardiac output using a new model of the circulation. Pharmacol. Rev. 33: 213–251, 1981.

30. Greenway, C.V. and Innes, I.R.: Effects of splanchnic nerve stimulation on cardiac preload, afterload and output in cats. Circ. Res. 46: 181–189, 1980.

31. Brunner, M.J., Shoukas, A.A. and MacAnespie, C.L.: The effect of the carotid sinus baroreceptor reflex on blood flow and volume redistribution in the total systemic vascular bed of the dog. Circ. Res. 48: 274–285, 1981.

32. Shoukas, A.A. and Brunner, M.C.: Epinephrine and the carotid sinus baroreceptor reflex. Influence on capacitive and resistive properties of the total systemic vascular bed of the dog. Circ. Res. 47: 249–257, 1980.

33. Bennett, T.D., Wyss, C.R. and Scher, A.M.: Changes in vascular capacity in awake dogs in response to carotid sinus occlusion and administration of catecholamines. Circ. Res. 55: 440–453, 1984.

34. Goldman, S., Olajos, M. and Morkin, E.: Control of cardiac output in thyrotoxic calves. J. Clin. Invest. 73: 358–365, 1984.

35. Ito, H. and Hirakawa, S.: Effects of vasodilators on the systemic capacitance vessels, a study with

the measurement of mean circulatory pressure in dogs. Jap. Circ. J. 48: 388–404, 1984.

36. Ogilvie, R.I.: Comparative effects of vasodilator drugs on flow distribution and venous return. Can. J. Physiol. Pharmacol. 63: 1345–1355, 1985.

37. Rothe, C.F., Stein, P.M., MacAnespie, C.L. and Gaddis, M.L.: Vascular capacitance responses to severe systemic hypercapnia and hypoxia in dogs. Am. J. Physiol. 249: H1061–H1069, 1985.

38. Rowell, L.B.: Reflex control of regional circulation in humans. J. Auton. Nerv. Syst. 11: 101–114, 1984.

39. Seaman, K. and Greenway, C.V.: Loss of hepatic venous responsiveness after endotoxin in anesthetized cats. Am. J. Physiol. 246: H658–H663, 1984.

40. Greenway, C.V., Burczynski, F. and Innes, I.R.: Effects of bromocryptine on hepatic blood volume responses to hepatic nerve stimulation in cats. Can. J. Physiol. Pharmacol. 64: 621–624, 1986.

41. Greenway, C.V.: Effects of sodium nitroprusside, isosorbide dinitrate, isoproterenol, phentolamine and prazosin on hepatic venous responses to sympathetic nerve stimulation in the cat. J. Pharmacol. Exp. Ther. 209: 56–61, 1979.

42. Greenway, C.V. and Innes, I.R.: Effects of arteriolar vasodilators on hepatic venous compliance and cardiac output in anesthetized cats. J. Cardiovasc. Pharmacol. 3: 1321–1331, 1981.

43. Barnes, R.J., Bower, E.A. and Rink, TJ.: Haemodynamic responses to stimulation of the cardiac autonomic nerves in the anaesthetized cat with closed chest. J. Physiol. (London) 299: 55–73, 1980.

44. Sarnoff, S.J., Gilmore, J.P. and Wallace, A.G.: The influence of autonomic nerve activity on adaptive mechanisms in the heart. In: Nervous Control of the Heart, ed. by W.C. Randall. Williams and Wilkins, Baltimore, pp 54–129, 1965.

20. Role of a changing venous capacitance in cardiovascular homeostasis

CARL F. ROTHE

Introduction

From his studies over the years, and as so well described in this paper, Greenway has helped to provide irrefutable evidence that the venous capacitance may be modified by the autonomic nervous system. A transfer of blood to the heart from the peripheral vasculature, induced by reflex changes in activity of smooth muscle of the vein walls, acts to modify right heart preload, and so significantly influences cardiac output.

Passive flow effects

The baro- and chemoreceptor reflexes are important, but let us not lose sight of the fact that *changes in blood flow* also influence the volume of blood in the peripheral tissue. In a recent series of experiments, we used the Rashkind-Shoukas venous-return reservoir, constant-cardiac output technique [1]. when we increased the perfusion rate from 110 to 140 ml $\cdot$ min^{-1} $\cdot$ kg^{-1}, about 10 ml/kg of blood left the reservoir and entered the dog (Fig. 20-1). Changing flow from 110 to 80 ml/min-kg caused a closely similar redistribution in the opposite direction. The slope of the line, the flow sensitivity, was about 0.27 ml/kg per 1 ml/min $\cdot$ kg BW. With reflexes intact, Numao and Iriuchijima [2] reported a flow sensitivity to changes in cardiac output of nearly 0.4 ml per ml/min. Attenuating the reflexes with 10 mg/kg of hexamethonium bromide reduced the response by about 30%. The resistance vessels, as revealed by the differences in arterial pressure at the same cardiac output, were more dramatically influenced by the blockade than the capacitance vessels (Fig. 20-2). A 50 ml/min-kg change in cardiac output, with *blocked reflexes*, produces about as much *passive* change in blood volume distribution (10 ml/kg) as *any* combination of *reflex* arterial baroreceptor pressure changes [1, 3, 4]. With reflexes blocked, the sensitivity to flow change is about 0.2 ml for *each* 1 ml/min change in flow. In the liver and intestine, the flow

228

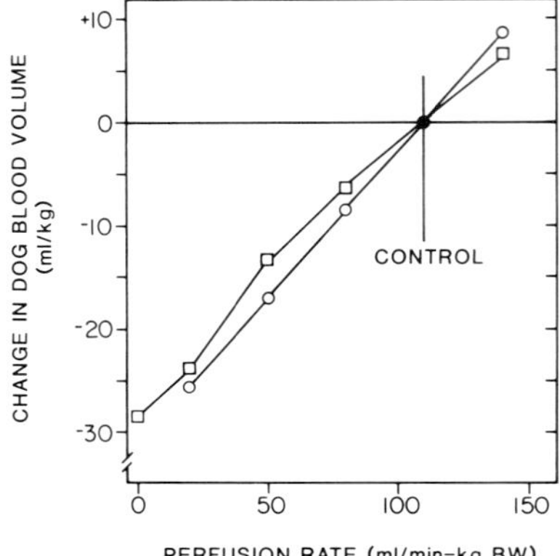

Figure 20-1. Change in dog blood volume following change in perfusion rate from a control of 110 ml · min⁻¹ · kg⁻¹. ○, preblockade; □, after reflex blockade with hexamethonium. Central venous pressure held at 3.1 mm Hg.

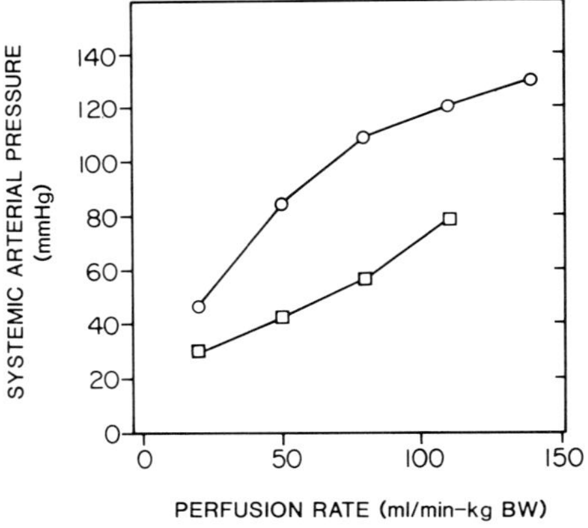

Figure 20-2. Systemic arterial pressure response to change in perfusion rate before (○) and after (□) reflex blockade with hexamethonium.

sensitivity is about 0.1 ml per 1 ml/min [5]. Why is the passive, total body response twice that of these major, highly compliant organs? The *passive flow effect* is a powerful, intrinsic, compensatory mechanism.

Spleen and other tissues

I fully agree that the splanchnic bed is the most dynamic and important bed for redistribution of blood volume. However, in his table of blood volumes that can be mobilized by the sympathetic system, most of the mobilized splanchnic volume is shown to be from the spleen (12% of the total blood volume) with only 6% from the liver and 3% from the intestinal bed. This large role of the spleen seems to be virtually unique to the dog and presents a problem if we are to extrapolate the data to the human. Our spleens are relatively small and unimportant. Furthermore, Shoukas et. al. [3] reported for the dog that changing the carotid sinus pressures between 50 and 200 mm Hg induced only a 2.5 ml/kg change in spleen volume. What other reflex mechanism might induce such a large (12% of blood volume or 9 ml/kg) change in the spleen volume? Nonetheless, even if the percent of the total blood volume mobilized by the sympathetic nervous system is only 20%, this amounts to about 15 ml/kg and is a substantial volume of great importance for short-term cardiovascular homeostasis.

In Greenway's Table, 31% of the total blood volume is in 'Other' tissues. Which tissues contain this volume? How is it controlled? How much of the volume in these tissues is available for *reflex* (or even passive-elastic blood volume) mobilization?

Unstressed volume

John Drees and I [6] reported about 15 ml/kg vascular volume difference between norepinephrine-stimulated and ganglionic-blocked dogs that had their spleens intact (Fig. 20-3). In that 1974 study, the difference is attributable to changes in unstressed volume, not changes in compliance – a result fully in agreement with the conclusions of Greenway in this paper and the 1973 studies of Shoukas and Sagawa [4]. Physiologists must measure 'unstressed volume' if they are to evaluate active (smooth muscle-induced) venoconstriction, *not just* compliance (the slope of the pressure–volume relationship).

Capacitance adrenergic receptors

Prof. Greenway showed that active contraction of the feline hepatic capacitance vessels is mediated by alpha-2 adrenoceptors. It has seemed clear [5, 7] that the venous system is activated primarily by alpha receptors. Others, however, support the concept of *beta-receptor* mediation [8] that may act by causing hepatic venous resistance relaxation [9–11] or hepatic venoconstriction by an indirect mechanisms [12]. Shoukas et al. [1] for example have found that epinephrine is a potent agent for inducing blood transfer from the capacitance vessels. Epinephrine is usually considered both an alpha *and* beta adrenergic receptor agonist. In some current pilot studies in which we use the constant cardiac output Rashkind-Shoukas technique, we found no significant change in reservoir volume in response to norepinephrine infusion (an alpha agonist) that caused marked

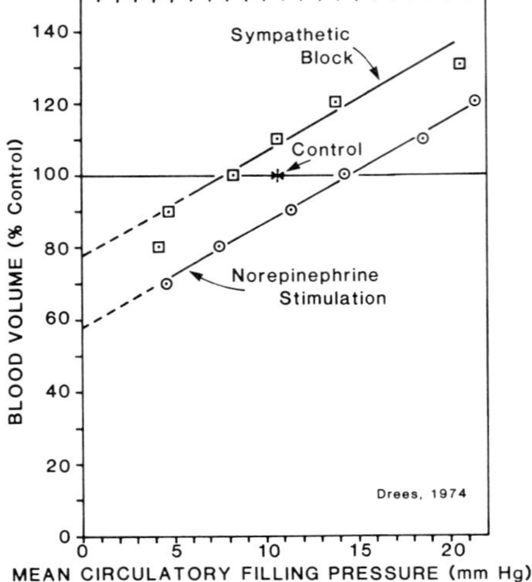

Figure 20-3. Changes in vascular capacitance. □, during reflex blockade with hexamethonium; ○, during infusion of norepinephrine ($1.5\,\mu g \cdot kg^{-1} \cdot min^{-1}$). (From Rothe, C.F. Physiology of venous return. *Arch. Int. Med.* 146: 977–982, 1986 with permission. Data from Drees and Rothe, 1974.)

(55 mm Hg) elevations in systemic arterial pressure. By contrast, isoproterenol infusions (a beta agonist) caused a 3.6 ml/kg increase in reservoir volume (venoconstriction) and a 40 mm Hg drop in arterial pressure. Some of the reservoir volume change was from changes in arterial bed volume following changes in systemic arterial pressure. Nonetheless, the beta adrenergic agonist caused venoconstriction. What *is the role of* capacitance vessel *beta receptors* in cardiovascular homeostasis?

References

1. Shoukas, A.A. and Brunner, M.C.: Epinephrine and the carotid sinus baroreceptor reflex: Influence on capacitive and resistive properties of the total systemic vascular bed of the dog. Circ. Res. 47: 249–257, 1980.
2. Numao, Y. and Iriuchijima, J.: Effect of cardiac output on circulatory blood volume. Jpn. J. Physiol. 27: 145–156, 1971.
3. Shoukas, A.A., MacAnespie, C.L., Brunner, M.J. and Watermeier, L.: The importance of the spleen in blood volume shifts of the systemic vascular bed caused by the carotid sinus baroreceptor reflex in the dog. Circ. Res. 49: 759–766, 1981.
4. Shoukas, A.A. and Sagawa, K.: Control of total systemic vascular capacity by the carotid sinus baroreceptor reflex. Circ. Res. 33: 22–33, 1973.
5. Rothe, C.F.: Venous system: Physiology of the Capacitance Vessels. In: Handbook of Physiology. The Cardiovascular System Sect. 2, vol. III, pt. 1, edited by J.T. Shepherd and F.M. Abboud. Am. Physiol. Society, Bethesda, MD 1983. Chapter 13, pp. 397–452.
6. Drees, JA. and Rothe, C.F.: Reflex venoconstriction and capacity vessel pressure–volume

relationships in dogs. Circ. Res. 34: 360–373, 1974.

7. Rothe, C.F.: Reflex control of the veins and vascular capacitance. Physiol. Rev. 63: 1281–1342, 1983.

8. Bennett, T.D., Wyss, C.R. and Scher, A.M.: Changes in vascular capacity in awake dogs in response to carotid sinus occlusion and administration of catecholamines. Circ. Res. 55: 440–453, 1984.

9. Rutlen, D.L., Supple, E.W. and Powell, W.J. Jr.: Beta-adrenergic regulation of total systemic intravascular volume in the dog. Circ. Res. 48: 112–120, 1981.

10. Rutlen, D.L., Supple, E.W. and Powell, W.J. Jr.: The role of the liver in the adrenergic regulation of blood flow from the splanchnic to the central circulation. Yale J. Biol. Med. 52: 99–106, 1979.

11. Green, J.F.: Mechanism of action of isoproterenol on venous return. Am. J. Physiol. 232: H152–H156, 1977.

12. Seaman, K.L. and Greenway, C.V.: Hepatic venoconstrictor effects of isoproterenol and nifedipine in anesthetized cats. Can. J. Physiol. Pharmacol. 62: 665–672, 1984.

General discussion of venous hemodynamics

The resistance and the capacitance elements in the venous circulation were discussed. It is clear that the two elements are independent and separable functionally. For example, sympathetic stimulation not only decreases venous resistance but also decreases unstressed volume, even though smooth muscle relaxation should increase unstressed volume. Also, in the liver histamine has no effect on unstressed volume but increases venous resistance. However, this is not to imply that the two elements are separate anatomically.

There was some discussion of the dynamic response of the venous circulation. While the response is slower than that of the arterial circulation precise data is lacking. Preliminary observations indicate the response of the liver is approximately 5–10 seconds while that of the spleen is in the order of minutes.

21. Principles of arterial hemodynamics

MICHAEL F. O'ROURKE

Introduction

The subject of haemodynamics is one of the most difficult in all physiology, requiring a knowledge of physical theory, engineering principles and mathematics as well as biology. It has in the past attracted a varied group of researchers from these different fields and from clinical medicine, as well with some (described by the late DA McDonald, one of the most colourful of all) 'measuring what could not be explained and others explaining what could not be measured' [1]. Controversy abounded on such fundamental issues as to whether wave reflection occurs in the arterial system (it does) and on whether it is valid to describe the pulse in the frequency, as well as in the time domain (it is). Researchers with different backgrounds spoke different languages and communication sometimes just did not exist. The field was not a comfortable one and traditional physiologists tended to eschew it. Clinicians in general did not dare enter. Consequently, the principles that arose and for which general agreement was ultimately reached have been slow to appear in text books of physiology or of medicine, and have not in the main been applied to clinical problems, despite their obvious relevance to arterial disease and the importance of this. Disease of arteries is directly responsible for between one third and one half of all deaths in the Western World.

The position now appears to have changed sufficiently for a broader and more confident exposition on 'Principles of Arterial Hemodynamics'. This chapter will attempt to review the field – and the history; with deference to their host department and in recognition of my own limitations, the emphasis will be on clinical implications and application.

History

The founder of arterial hemodynamics was an English clergyman, Stephen Hales, whose major work was performed during the early part of the 18th Century. Hales' principal interest [2] was to apply the new advances in physics which had been developed by Isaac Newton to the circulation; Hales' famous book 'Haemastatics' [3] was published under the authority of Newton as President of the Royal Society. He was the first to measure arterial pressure and to formulate the concept that vascular resistance to blood flow is in the short and narrow arterioles and capillaries. Hales emphasised the importance of arterial elasticity aiding in acceptance of pulsatile flow from the ventricle of the heart, and converting this into steady flow through the smallest high resistance vessels.

He likened the arterial system to the air filled dome of the contemporary fire engine; in German translations of his book, this became 'Windkessel', a term which is still used to day to describe the cushioning functions of arteries.

As an animal body consists not only of a wonderful texture of solid parts but also of a large proportion of fluids which are continually circulating and flowing thro' an inimitable embroidery of blood vessels and other inconceivably minute canals; and as the healthy state of an animal principally consists in the maintaining of a due equilibrium between those solids and fluids; it has ever since the important discovery of the circulation of the blood been looked upon as a matter well worth enquiring into to find the force and velocity with which these fluids are impelled; as a likely means to give a considerable insight into the animal oeconomy.

Stephen Hales 1769 [3]

Thomas Young [4] had a similar aim to Hales in the work he presented at the beginning of the 19th Century. This had followed the studies of hydrodynamics for ideal fluids by Euler, Bernouilli, and others. Both Young and Bernouilli were medical graduates and interested in application of physical laws not only to biology but also to medicine. Young's principal contribution was to elastic properties of materials in general, and of arteries in particular. He stressed the importance of travelling waves in arteries and of the relationship between arterial elasticity and pulse wave velocity. The precise relationship between pulse wave velocity and vascular properties was established by Moens and Korteweg following earlier work on wave transmission and reflection by the brothers Weber. In the mid 19th century Euler's equations of motion had been modified by Navier and by Stokes to take account of blood viscosity [7].

The importance of fluid viscosity was established by Poiseuille [5, 6] who extended Hales' work on the concept of peripheral resistance and on low resistance conduit arteries. Throughout the 19th century advances in theory, measurement and medical application occurred together. Marey, in Paris, developed the sphygmograph and an accurate flow meter. Mahomed [8] improved the sphygmograph and used it to determine abnormalities of the pulse and of arterial pressure in man. By 1874 he had extended Bright's work on arterial pressure and kidney disease and had described in some detail the natural history of the clinical condition we now know as essential hypertension.

The method of arterial pressure measurement that is used today was developed by Riva-Rocci and by Korotkov [9]. While this enabled non-invasive, easy and reasonably accurate determination of arterial pressure in man, it led to a careless and simplistic approach to arterial hemodynamics with systolic and diastolic pressures seen as having particular physiological significance, rather than the extremes – the peak and nadir – of the arterial pressure wave in one artery [10]. Systolic pressure was equated with cardiac strength and diastolic pressure with arteriolar tone. The idea, still current, evolved that elevation of diastolic pressure is the hallmark of hypertension and that elevation of systolic pressure is innocuous [10].

Otto Frank dominated the studies of arterial hemodynamics in the latter part of the 19th, and early part of the 20th Century. Frank [11–12] tried to reconcile the Windkessel theory (which considered elasticity to be 'lumped' at the one point) with the theory of wave travel and reflection. His aim was to measure flow, and cardiac output, from measurements of arterial pressure; he had previously perfected a mechanical manometer, obtaining pressure waves virtually as accurate as any determined today. Frank's work and that of his colleagues in Europe was disrupted by the First World War and by its sequelae. The 20th century however marked the emergence of the United States of America as the dominant site of scientific and biological medical research, initially under the influence of philanthropic foundations [13]. Advances in manometric instrumentation were made by Hamilton and others, and in interpretation by his group, by Katz, Wiggers and many others. Kolin and Wetterer (the latter in Germany) introduced the electromagnetic flowmeter before war again intervened [7, 14]. Following World War Two the success of pioneering cardiac surgery necessitated cardiovascular diagnostic laboratories for human studies. The subsequent application of physiological measurements to clinical diagnosis and monitoring is well known to all. It has been aided by improvements in technology including use of computer science.

The major advance in arterial hemodynamics since World War Two has been in the concept of steady state analysis of the arterial pulse. The pioneering work was conducted by a physiologist, DA McDonald, and the mathematician, JR Womersley, working together in London between 1952–1957. Womersley examined and quantified assumptions used in applying a linearised solution of the Navier/Stokes equation to an arterial segment, and showed that errors were small enough to be ignored – to a first approximation [15, 16]. The work was pursued with the arterial pulse broken down into its component harmonics, and the concept of longitudinal impedance developed. This concept was extended by MG

236

Taylor in McDonald's department through consideration of complex wave velocity, enabling the relationship between flow and absolute pressure to be described and explained as input impedance of a vascular bed [17]. Taylor's subsequent theoretic studies on input impedance were conducted in conjunction with experimental determinations [17–22] and permitted the concept to be validated. This work is described in greater detail elsewhere [17, 14]. The past 20 years has seen extension of these studies in describing arterial pressure wave transmission and pressure/flow relationships in experimental animals and in man. The basic principles are now well established and accepted. However, acceptance of clinical implications has been slow. For instance, clinicians still speak of 'the' systolic and 'the' diastolic pressure as though these were the same in all arteries of man under all conditions as in the brachial – ignoring the gross alterations that often occur to the amplitude of the pressure wave during propagation from central to peripheral arteries. Left ventricular 'afterload' is described in terms of brachial systolic pressure without consideration of pressure wave amplification between the ascending aorta and brachial artery. In addition, the complications of arterial stiffening with age have really not been addressed. I would contend that application of physiologic theory to arterial disease is still in its infancy.

Structure and functions of the arterial system

The systemic arterial system is a branching network of tubes which accepts pulsatile flow from the left ventricle of the heart and passes this on in an almost steady stream into the arterioles. The arterial system thus has two functions – to distribute blood to bodily organs and tissues (its conduit function) and to dampen out the fluctuations which are consequences of intermittent ventricular ejection (its cushioning function). Hales saw these two functions as anatomically discrete with the central aorta acting as pressure chamber or windkessel and peripheral arteries acting as conduit vessels (Fig. 21-1).

To an extent Hales was correct in that the central aorta is relatively more distensible than are peripheral arteries, but it is clear that the aorta is a conduit as well as a cushion and peripheral arteries likewise. The functions cannot be separated anatomically. But they can be separated in terms of measured pressure and flow waves. The waves comprise mean and pulsatile components. McDonald and Womersley [15, 16] justified this separation in establishing the concept of steady state analysis as discussed previously. The conduit function then can be described in terms of steady pressure and flow and the cushioning function in terms of pressure and flow pulsation.

The efficiency of the arterial system can be gauged in terms of mean pressure and flow (for conduit function) and pulsatile pressure and flow (for cushioning function). Efficient conduit function is responsible for the absence of detectible mean pressure gradient between the ascending aorta and small peripheral arteries

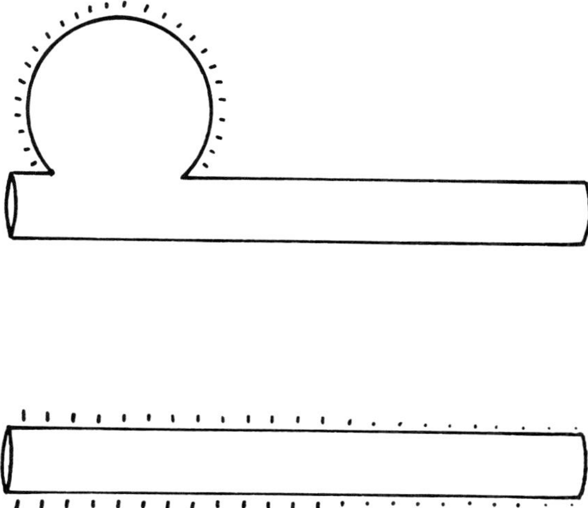

Figure 21-1. The cushioning and conduit functions of the arterial system may be represented separately by a Windkessel and distributing tube (above), or by a single distensible tube (below) in which both functions are combined. From O'Rourke 1982 [14].

(Fig. 21-2) [5]. There must, of course, be a gradient, but under normal resting conditions this is rarely more than 4 mm Hg over a distance of 1 meter or more in normal man. Efficient cushioning function is apparent in the low amplitude of ascending aortic pulse pressure, and in the small differences between mean systolic and mean diastolic pressure in the ascending aorta [23]. It is possible to measure the relative proportions of steady and of pulsatile energy lost in the systemic circulation; under normal conditions the pulsatile component is approximately 10% of the steady component [23]. This is another indication of efficient cushioning function.

While it is possible to describe overall function of the arterial system in terms of conduit and cushioning function, the details of function and of arterial structure are almost infinitely complex. The lengths and branching patterns of arteries are variable (though relatively consistent in adults of the same species), incremental Young's modulus of the wall at a given pressure increases progressively between the central aorta and peripheral arteries, but the wall at any point shows markedly nonlinear stress/strain relationships – as would be expected from its predominantly two phase composition. Activation of smooth muscle in the arterial wall alters calibre of the vessels and changes the distribution of tension to load-bearing elements [24]. The arterial wall contains blood – a suspension of cells, with viscosity dependent on calibre of vessel and on rate of shear.

It would be impossible to devise a truly realistic model of the arterial system. Many, of course, have been proposed [25–28]. It is surprising that relatively simple models can give a realistic approach to arterial behaviour, given the

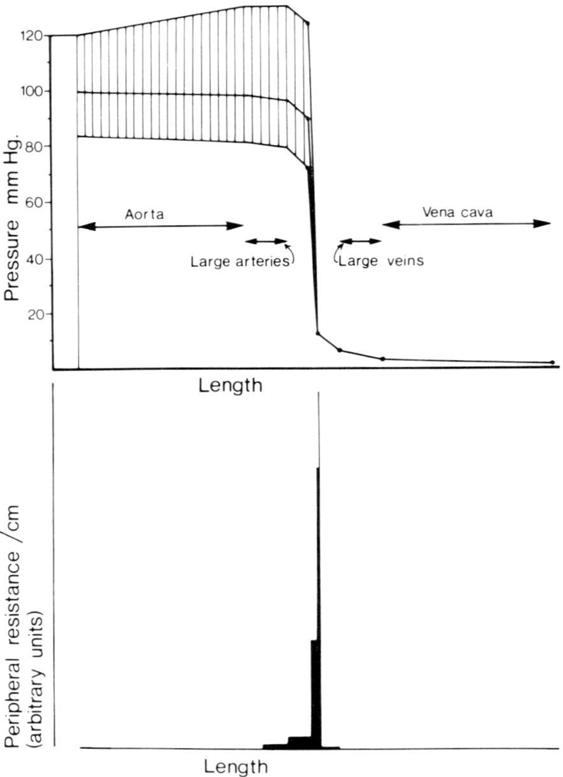

Figure 21-2. (Top) Changes in mean pressure and in pulsatile pressure generated by the left ventricle between the ascending aorta and vena cava. (Bottom) Resistance in corresponding segments of the vascular bed. From O'Rourke 1982 [14].

known complexities. Albert Einstein is quoted as advising 'make everything as simple as possible, but not simpler'. With respect to arterial function, the opportunity certainly exists. Hopefully the temptation to oversimplify can be avoided.

Pressure and flow waves in arteries

The contour of the ascending aortic flow wave is surprisingly similar in different animals, at different heart rates, and under different conditions (Fig. 21-3). This bespeaks for fundamental similarities in left ventricular function. Peak flow is achieved early, within the first third of systole, with flow velocity falling slowly thereafter. At normal resting heart rates, the duration of systolic flow is approximately 40% of the whole cycle. The total period of systolic flow varies widely in different species, being short in rats and rabbits (approximately 120 msec), and

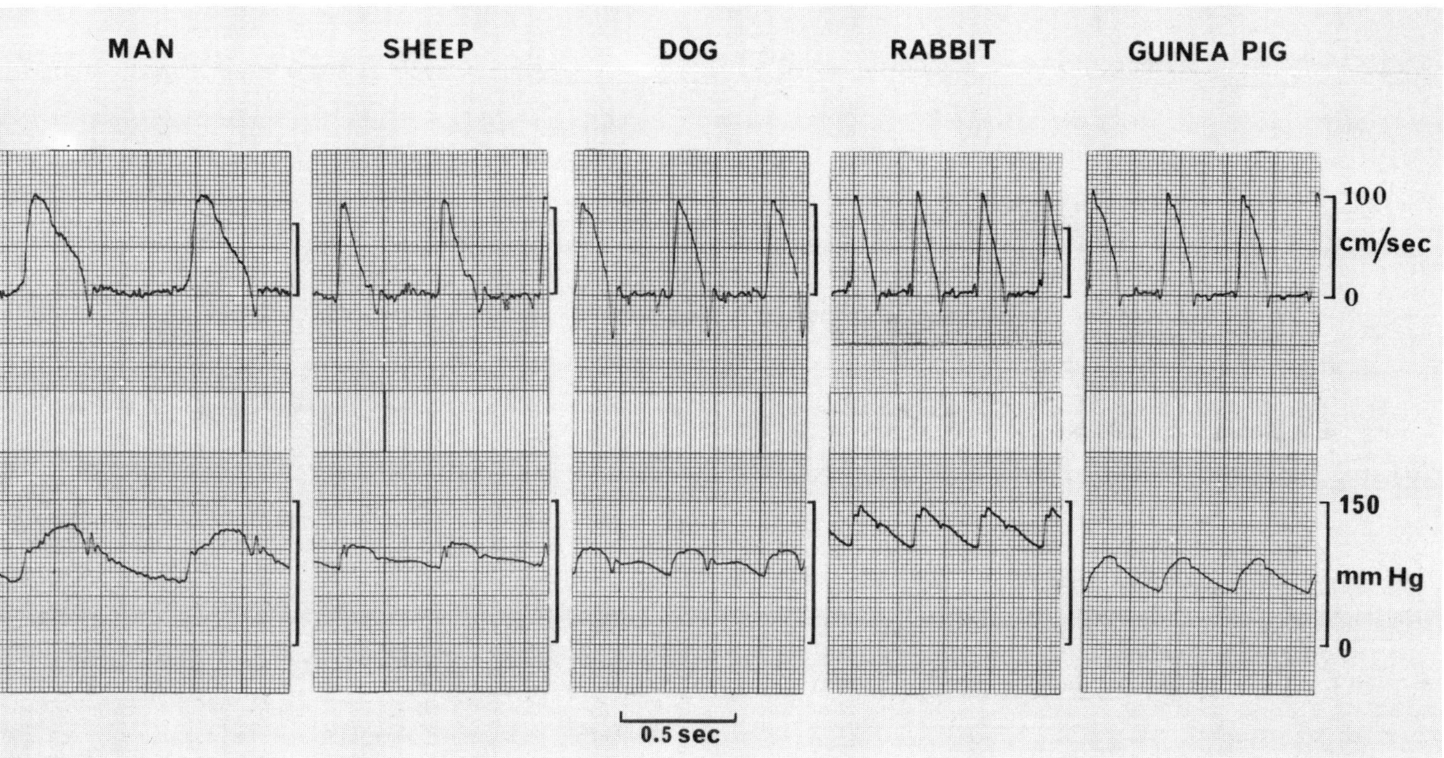

Figure 21-3. Flow waves (above) and pressure waves (below) in the ascending aorta of five different mammals. Flow calibration (different for each animal) is 100 cm/sec. Pressure and time calibration are the same for each mammal. From O'Rourke 1982 [14].

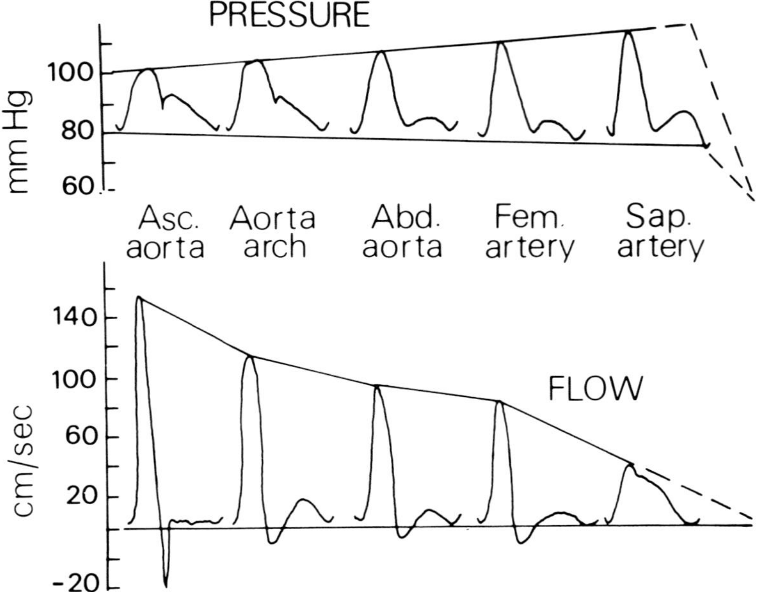

Figure 21-4. Diagrammatic representation of change in pressure (above) and flow (below) patterns between the ascending aorta and peripheral arteries. The most distal pressure and flow patterns illustrated are those in the saphenous artery. Beyond this site, dotted lines indicate the steep fall in systolic pressure, diastolic pressure and pulse pressure and further attenuation of pulsatile flow within the arterioles downstream. After McDonald (1960) [7].

relatively long in man (approximately 300 msec); this corresponds to the smaller animals.

Between the ascending aorta and peripheral arteries, the flow wave is gradually attenuated, with a fall in peak flow velocity, a lengthening in the duration of forward flow and reduction in flow oscillation (Fig. 21-4). However, flow oscillations often become particularly prominent close to the heart in the aortic arch branches – the innominate, common cartoid and subclavian arteries and in the descending thoracic aorta [14]. In these vessels, reciprocal flow oscillations between upper and lower parts of the body are usually very obvious [9]. These suggest the presence of wave reflection between upper and lower body sites with generation of a type of damped resonance (Fig. 21-5).

The typical ascending aortic pressure wave (Fig. 21-4) shows a more rounded systolic peak than does flow, followed by a notch referred to variously as the incisura or dicrotic notch, then by a low wide secondary wave in early diastole usually called the dicrotic wave. There is far more variability in the contour of the ascending aortic pressure wave than there is in ascending aortic flow (Fig. 21-3). This typical pattern as described is seen in most experimental animals and in children and young human adults [14]. It is not seen in most adult humans, nor in some particular experimental animals – guinea pigs or snakes. Here there is no

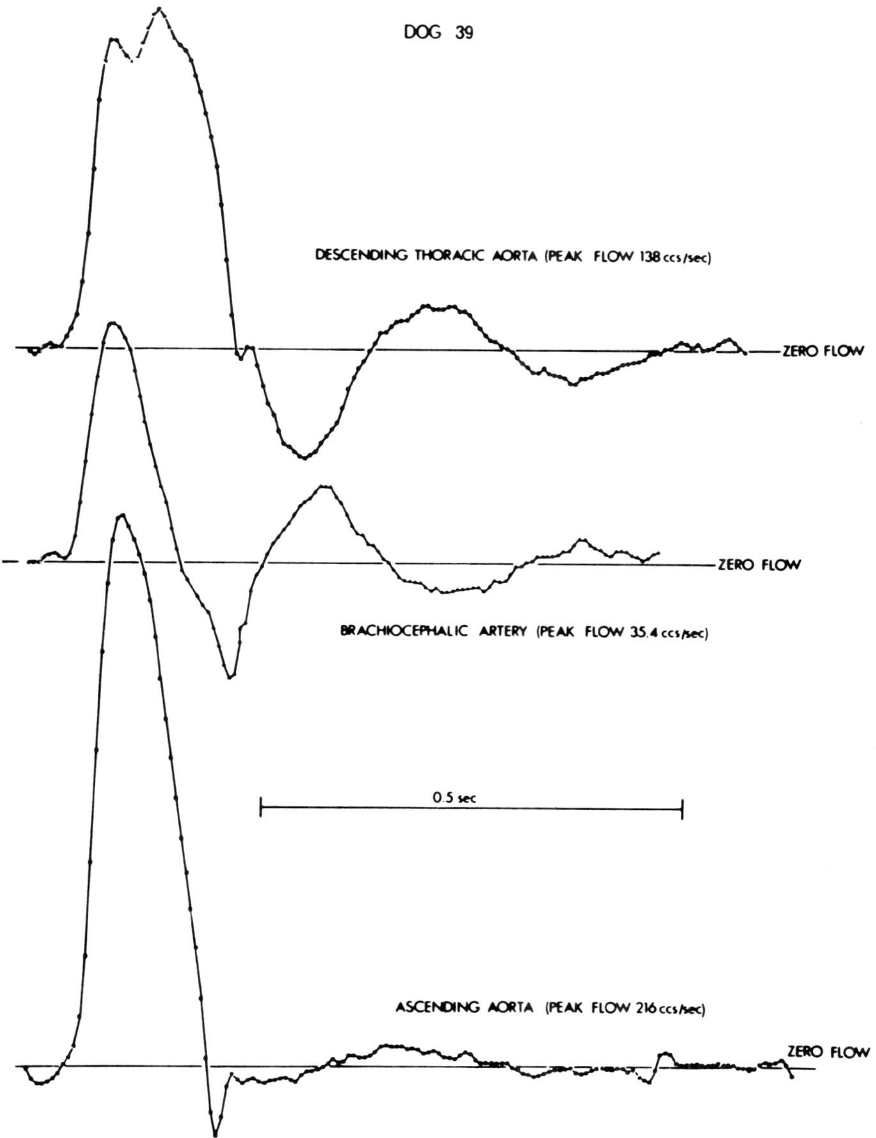

Figure 21-5. Flow waves recorded in the descending thoracic aortic, brachiocephalic artery and ascending aorta of a dog. From O'Rourke [24].

diastolic wave and the rounded systolic peak is replaced by a sharper peak in late systole. These differences must be due to vascular properties since aortic flow, and hence ventricular ejection patterns, are similar. They are explicable on the basis of differences in wave reflection. In adult humans, and in guinea pigs, wave reflection from a functionally discrete peripheral reflecting site appears to return

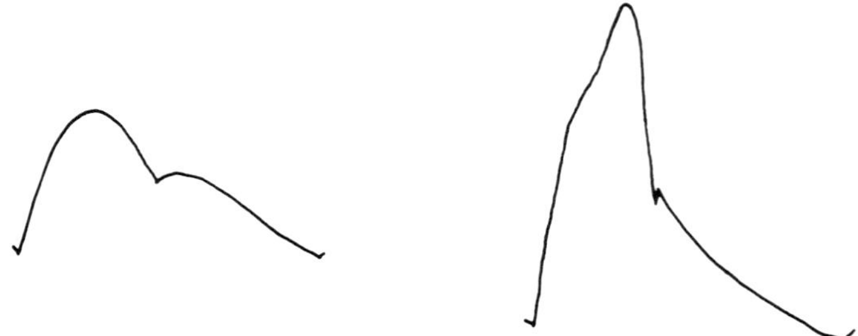

Figure 21-6. Typical ascending aortic pressure waves in a child (left) and adult human (right). Changes with age are explicable on the basis of increased aortic stiffness and early return of wave reflection.

earlier than is usual (in humans due to short body length), causing the secondary wave to move from diastole into systole and so generate the late systolic peak (Fig. 21-6) [14]. In snakes it appears that wave reflection is far more diffuse, with no functionally discrete reflecting site, and so no discrete diastolic wave; this behaviour is predictable on the basis of the long tapering body and arterial branching patterns [29].

The arterial pressure wave usually changes markedly between the ascending aorta and peripheral arteries. Mean pressure falls slightly as described, and the foot of the wave is delayed (because of finite wave travel), but the wave itself undergoes amplification with increase in the systolic peak and lesser reduction in diastolic pressure (Fig. 21-7). At the same time the diastolic wave becomes more apparent in the peripheral artery.

Most studies of wave transmission have been performed along the aorta between ascending aorta and femoral artery, but similar changes are seen between the aortic arch and brachial or radial artery [30]. In adult man, these changes in pulse contour and amplitude are often less apparent than in children but they have been shown to vary with different physiological maneouvres and with exercise [14, 31]. The general phenomenon of peripheral pulse wave amplification is attributable to wave reflection and to the greater stiffness of peripheral arteries; differences in amplification under different conditions can be explained on the basis of differences in intensity and timing of wave reflection [14].

Steady state analysis of arterial pressure and flow waves

The rationale for this approach was established by McDonald and Womersley [7, 15, 16]. The approach had been used previously, but not pursued, by Frank and by Aperia [32]. Figure 21-8 shows pressure and flow waves recorded in the femoral artery of a dog, broken down into component harmonics, with corresponding terms related to give impedance modulus (amplitude of pressure harmonic/ amplitude of flow harmonic at the same frequency) and phase (delay between

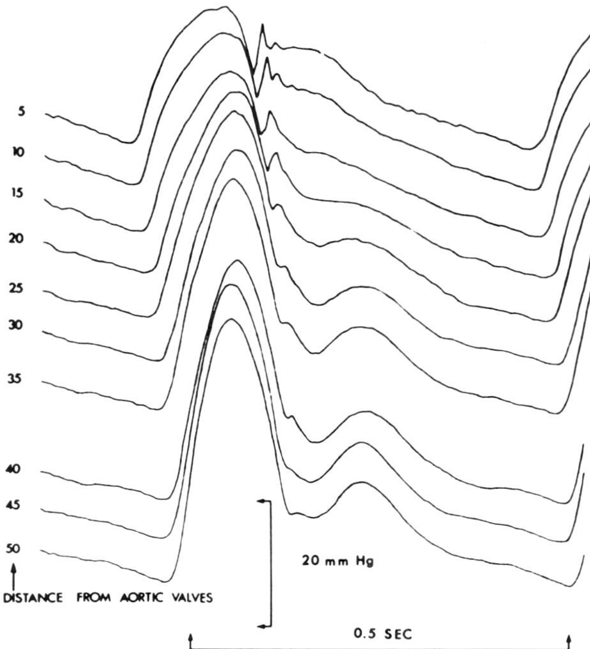

Figure 21-7. Pressure waves recorded successively at 5 cm intervals between the aortic arch (above) and external iliac artery (below) in a 16.5 kg wombat, through a catheter inserted in the femoral artery. The wombat (Wombat hirsuitis) is a native Australian marsupial, similar in size to a dog, but having a thick head, and short, stubby limbs. From O'Rourke 1967 [24].

harmonic of pressure and corresponding harmonic of flow), plotted against frequency. The zero frequency term for modulus is the resistance: mean pressure/ mean flow. Analysis of waves such as those in Fig. 21-8 gives values of impedance modulus at heart frequency and at multiples of this (corresponding to the second and higher harmonics).

It is possible to obtain values for intervening frequencies by pacing the heart at different rates (Fig. 21-9), or by applying a related analytical technique (frequency spectrum analysis) for pressure and flow waves recorded with the heart beating irregularly [33]. Data obtained with these different techniques is presented in Figs. 21-9–21-13. Figure 21-9 shows a typical plot of impedance values in the femoral artery of a dog. The consistency of results supports the concept of linearity: similar values of impedance were obtained from the third harmonic of waves recorded with the heart beating at 60/min as from the first harmonic of the waves recorded with a heart rate of 180/min. Impedance patterns are similar in different arteries (except the ascending aorta which is discussed separately).

The impedance modulus falls from a relatively high value of zero frequency to a minimal value – in the femoral artery at around 10 to 12 Hz – then rises again to settle around a reasonably steady value at high frequencies. Impedance phase

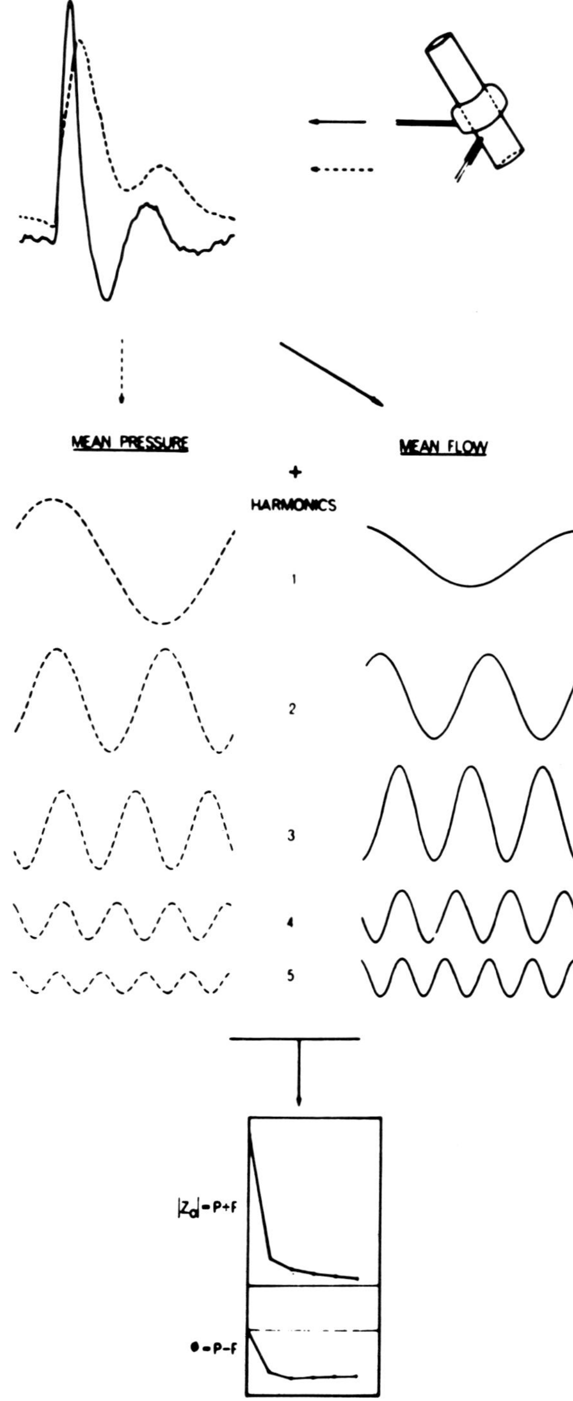

Figure 21-8. Pressure (broken line) and flow (solid line) waves in the femoral artery of a dog, broken down into mean terms and Fourier series, the first 5 components of which are shown. From mean values and corresponding harmonics, impedance modulus (Z_o) and phase (θ) may be determined as a function of frequency (bottom) – modulus as the amplitude of pressure harmonic divided by amplitude of corresponding flow harmonic and phase as the delay between corresponding harmonics. From O'Rourke and Taylor 1966, with permission American Heart Association Inc. [21].

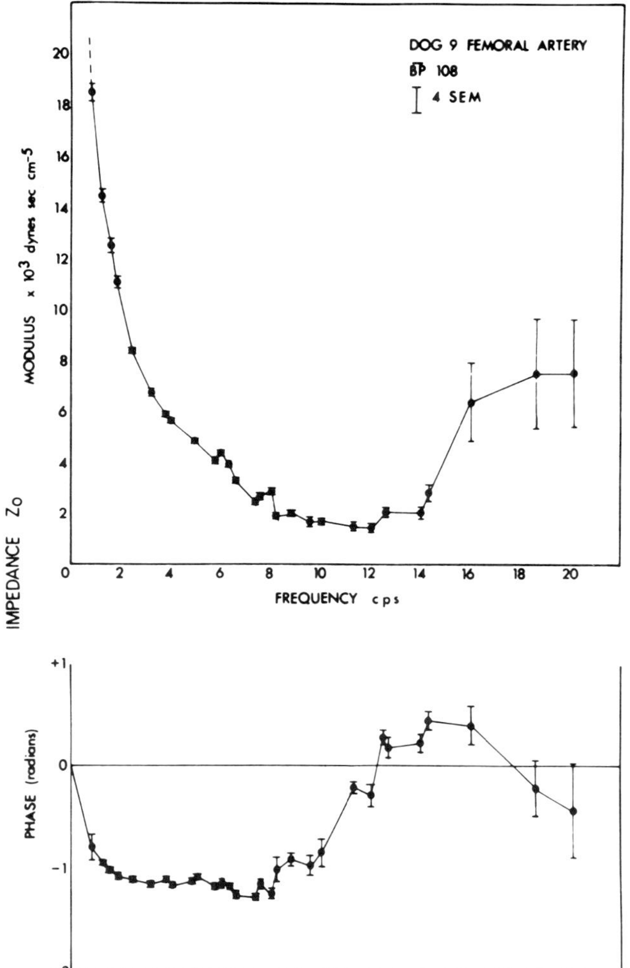

Figure 21-9. Vascular impedance under control conditions in the femoral artery of a dog, with modulus (above) and phase (below) plotted against frequency. Impedance was determined from Fourier analysis of a series of 57 waves recorded in a dog with heart block, whose heart was paced at different frequencies. Abscissa Hertz. From O'Rourke and Taylor 1966, with permission American Heart Association Inc. [21].

becomes negative at low frequencies (flow preceding pressure), then crosses zero to become positive, before settling around zero. Taylor [20, 21] applied his multibranched model of a vascular bed to interpret impedance patterns under normal conditions and during elevation of arterial pressure, and with intense vasoconstriction and vasodilation of the vascular bed induced by intra-arterial injection of acetycholine and of noradrenalin respectively (Fig. 21-10).

He showed that the normal patterns were attributable to high resting vasomo-

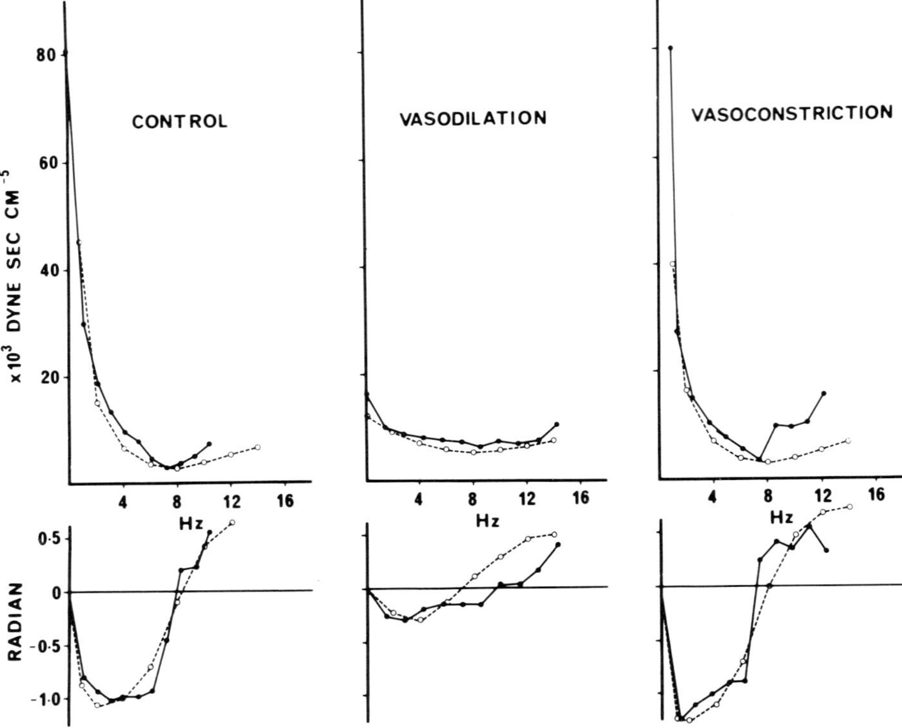

Figure 21-10. Solid lines: Experimentally determined values of impedance modulus and phase in the femoral artery of a dog under control conditions and during intra-arterial injection of acetylcholine (centre) and norephinephrine (right). Dashed lines: Impedance at the input of Taylor's model of the femoral vascular bed with reflection coefficient 0.8 (left), 0.95 (right). From O'Rourke 1982 [14].

tor tone with wave reflection approximately 80% at individual peripheral arterial terminations and that the pattern seen with increased arterial pressure (Fig. 21-11) – shifting of curves bodily to the right – is attributable to higher increased arterial tension and increased pulse wave velocity, with earlier return of echoes from the peripheral terminations. The changes induced by intra-arterial acetylcholine were attributable to marked reduction (to near zero) in peripheral reflection coefficient (with the position of the reflecting sites unchanged) while the relatively modest change induced by intense vasoconstriction was due to the small difference between normal 80% and 95% reflection coefficient with vasoconstriction.

The femoral vascular bed was very suitable for such experimental determination; it was possible to increase arterial pressure with trivial changes in peripheral resistance of the bed, and to cause profound vasodilation without causing a

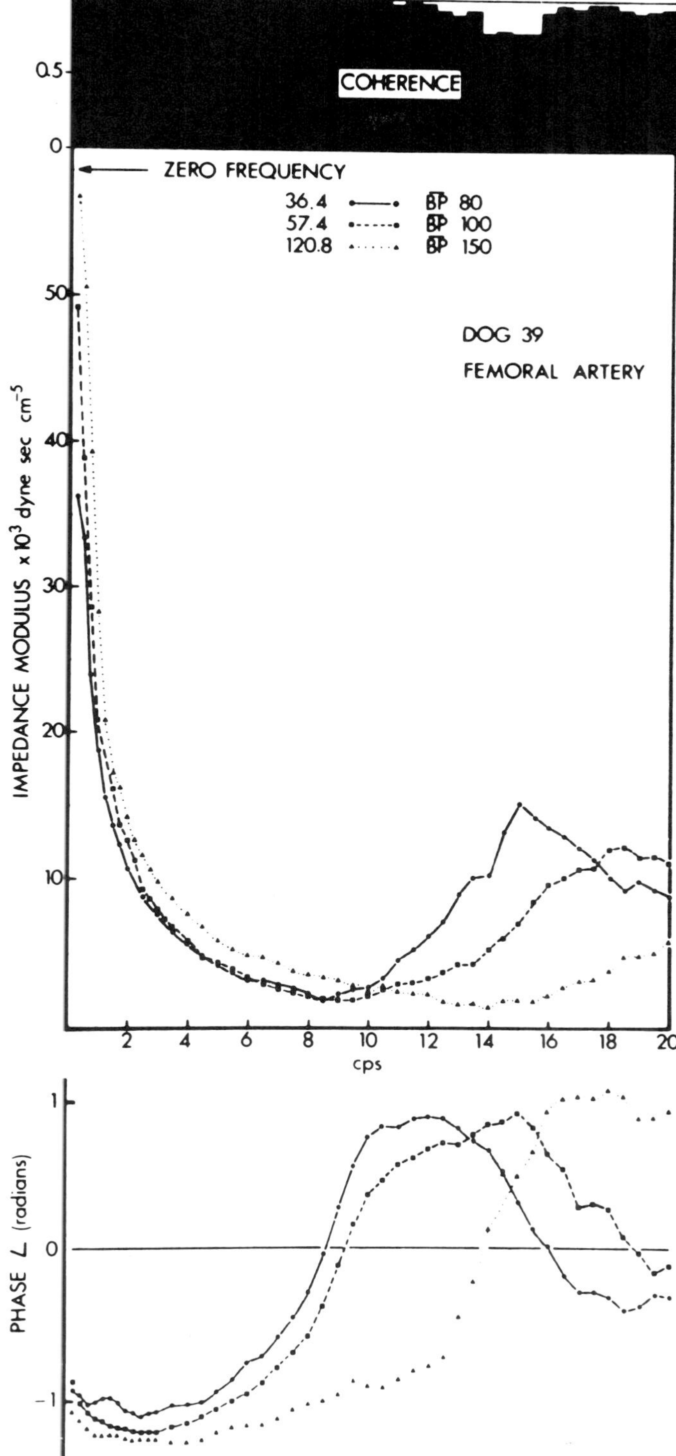

Figure 21-11. Vascular impedance in the femoral artery of a dog under control conditions with mean arterial pressure 80 mm Hg, and during infusion of norepinephrine at mean arterial pressure 100 mm Hg and 150 mm Hg. Peripheral resistance, initially 36.4 dyne · sec · cm⁻⁵, rose to 57.4 then 121 dyne · sec · cm⁻⁵. Shift of impedance curves to the right is attributable to increase in mean pressure and in pulse wave velocity. From O'Rourke 1970, with permission American Heart Association Inc [21].

248

marked drop in mean arterial pressure. There is no reason to believe the same principles do not apply to other vascular beds. The effects of intra-arterial acetylcholine is of particular interest. The experiment showed that wave reflection could be eliminated by intense vasodilation, suggesting vascular tone was responsible for the high resting reflection coefficient – not the arterial branching pattern – which is, of course, not altered by a vasodilator agent. Wave reflection can arise from any discontinuity or change of impedance or resistance in the vascular bed. While branching points are potential sites of wave reflection, it appears that the dominant sites in a vascular bed are the individual junctions of low resistance arteries and high resistance arterioles.

Differences between impedance patterns in other arteries are readily explained on the basis of principles established for the femoral vascular bed. The distance to peripheral reflecting sites determines the frequency of modulus minimum and phase crossover; hence this frequency is lower in central than in peripheral arteries and impedance modulus appears to fall more steeply in the central vessel (Fig. 21-12). The degree of fluctuation in modulus and phase is lower than in the femoral artery. In central arteries the first minimum of modulus and phase crossover is usually followed by a second maximal value of modulus at near twice the frequency of the original minimum and a second phase crossover; this again is what one would predict in the presence of single peripheral reflecting site [22, 24]. However, at higher frequencies values of impedance modulus tend to remain relatively stable; this represents the characteristic impedance – the value of modulus uninfluenced by wave reflection [14, 22].

Patterns of impedance modulus in the ascending aorta are different to those seen in other arteries (Fig. 21-13). The first minimum of modulus occurs at a lower frequency than in any other artery of the same animal (as would be expected) but there are often two minimal values of impedance at close frequency, or a single broad minimum and two fluctuations of phase [7, 14, 22].

These impedance patterns are attributable to the interacting effects of two separate vascular beds in parallel, with two functionally discrete reflecting sites – one in the lower part of the body corresponding to the sum total of the individual reflecting sites in the trunk and lower limbs, and the other closer at hand in the upper body corresponding to the sum total of reflecting sites in the head, neck and upper limbs [20, 22]. Just as with pressure and flow waves recorded at the same point, it is possible to relate the corresponding frequency components of pressure waves recorded at different sites between central and peripheral arteries (Fig. 21-14). These plots show progressive increase in modulus up to the more distal sites, with fluctuation of the higher harmonics in the proximal sites. This behaviour is what would be expected from peripheral wave reflection, and supports the interpretations of the pressure waves, flow waves, and impedance patterns [7, 14].

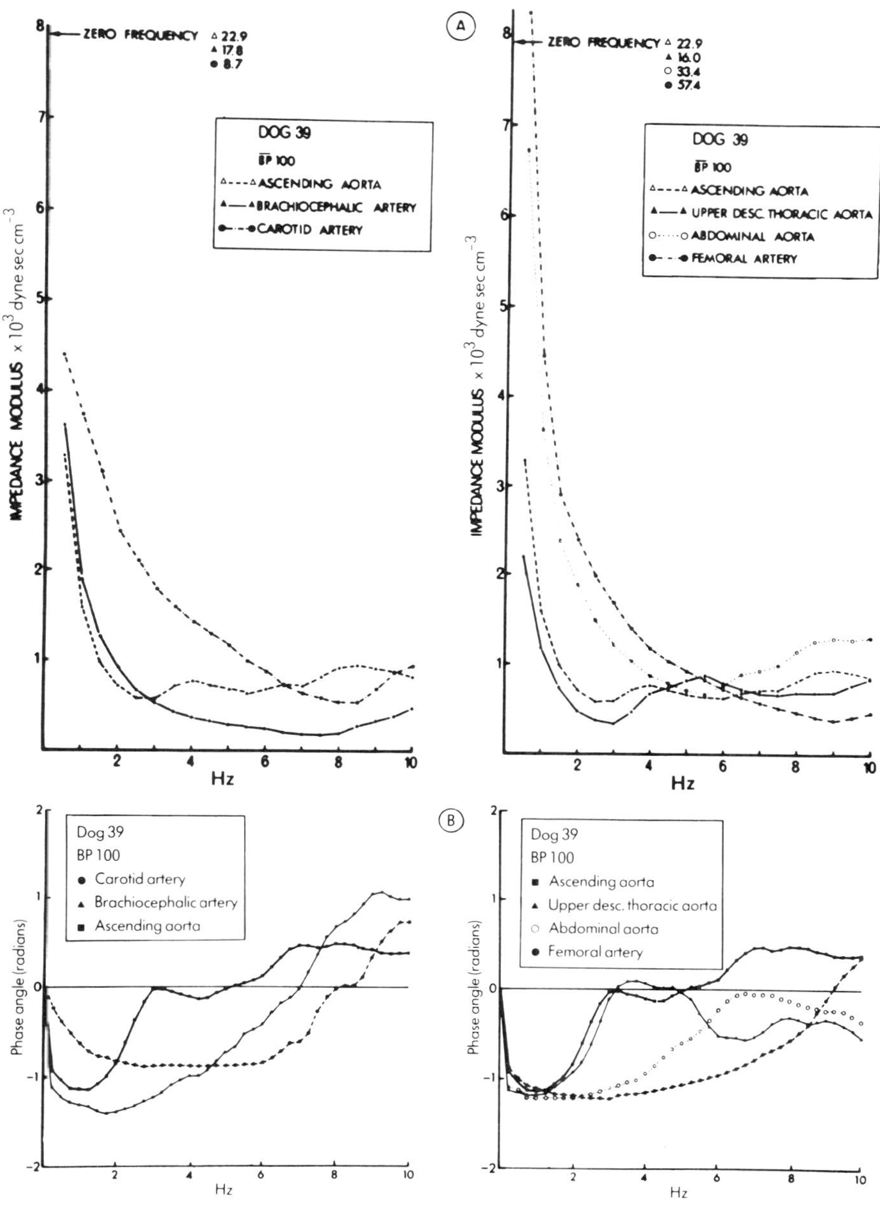

Figure 21-12. A: Changes in modulus of vascular impedance between the ascending aorta and carotid artery (left) and between the ascending aorta and femoral artery (right) of a 21 kg dog. Modulus expressed in terms of linear flow velocity. Peripheral resistance shown above. B: Changes in impedance phase angle between the ascending aorta and carotid artery (left) and between the ascending aorta and femoral artery of the same dog. From O'Rourke 1967 [24].

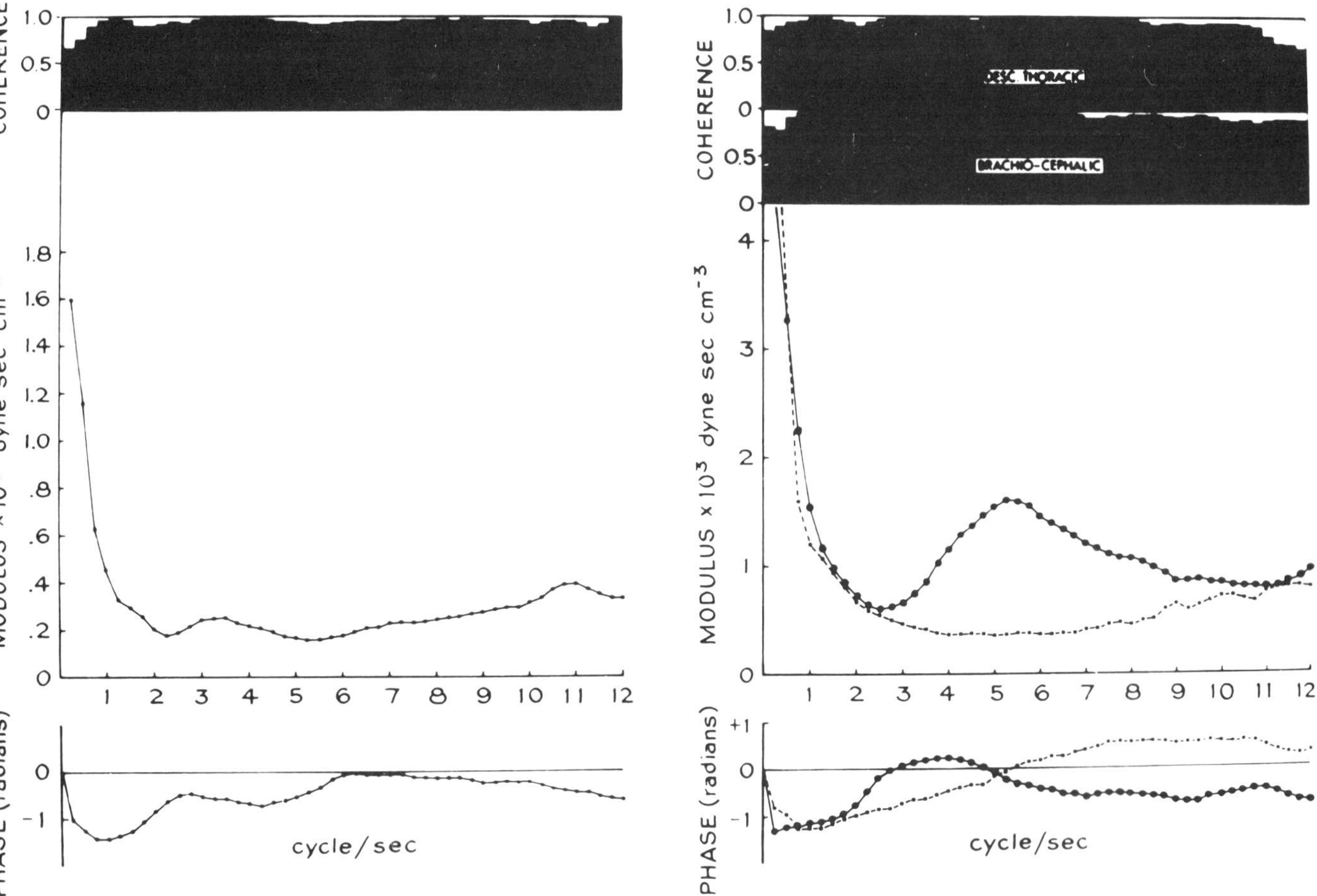

COHERENCE
MODULUS x 10³ dyne sec cm⁻⁵
PHASE (radians)
cycle/sec
COHERENCE
DESC. THORACIC
BRACHIO-CEPHALIC
MODULUS x 10³ dyne sec cm⁻³
PHASE (radians)
cycle/sec

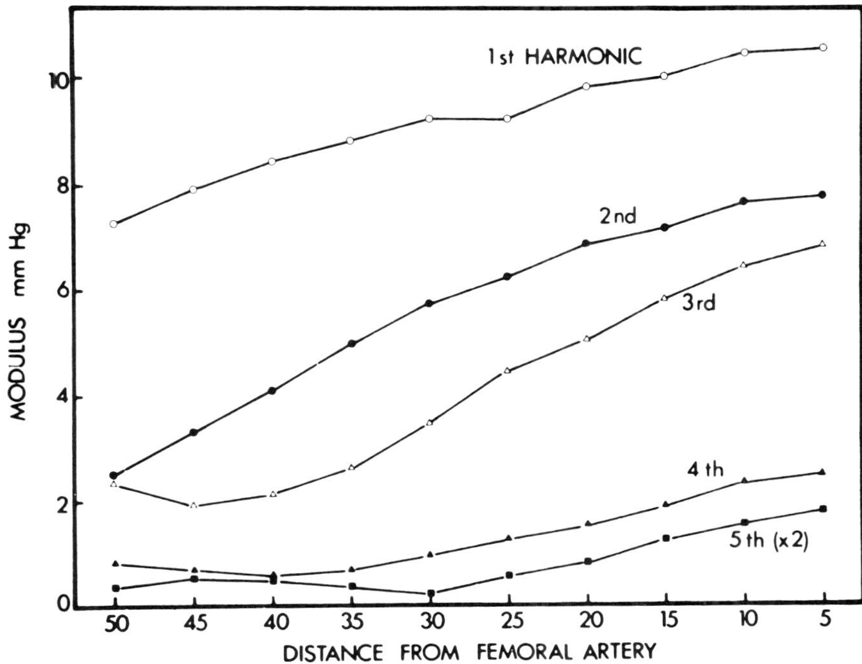

Figure 21-14. Amplitude of the first five harmonics of pressure waves recorded between the aortic arch (position 50) and femoral artery of a wombat. Individual waves are shown in Figure 7. From O'Rourke 1967 [24].

Wave reflection

There is now overwhelming evidence of wave reflection – and of strong wave reflection – in the arterial tree. The fluctuations of impedance modulus and phase are the most precise indicators of this; analysis of impedance patterns under different conditions in experimental animals and in vascular models gives accurate information on position, site, and intensity and mechanics of this, but the evidence is apparent in the pressure wave harmonics and in the pressure and flow waves themselves. Given the known damping of waves travelling in arteries and the particularly high attenuation in the smallest vessels [7], it is surprising that wave reflection is so prominent. Even more surprising is that wave reflection appears to be so discrete, and that it appears to come from lumped peripheral

←

Figure 21-13. Vascular impedance at three sites in a 23 kg dog at the same mean arterial pressure (100 mm Hg). Left, ascending aorta; Right, upper descending thoracic aorta (solid line) and proximal brachiocephalic artery (broken line). From O'Rourke and Taylor 1967, with permission American Heart Association Inc [23].

252

reflecting sites. With the different distances to peripheral reflecting sites, one would expect a great deal of dispersion and cancellation of reflected waves [20].

This certainly is seen in snakes [29], but in other animals and in man, the apparent functionally discrete peripheral reflecting sites may be due to the concentration of arterial terminations in large localised muscle groups [14]. The ascending aortic impedance results (Fig. 21-13) indicate that there are two peripheral functionally discrete reflecting sites – one in the upper and the other in the lower body. The study suggested that the systemic circulation may be represented by an asymmetric T tube (Fig. 21–12) – with a short limb representing all arteries supplying the upper body – and its end, their multiple terminations, and with the long limb representing the descending aorta and lower limb arteries with the longlimb representing the sum of all arterial terminations in the lower part of the body. While the model was suggested by the impedance results, it provided a better explanation than had previously been available for the patterns of pressure waves and the flow waves in the aorta and large arteries and especially for the reciprocal fluctuations of pressure and of flow between the upper and lower parts of the body (Figs. 21-5, 21-7) [14]. Westernof and colleagues have suggested a different approach to study of wave reflection, and it has recently been applied by Laskey, Kussmaul and colleagues [36] from Philadelphia in the study of cardiomyopathy and its management in man.

Vascular impedance and cardiac load

The ascending aortic impedance characterstics the hydraulic load presented to the left ventricle of the heart by the whole systemic circulation [7, 14, 22]. Milnor [37] has argued that impedance is ventricular afterload, one has to recognise that it is a complex quantity having modulus and phase and that it is also frequency-dependent. One can describe a change in afterload as impedance but one has to specify at what frequency and with which phase. It is insufficient to regard characteristic impedance as afterload, since this value is only relevant to very high harmonics of the arterial pulse, not to the first three harmonics which contain the greatest proportion of the wave. Studies of ascending aortic impedance have shown how the arterial system has adapted to its role of accepting pulsatile flow from the heart [14, 22, 23]. From its resistive value at zero frequency, impedance modulus fall steeply to a trough. Its lowest value is one fiftieth or less of resistance (Fig. 21-13). At normal heart rate frequencies, the first three harmonics of the aortic flow wave fall within this trough and so generate relatively small pressure fluctuations – so small that the extra energy lost in the circulation on account of pulsatile input is only about one tenth of that expended in maintaining steady flow. There is a 'match' between the output from the heart and the circulation's input impedance (Fig. 21-16).

The circulation is 'tuned' to the normal heart frequency; 'tuning' probably

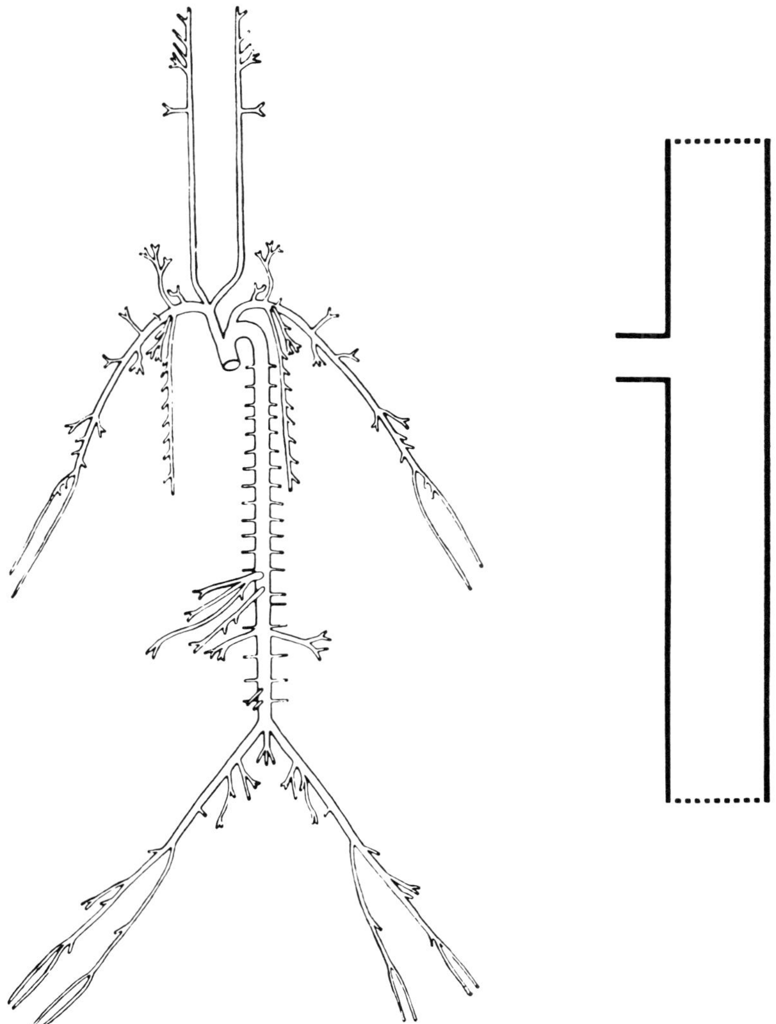

Figure 21-15. The systemic arterial system of a dog represented by a single tube, incompletely occluded at both ends, which receives blood from the heart one third of the way along its length.

improves further when heart rate increases during exercise [14]. The factors responsible for favourable match involve low ascending aortic impedance, wave reflection, differential reflection between upper and lower body, and an appropriate relationship between heart rate and body length [23]. The last factor is probably responsible for the inverse relationship between heart rate and body length in mammals [14, 38]. It must be clear, however, that the match – the fine tuning – is delicate and will be upset by anything which alters the frequency of

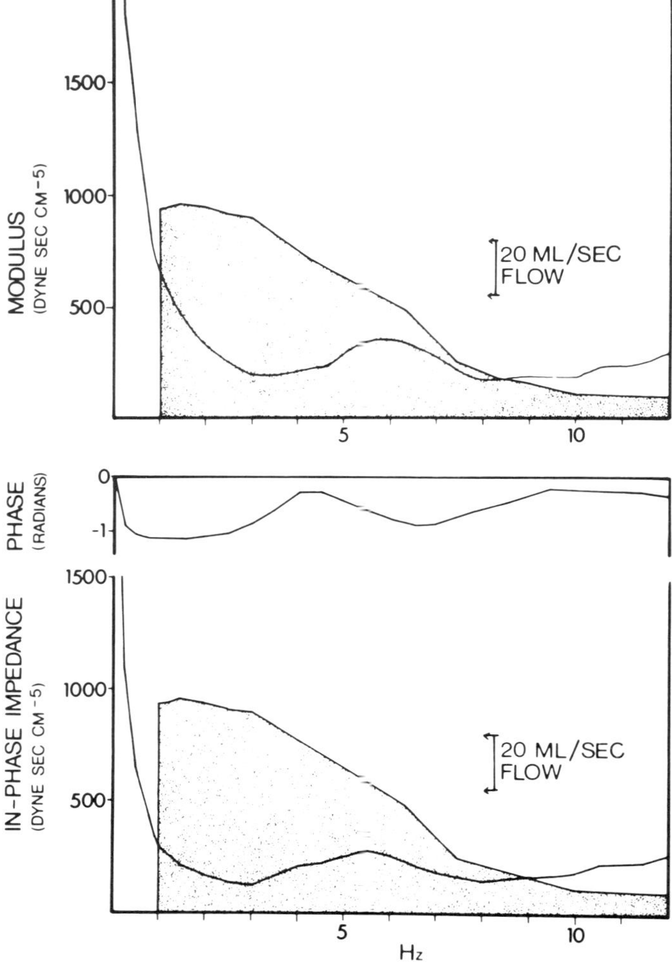

Figure 21-16. Top: Relationship between impedance modulus in the ascending aorta of a dog and amplitude of harmonics of ventricular ejection (flow) waves (stippled area) as determined in an animal of similar size. Bottom: Relationship between inphase impedance (Z cosine O) in the ascending aorta of the same dog and amplitude of harmonics of ventricular ejection (flow) waves (stippled area). From O'Rourke 1982 [14].

impedance and highest values of flow harmonics. Change in timing of wave reflection thus can readily disturb this delicate match.

Man

There are important differences in arterial parameters between adult man and other experimental animals. These were known and their significance described well before modern instruments had been introduced to record arterial pressure waves. CS Roy in 1880 stated 'only in the case of young children do we find the elasticity of arteries is so perfectly adapted to the requirements of the organism as it is in the case of the lower animals' [39], and Mahomed [8] in 1874 had described change in contour of the arterial pressure wave, with development of a late systolic peak and absent diastolic wave in subjects with stiffened arteries, with development of a late systolic peak and absent diastolic wave in subjects with subjects with stiffened arteries, with high arterial pressure, and in the elderly (Fig. 21-6).

Changes in arterial shape with aging were described again 90 years later by Freis and colleagues [40], and by ourselves [41]. The changes are attributable to early return of wave reflection so that the secondary diastolic wave moves into systole; this augments the pressure in systole and causes relative decrease of pressure during diastole. The pressure wave illustrated in Fig. 6 is typical of that seen in a 40 year old human adult, not just in an elderly subject. The change of pressure wave shown in man with age is associated with change in ascending aortic impedance patterns [42]. This has not been stressed by previous workers, who compared the human result with those in dogs and rabbits. The data are in many ways similar, with the first minimum of modulus reached at around 4 Hz. One would however expect this to be different since rabbits and dogs are far smaller than man. The ascending aortic impedance values are inappropriate for man in relation to body length, and in relation to ventricular ejection. Heart rate in man is slower and duration of ejection longer than dogs and rabbits. Hence in man the appropriate match between ventricular ejection and vascular impedance is lost. The tuning is grossly disturbed. Values of impedance modulus are inappropriately high at the frequencies of the important flow harmonics (Fig. 21-17) [42, 44].

What is responsible for these changes in man with age? One factor is the progressive increase of arterial stiffness that occurs with age in man and which is not seen in other animals during the normal life span. This increased stiffness is manifest as increase in pulse wave velocity by about 50% between the age of 10 and 50 years (Fig. 21-18) [45, 46, 47]. Another factor may be the proximal aortic dilation which occurs with age [48] and results in an impedance mismatch and so generation of wave reflection in the abdominal aorta [49].

These points are of more than passing academic interest. They are relevant to the management of conditions such as cardiac failure and angina pectoris where one wishes to optimise the interaction between heart and vascular system. Wave reflection may be beneficial for experimental animals and for children, but its effects are detrimental to adult man. Ability to delay or reduce peripheral wave reflection in man is clearly an important therapeutic strategy.

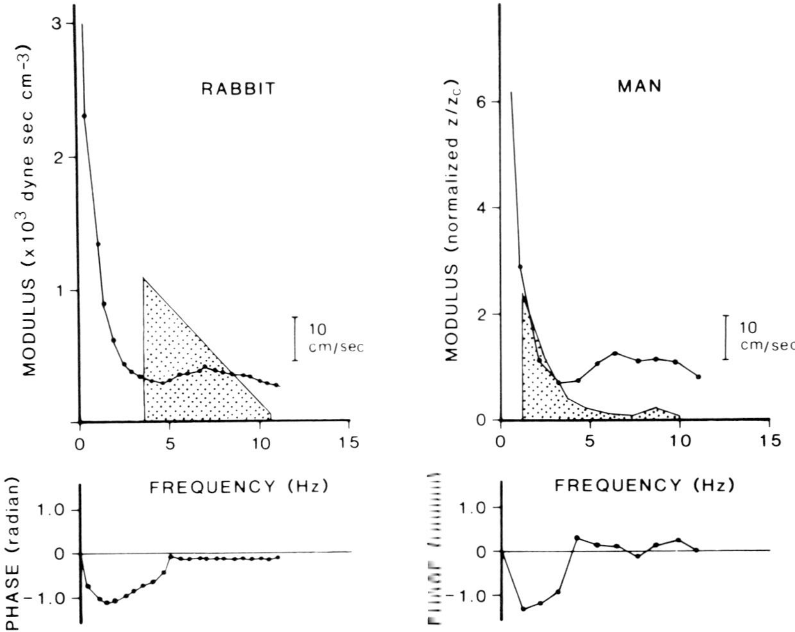

Figure 21-17. Ascending aortic impedance in a group of rabbits of average weight 3.0 kg (left) and in a group of middle aged humans of average weight 72 kg (right). Inset is the amplitude of lower harmonics of typical ascending aortic flow waves in rabbit and man. In rabbits there is a match between heart rate and minimal value of impedance modulus. The match is distorted in adult man. Date from reference 14 and 43.

Conclusions

The noted bank robber, Willie Sutton, when asked 'Why rob banks?' is reported to have answered 'That's where the money is'. The 'money' in more than one sense appears to be in clinical application of arterial hemodynamics – to erroneous concepts of systolic and diastolic pressure in hypertension, to the distorted wave reflection of adult man, to modification of wave reflection in angina pectoris and in heart failure. The 'money' is in the most common serious conditions afflicting adult man. The principles of hemodynamics are now sufficiently established for such to proceed expeditiously and smoothly.

References

1. McDonald, D.A.: Hemodynamics. Ann. Rev. of Physiol. 30: 526–56, 1968.
2. McDonald, D.A. and Taylor, M.G.: The hydrodynamics of the arterial circulation. In Prog. Biophys. 9: 107–73, Pergamon, London, 1959.

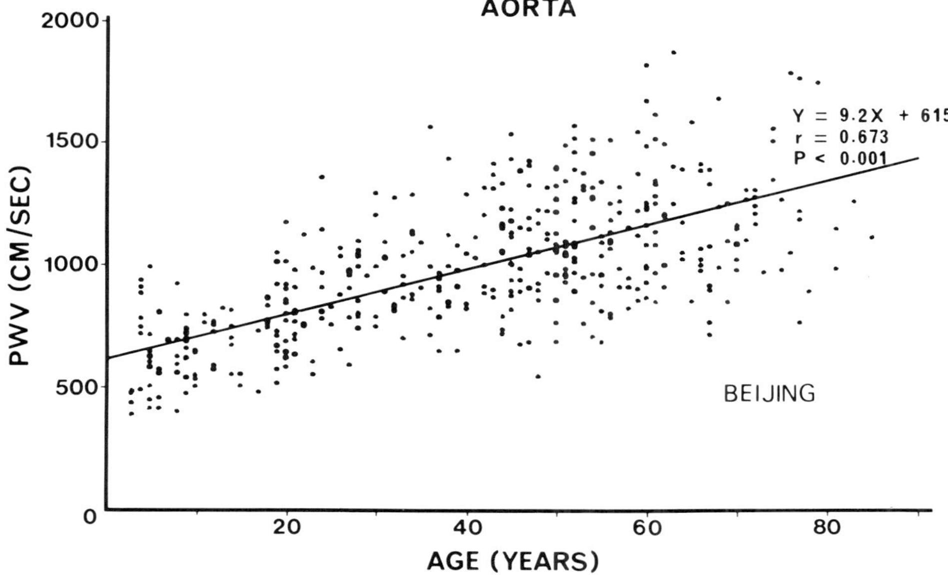

Figure 21-18. Aortic pulse wave velocity determined non invasively in a group of 480 apparently normal healthy subjects in urban Beijing. Prevalence of atherosclerosis was very low in this society. From Avolio et al 1983 [47].

3. Hales, S.: Statical essays containing haemastatics. 3rd ed Wilson and Nichol, London, 1769.

4. Young, T.: On the functions of the heart and arteries. The Croonian Lecture Phil. Trans. Roy. Soc. 99: 1–31, 1808.

5. Poiseuille, J.M.: Recherches sur la force de coeur aortique. In Ruskin A, Classics in arterial hypertension. Thomas Springfield, 1956.

6. Poiseuille, J.M.: Recherches experimentals sur le mouvement des liquides dans les tubes de tres petits diametres. Comptes Rendus Hebdomadaires des seances de L'Academie des Sciences. 11: 961–67, 1041–1048, 1840.

7. McDonald, D.A.: Blood flow in arteries. Arnold, London, 1974.

8. Mahomed, F.: The aetiology of Bright's disease and the prealbuminuric stage. Med. Chir. Trans. 57: 197–228, 1874.

9. Ruskin, A.: Classics in arterial hypertension. Thomas Springfield, 1956.

10. O'Rourke, M.F.: Hypertension is a myth. Aust. NZ. J. Med. 13: 84–90, 1983.

11. Frank, O.: Der puls in den Arterien. Z. Biol. 46: 441–553, 1905.

12. Frank, O.: Die Theorie der Pulswellen. Z. Biol. 85: 91–130, 1927.

13. Berliner, H.S.: A system of scientific medicine: philanthropic foundations in the Flexner Era. New York, Tavistock.

14. O'Rourke, M.F.: Arterial function in health and disease. Churchill, Edinburgh, 1982.

15. McDonald, D.A.: The relation of pulsatile pressure to flow in arteries. J. Physiol. (London) 127: 533–52, 1955.

16. Womersley, J.R.: The mathematical analysis of the arterial circulation in a state of oscillatory motion. Wright Air Development Center Technical Report, WADC – TR, 56–614, 1957.

17. Taylor, M.G.: An approach to an analysis of the arterial pulse wave. I. Oscillations in an

attenuating line. Phys. Med. Biol. 1: 258–69, 1957

18. Taylor, M.G.: An approach to an analysis of the arterial pulse wave. II. Fluid oscillations in an elastic tube. Phys. Med. Biol. 1: 321–9, 1957.

19. Taylor, M.G.: Wave travel in arteries and the design of the cardiovascular system. In Pulsatile Blood Flow ed Attinger EO, New York, McGraw p 343–67, 1964.

20. Taylor, M.G.: The input impedance of an assembly of randomly-branching elastic tubes. Biophys. J. 6: 29–51, 1966.

21. O'Rourke, M.F. and Taylor, M.G.: Vascular impedance of the femoral bed. Circ. Res. 18: 126–139, 1966.

22. O'Rourke, M.F.and Taylor, M.G.: Input impedance of the systemic circulation. Circ. Res. 20: 365–380, 1967.

23. O'Rourke, M.F.: Steady and pulsatile energy losses in the systemic circulation under normal conditions and in simulated arterial disease. Cardiovasc. Res. 1: 313–26, 1967.

24. O'Rourke, M.F.: Pressure and flow waves in systemic arteries and the anatomical design of the arterial system. J. Appl. Physiol. 23: 139–49, 1967.

25. Kenner, T.: Models of the arterial system. In The Arterial System. Eds Bauer RD, Busse R, Springer, New York p 80–88, 1978.

26. Noordergraaf, A., Jager, G.N. and Westerhof, N. eds): Circulatory analog computers. Amsterdam, North Holland, 1963.

27. Westerhof, N., Bosman, F., de Vries, G.J. and Noordergraaf A.: Analog studies of the human systemic arterial tree. J. Biomech. 2: 121–143, 1969.

28. Avolio, A.P.: Hemodynamic studies and modelling of the mammalian arterial system. PhD Thesis, University of New South Wales, 1976.

29. Avolio, A.P., O'Rourke, M.F. and Webster, M.E. Pulse wave propagation in the arterial system of the diamond python (Morelia spilotes). Am. J. Physiol. 245: 831–36, 1984.

30. Remington, J.W.: The physiology of the aorta and major arteries. Handbook of Physiology, American Physiological Soc., Washington DC, Vol 2 Circulation 2 pp 799–838, 1965.

31. Rowell, L.B., Brengelman, G.I., Blackman, J.R. Bruce, R.A. and Murray, J.A.: Disparities between aortic and peripheral pulse pressures induced by upright exercise and vasomotor changes in man. Circulation 37: 954–964, 1968.

32. Aperia: Haemodynamical studies. Scand. Arch. Physiol. 83 Suppl I: 1–230, 1940.

33. Taylor, M.G.: Use of random excitation and spectral analysis in the study of frequency-dependent parameters of the cardiovascular system. Circ. Res. 18: 585–95, 1966.

34. Taylor, M.G.: Haemodynamics. Ann. Rev. Physiol. 35: 87–114, 1973.

35. Westerhof, N., Sipkema, P., Van der Bos, G.C., Elzinga, G.: Forward and backward waves in the arterial system. Cardiovasc. Res. 6: 648–656, 1972.

36. Laskey, W., Kussmaul, K.G., Martin, J.L., Kleaveland, J.P., Hirshfield, J.W. and Stiroff, S.: Characteristics of vascular hydraulic load in patients with heart failure. Circulation 72: 61–71, 1985.

37. Milnor, W.R.: Arterial impedance as ventricular afterload. Circ. Res. 36: 565–570, 1975.

38. Gow, B.S. and O'Rourke, M.F.: Comparison of pressure and flow in the ascending aorta of different mammals. Proc. Aust. Physiol. Pharmacol. Soc. 1: 68, 1970.

39. Roy, C.S.: The elastic properties of the arterial wall. J. Physiol. (London) 3: 125–159.

40. Freis, E.D., Heath, W.C., Luchsinger, P.C. and Snell, R.E.: Changes in the carotid pulse which occur with age and hypertension. Am. Heart J. 71: 757–765, 1966.

41. O'Rourke, M.F., Blazek, J.V., Morreels, C.L. Jr and Krovetz, L.J.: Pressure wave transmission along the human aorta: changes with age and in arterial degenerative disease. Circ. Res. 23: 567–579, 1968.

42. Nichols, W.W., O'Rourke, M.F., Avolio, A.P., Yaginuma, T., Murgo, J.P., Pepine, C.J. and Conti, C.R.: Effects of age on ventricular/vascular coupling. Am. J. Cardiol. 55: 1179–1184, 1985.

43. Murgo, J.P., Westerhof, N., Giolma, J.P. and Altobelli, S.A.: Aortic input impedance in normal

man: relationship to pressure waveshapes. Circulation 62: 105–116, 1980.

44. O'Rourke, M.F., Yaginuma, T. and Avolio, A.P.: Physiological and pathophysiological implications of ventricular/vascular coupling. Ann. Biomed. Eng. 12: 119–134, 1984.

45. Bramwell, J.C. and Hill, A.V.: The velocity of the pulse wave in man. Proc. Roy. Soc. 93: 298–306.

46. Ho, K.: Effects of aging on arterial distensibility and left ventricular load in an Australian population. BSc (Med) Thesis, University of New South Wales, 1982.

47. Avolio, A.P., Chen, S.G., Wang, R.P., Zheang, C.L., Li, M. and O'Rourke, M.F.: Effects of aging on arterial compliance and left ventricular load in a northern Chinese urban community. Circulation: 50–58, 1983.

48. Langewouters, G.J.: Visco-elasticity of the human aorta in vitro in relation to pressure and age. PhD Thesis, Free University of Amsterdam, 1981.

49. Latham, R.D., Westerhof, N., Sipkema, P., Rubal, B., Reuderink, P. and Murgo, J.P.: Regional wave travel and reflections along the human aorta: a study with six simultaneous micromanometric pressures. Circulation 72: 1257–69, 1985.

22. Arterial dynamics: a comment on arterial wave reflections

RICKY D. LATHAM

Introduction

We have been privileged to hear the thorough general discussion of arterial dynamics by Dr. Michael O'Rourke. Whereas this field lends itself to many areas of intensive investigation, I will limit my comments to that of arterial wave reflections and modeling the systemic arterial tree. Since the early part of this century when Hamilton and Dow [1] proposed the presence of standing waves in the aorta, numerous studies have been performed to investigate the phenomenon of reflections in the systemic circulation with attempts to hypothesize simplified models of the reflective systemic circulation [2–5]. Much of this previous work has focused on determining the site(s) of origin of reflections.

Our laboratory has recently reported a study which was designed to investigate the regional pulse wave transmission characteristics along the human aorta in normal man [5]. Multisensor micromanometric catheterization techniques were utilized. A custom-designed catheter mounted with six micromanometric transducers at 10 cm intervals was positioned along the descending aorta such that the tip was in the distal external iliac and the proximal transducer was located in the aortic arch. Pressures in the left ventricle and ascending aorta were simultaneously recorded prior to insertion of the six-sensor catheter. The study protocol consisted of recording pressures at baseline control, during a Valsalva and then a Mueller maneuver, and finally during femoral artery occlusion by bilateral manual compression. We found that the proximal aortic waveshape in the control condition characteristically revealed a mid-to-late secondary systolic peak separated from the early systolic upstroke by a definite point of inflection (representing the foot of the reflected wave). As pressures were recorded distally, this point of inflection occurred earlier on the systolic waveform until it was obscured in the upstroke on the pressure contour recorded just above the origin of the renal arteries. A secondary inflection was noted in more distal waveforms. These data, along with alterations in the apparent phase velocity profiles (as a function of frequency), led to the conclusion that a site of prominent reflection was probably located in the aortic region incorporating the branches of the celiac, mesenteric and renal arteries. This was further suggested on arteriography which showed a significant, sudden decrease in aortic dimension from a level proximal to the renal arteries compared with the diameter of the segment distal to these branches. The reflection coefficient across the junction of the branches of the renal arteries from the descending aorta was calculated at approximately 0.40.

Finally, we demonstrated that physiologic maneuvers significantly affected wave reflections, with an increase in the returning reflected wave manifested during the Mueller maneuver and femoral artery occlusion, and the amplitude significantly decreased during the Valsalva maneuver. We concluded that there are at least two major sites of reflections affecting the proximal aortic pressure wave contour which arise from the lower part of the body. The first appears to be at the aortic level incorporating the branches of the celiac, mesenteric, and renal arteries, and the second site distal to the terminal aortic bifurcation. Therefore, these data suggest that the reflective systemic circulation in man may be modeled by two non-homogenous tubes in series (see Figure), in contrast to the asymmetric T-tube model previously discussed.

We have carried this investigation a step further in a population of normotensive baboons (papio anubis) to overcome some of the limitations of our previous study and the ethical constraints involved with human investigations. We selected a species phylogenetically close to man to test if the pulse transmission characteristics in this species would be similar to normal man. These animals were catheterized in the anesthetized state utilizing the same multisensor catheters from our previous study. Simultaneous pressures along the aorta were recorded at baseline normotensive pressure, during hypotension induced with nitroprusside infusion, and hypertension attained with phenylephrine infusion. The aorta was occluded at selected sites using a balloon-tipped catheter filled with a Renografin-saline mixture. Occlusions were performed at the terminal aortic bifurcation, the level approximating the renal artery origins, midthoracic and proximal descending aorta, and bilateral carotid occlusion (left brachiocephalic-right carotid). The objective was to determine the presence and significance of reflections from the upper extremity as opposed to the lower extremity, and the influence of changes in the mean aortic pressure upon these reflected waves during occlusion.

We found that during the abdominal aortic occlusion, there was a significant prolongation of the ejection period and some alteration in the proximal aortic waveforms. The effect on the wave contours is much exaggerated when the occlusion is performed at a more proximal site. In contrast, bilateral carotid occlusion induced no distortion of the proximal aortic wave shapes. During nitroprusside infusion, changes during occlusion on the aortic pressure contours were more pronounced than alterations observed at normotensive levels. Again, no significant changes in the proximal aortic wave shapes occurred with bilateral carotid artery occlusion. We feel these data support a model of circulation

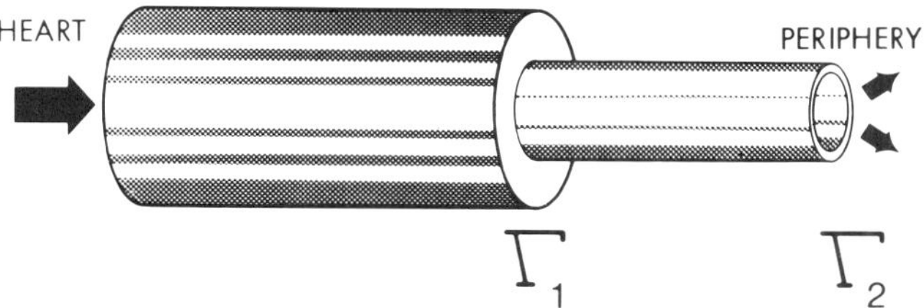

Figure 22-1. Two non-homogenous tubes in series as a model for the reflective systemic circulation.

resembling two non-homogenous tubes in series in which the dominant sites of wave reflection occur in the descending aorta and lower body. We have not found data in our studies in man and primates to support significant reflections from the head and upper extremities affecting the proximal aortic wave shapes.

It is reasonable to assume that reflections may arise from different sites and be manifested on pressure waveforms in a variety of ways, depending upon the species studied. It is also probable that one 'reflective model' for the systemic circulation is not valid for all species. A study of the arterial wave reflection phenomenon provides understanding of the hydraulic properties of the systemic circulation under investigation. It is interesting to consider that the significance of wave reflections may be more important as a marker for the physical properties/ condition of the macrovasculature in the system in which they are observed, analogous to use of the heart rate to describe the chronotropic state of the heart. The amplitude of reflected waves is readily changed by alterations in the stiffness of the aorta, and thus they may have a role as a marker for changes in central aortic compliance. Further studies are needed in this area.

References

1. Hamilton, W.F. and Dow, P.: An experimental study of the standing waves in the pulse propogated through the aorta. Am. J. Physiol. 125: 48–59, 1939.
2. Luchsinger, P.C., Snell, R.E., Patel, D.J. and Fry, D.L.: Instantaneous pressure distribution along the human aorta. Circ. Res. 15: 510, 1964.
3. O'Rourke, M.F.: Pressure and flow waves in systemic arteries and the anatomical design of the arterial system. J. Appl. Physiol. 23: 139, 1967.
4. Van den Bos, G.C., Westerhof, N., Elzinga, G. and Sipkema, P.: Reflection in the systemic arterial system: effects of aortic and carotid occlusion. Cardiovasc. Res. 10: 565, 1976.
5. Latham, R.D., Westerhof, N., Sipkema, P., Rubal, B.J., Reuderink, P. and Murgo, J.P.: Regional wave travel and reflections along the human aorta: a study with six simultaneous micromanometric pressures. Circ. 72: 1257, 1985.

264

General discussion of arterial hemodynamics

It was noted that the contribution of the large, proximal arterial branches was minimal and less than might have been supposed, suggesting very favorable impedance matching.

There was interest in the effects of exercise on wave reflection but such studies are limited by practical considerations since it is not feasible to study patients during upright exercise.

The significance of these findings was questioned in light of the textbook view that external work accounts for only 25% of oxygen consumption and the oscillatory component only 15% of this. In reply, the accuracy of these estimates were challenged in that they might depend on unrealistic assumptions.

23. Control of the circulation

KIICHI SAGAWA, KENJI SUNAGAWA, DANIEL BURKHOFF and
JOE ALEXANDER, JR

Introduction

This symposium focuses on the mechanics of heart muscle contraction, ventricular pump function, and central hemodynamics. Therefore, despite the title, this chapter confines itself to discussions on the mechanical interactions between the heart and the vasculature with special reference to physiological optimizations of their coupling. Such basic knowledge on the interactions is prerequisite for quantitative understanding of the neural and humoral controls of the circulatory system. Take arterial baroreceptor reflex control of ventricular contractility for example. It has repeatedly been observed that reduction of pressure in the isolated baroreceptor does not significantly increase cardiac output even though there is an obvious reflex pressor response. This apparent lack in cardiac response may only be apparent because the reflex augmentation of the contractility may be just enough to overcome the reflex-induced increase in peripheral resistance and hence to maintain cardiac output [1]. Only when the basic mechanics of the interaction between the ventricle and the arterial system are clearly understood, can the true reflex effect on cardiac contractility be appreciated from the measured change in cardiac output.

Before discussing the mechanical interactions between the heart and vasculature, we will briefly review the fundamental task assigned to the heart. The review will lead to the energetic basis of cardiac pump function.

Metabolic requirement of circulatory activities

The circulatory system subserves the homeostasis of the body by circulating blood at an adequate rate and with a proper distribution throughout the body to meet its metabolic demands. Among many substances transported via blood oxygen has been considered to be the key controlled variable for the reason that its severe shortage quickly impairs cerebral and myocardial function. The whole body oxygen balance and consequent requirements of the energy output from the cardiac pump and of coronary flow to support this myocardial activity are shown in Fig. 1.

In contrast to ordinary physiological diagrams which indicate the flow of actions among the components of the system, this diagram begins with the oxygen demand of the body (shown in the upper left corner) and indicates the flow of demands successively placed on the respiratory and circulatory functions. The body's oxygen demand is roughly .25 l/min for a 70-kg man at rest and may increase to 1 l/min during exercise. Because the tissues utilize, on an average, only 20% of oxygen carried to them by arterial blood, an oxygen flow of as much as 1 to 4 l/min must be available to the tissues under ordinary circumstances. To accomplish this oxygen supply, a flow of fully oxygenated arterial blood of 5 to 20 l/min must be generated by the heart. The normal total vascular resistance is such that mean arterial pressure will be approximately 100 mm Hg at this cardiac output. This means that the left ventricle must liberate a mechanical power as much as 66 joules/min (1 mm Hg $\cdot$ ml = $1 \cdot 33 \cdot 10^{-4}$ joule), or, assuming a heart rate of 66 beats/min, a stroke energy of 1 joule at rest. For the entire heart, the oxygen consumption can be roughly doubled (i.e. 2 watts at rest and 10 watts during heavy exercise). This includes the oxygen required for basal metabolism and for excitation-contraction coupling of both atria and ventricles.

As Dr. Gibbs expertly reviewed the so-called mechanical efficiency of the cardiac pump (external work/unit oxygen consumption/beat) is quite variable with the type of physical activity and hemodynamic loading. As a ballpark figure, an efficiency of 15% was used for the diagram, which means that the heart needs a fuel supply of 13 to 66 watts, or 780 to 4000 joules/min. Conventionally, 1 ml of oxygen is considered to produce about 20 joules of energy. Therefore, the heart requires 40 to 200 ml/min O_2 supply. Thanks to the high oxygen utilization (75%) this much oxygen can be delivered to the myocardium by a coronary blood flow of 266 to 1330 ml/min. This requirement is easy to meet at rest. The requirement during a severe exercise may be quite difficult to meet even for a healthy heart when heart rate is high, and consequently, the duration of diastole, an important determinant of coronary flow, is markedly shortened. If the coronary bed is constricted for one reason or another, oxygen delivery to the myocardium will become severely compromised.

Interactions at veno-atrio-ventricular junction

For the ventricle to generate the required amount of stroke energy, it must first be filled in diastole to a proper volume. With the normal diastolic compliance, this extent of ventricular filling is achieved by a transmural pressure of 3 to 4 mm Hg for the right ventricle and 6 to 8 mm Hg for the left ventricle. The transmural ventricular pressure in vivo is extremely difficult to measure accurately because

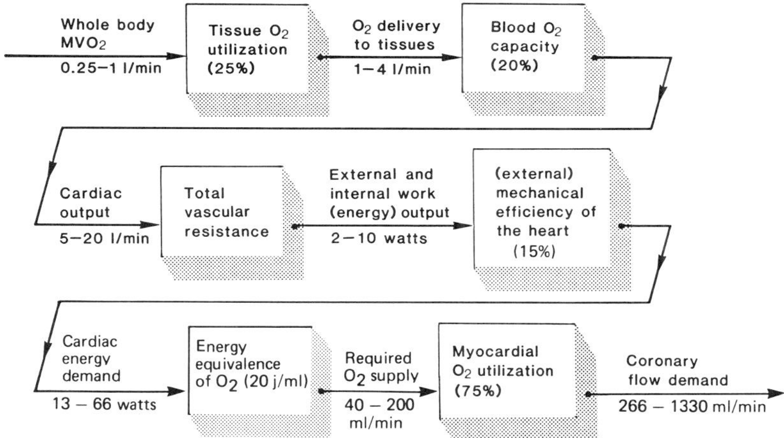

Figure 23-1. Demand flow chart from bodily O_2 consumption to cardiac work and coronary blood flow.

the extracardiac pressure is dependent on so many factors, including intrapleural pressure and intrapericardial pressure, and these pressures consist of not only uniform fluid pressure, but also of regional solid (contact) force exerted by the lung and pericardial tissues. Dr. Tyberg illustrated this complex reality and presented practical approaches to deal with it. Dr. Smith also discussed the transseptal interactions between the ventricular chambers of the heart which are amplified in vivo by the pericardial constraints. Their discussion cautions those who tend to interpret cardiac chamber mechanics solely on the basis of knowledge on isolated cardiac muscle and ventricular mechanics.

Another point often neglected and missing in our quantitative understanding is the contribution of atrial contraction. We [2, 3] have recently studied left atrial contraction in an isolated canine heart preparation with computer-simulated physiological loading. A balloon was fit to the atrial cavity and connected to a servo-controlled piston pump so that the atrium can be filled and can eject as if it were in vivo. The pulmonary venous return to the left atrium was modelled by combining a constant source pressure (P_v) with a C-L-R circuit as shown in Fig. 23-2. Diastolic filling of the left ventricle was also modelled by connecting the atrium with a sinusoidally time-varying ventricular elastance through a valve, an inertance, and a resistance. The experimental results from 6 atria indicated that the end-systolic atrial elastance ($E_{es,a}$) was indeed insensitive to loading conditions. That is, whether the atrium is physiologically ejecting or isovolumically contracting, the atrial end-systolic pressure-volume relationship (ESPVR) can be described as:

$$P_{es,a} = E_{es,a} (V_{es,a} - V_{o,es,a}) \tag{1}$$

in which $P_{es,a}$ and $V_{es,a}$ are end-systolic atrial pressure and volume and $V_{o,es,a}$ is the volume axis intercept of the end-systolic pressure-volume relationship (the ESPVR line).

An example of the atrial P-V diagrams is shown in Fig. 23-3, where both isovolumic and ejecting contractions at different volumes come to a similar ESPVR line. In fact, the entire systolic portion of the instantaneous atrial elastance curve was far less dependent on afterloading condition than was the ventricle. The onset of atrial relaxation was independent of the systolic loading condition as has previously been observed by Coutteney et al. [4]. The systolic phase of atrial contraction can therefore be described by a simple (instantaneous) P-V relationship similar to Equation 1. By contrast, the onset and time course of ventricular diastolic elastance is very complex being a function of three major factors as reviewed by Brutsaert et al. [5].

The C-R-L circuit for pulmonary venous return (Fig. 23-2) is based on a preliminary experimental finding on the input impedance of the systemic venous bed (seen inversely from the right atrial port). The impedance spectrum shown in Fig. 23-4 was obtained by applying pseudo-random flow perturbations at the vena caval junction and cross-correlating the flow perturbation signal with the venous pressure response (white noise approach). Of considerable interest is the finding that the venous impedance modulus (the mid panel) gradually increased with frequency from a value of about 0.2 mm Hg - sec/ml to a value nearly 10 times as large at 8 Hz. The increase in modulus was associated with an exponential attenuation of the phase lag (bottom panel). The behaviour of the venous impedance modulus spectrum is opposite to that of arterial input impedance (which is large in the low frequency region and decreases with frequency). The large venous impedance moduli at high frequencies may be important in preventing a large backflow of blood into the veins during atrial contraction (at a greater velocity than the ventricle). This preliminary finding warrants further experimental studies on systemic and pulmonary venous input impedance.

Before concluding this section, we have to emphasize the importance of the baseline filling pressure(BFP) of the systemic and pulmonary vascular beds for diastolic filling of the right and left ventricle. The baseline filling pressures (mean systemic and mean pulmonary pressures of Guyton [6]) then are determined by the blood volume and the vascular pressure-volume relationships in the systemic and pulmonary vascular bed. Dr. Greenway discussed these aspects in individual regions of the splanchnic bed – in particular, the hepatic bed – with reference to their neural and humoral control. In recapitulation, we want to draw your attention to the fact that whenever systemic arterial pressure increases, whether by increase in cardiac output or by increase in arterial resistance, the hypertension is bound to shift an amount of venous blood into the systemic arterial bed and thus decrease central venous pressure. This decrease in central venous pressure can be counteracted if the systemic venous capacity (unstressed volume and/or compliance) diminishes at the same time. This was indeed found in the case of

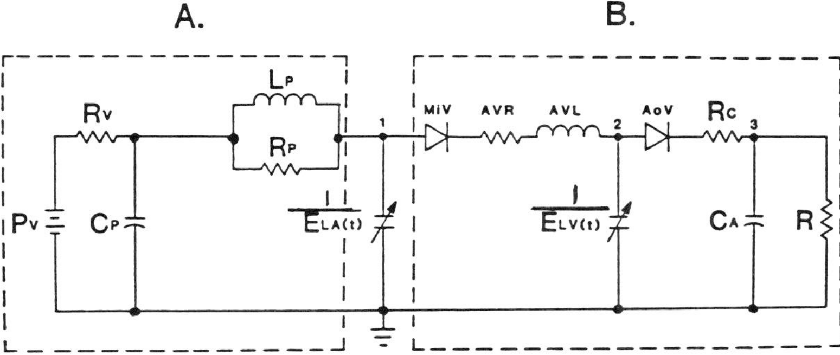

Figure 23-2. Electrical analogue of the left atrial preloading circuit (A) and the afterloading system, i.e., the diastolic and systolic left ventricular properties (B). E_{LA} (t) and E_{LV} (t) represent the time-varying elastance of the left atrium and left ventricle, respectively. E_{LA} (t) is that of the real (measured) atrium, whereas E_{LV} (t) is that of an LV model based on previous studies and assumed to vary between 0.25 and 5.0 mm Hg/ml during each cardiac cycle in a sinusoidal fashion. P_V = pulmonary venous source pressure for ventricular filling assumed to be constant. R_v = source resistance, L_p = pulmonary inertance, AVR = atrio-ventricular resistance, AoV = aortic valve, R_c = characteristic impedance of the systemic vascular bed. C_A = systemic arterial compliance, R = systemic arterial resistance. The physiological systems in Panel A and Panel B were simulated on-line by a digital computer during experimental determination of E_{LA} (t) in an excised perfused canine heart. Reproduced from the Ph.D. thesis by J. Alexander, Jr. [3].

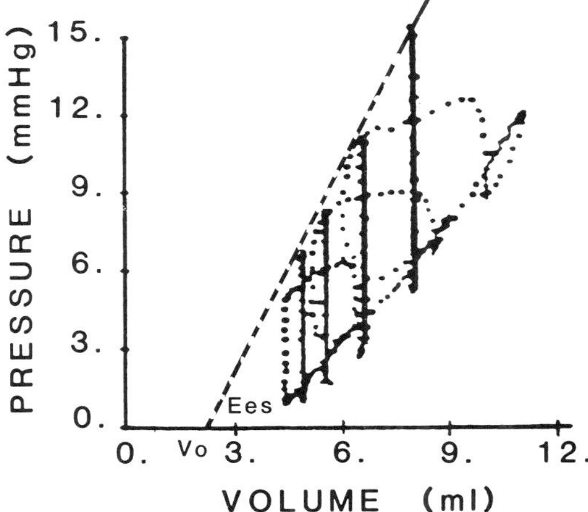

Figure 23-3. Pressure-volume trajectories of left atrial contractions. The 4 solid lines represent isovolumic contractions, whereas the dotted curves represent physiologically ejecting contractions realized with the computer-simulated loading system shown in Fig. 2. Note the superposition of the linear end-systolic pressure-volume relationships for the two contraction modes. Reproduced from the Ph.D. thesis by J. Alexander, Jr. [3].

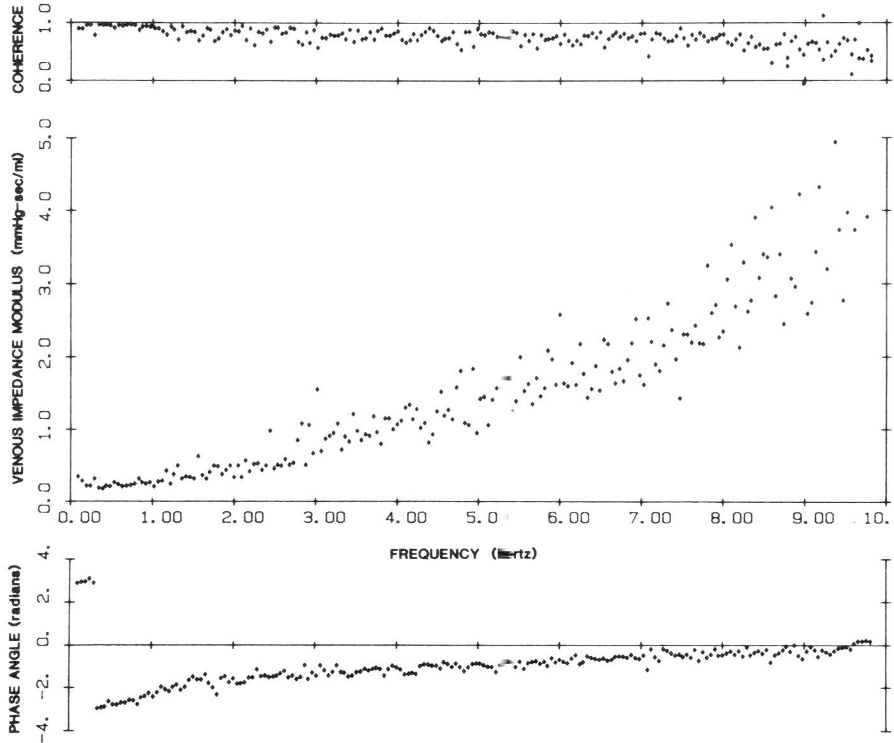

Figure 23-4. Frequency spectrum of the systemic venous input impedance studied by pseudo-random perturbation of systemic venous return. The top panel is the coherence function which expresses the strength of correlation between the pulmonary venous flow and pressure at the respective frequency. Note the frequency-dependent increase in the modulus (2nd panel) as opposed to its decrease with frequency in the arterial input impedance. See text for further explanation. Reproduced from the Ph.D. thesis by J. Alexander, Jr. [3].

reflex hypertension mediated by the carotid sinus baroreceptors [7]. In addition, blood can shift to the cardiopulmonary bed from the systemic bed under the influence of mediated by adrenergic mechanisms [8]. These mechanisms tend to maintain right ventricular filling during the systemic arterial pressor reflex.

We also must emphasize the importance of venous resistance in controlling ventricular filling and cardiac output. Although small in magnitude, venous resistance lowers ventricular filling pressure from the baseline vascular filling pressure in proportion to cardiac output [9]. Thus, cardiac output exerts an important negative feedback on itself throughout venous resistance, which had not been clearly understood until Guyton illustrated it by the venous return-cardiac output equilibrium diagram [6]. This negative effect of cardiac output is shown by the curve labelled venous pressure in Fig. 23-5. It originates at the baseline vascular filling pressure (B.F.P.) on the ordinate and courses rightward and downward with increasing cardiac output to a point on the zero pressure line. Cardiac output cannot increase beyond this point due to collapse of the veins.

Interactions at the ventriculo-arterial junction

A linearized relationship of mean arterial pressure with cardiac output is also shown in Fig. 23-5. It originates at the B.F.P. and terminates at the cardiac output that causes the venous collapse. We must add, however, that the zero-flow pressure actually seen at the arterial port after stopping cardiac contraction may not be the same as the B.F.P. seen at the venous port due to a number of factors [10, 11]. Understanding the mechanics behind this nonlinearity is probably highly desirable so that we can accurately define afterload resistance to ventricular ejection.

Moreover, an increase in cardiac output will cause a proportional increase in mean arterial pressure which in turn will immediately counteract the increase in cardiac output that caused the pressure to rise. Thus, it is interesting to recognize that the heart is provided with a negative feedback mechanism at its arterial junction as well as at the venous port. Dr. Elzinga has shown this afterload effect on cardiac output in his ventricular pump function graph. We have shown the effect by the slope (E_{es}) of the end-systolic P-V relationship [12]. In either curve, a stronger ventricle can be represented by a steeper slope of these relationships which means a smaller outflow reduction by a given increase in afterload pressure. In other words, the negative feedback through the arterial resistance works more strongly for a weak ventricle than for a strong ventricle. This explains why drugs that reduce afterload cause a much greater increase in cardiac output in diseased hearts than in a normal heart.

A number of involved analyses have been performed to understand arterial pressure-flow dynamics and its effect on ventricular ejection. For example, some investigators have explored, theoretically, an ejection pattern which minimizes stroke work or minute power [13, 14]. Others have analyzed the relationship among the animal size, heart rate, and arterial pressure and flow wave forms [15]. Dr. O'Rourke presented an elegant review on these and other comparative physiological aspects of arterial hemodynamics with emphasis on the concept that with increasing age the reflected pressure wave is accelerated which enhances ventricular work and decreases coronary flow.

Dr. Elzinga lucidly explained how the relation between mean ventricular pressure and mean outflow describes the characteristics of the ventricular pump. He then showed that in anesthetized open-chest cats, the left ventricle worked at such a combination of contractility and afterload that the left ventricle transferred a maximal power to the arterial system [16]. It is tempting to regard this finding and the similar finding for the right ventricle by Piene and Sund [17] as a beautiful example of the use of the general physical principle that a maximal rate of energy

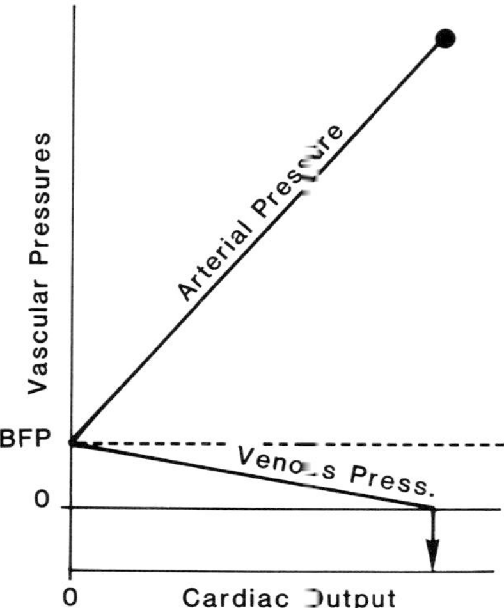

Figure 23-5. Relationship of cardiac output to systemic arterial pressure and venous pressure. BFP: baseline vascular filling pressure (i.e., Guyton's mean systemic pressure). See text for further explanation.

transfer occurs when the load impedance equals the source impedance. However, Dr. Elzinga warned us about a number of questions that must be answered before we completely accept this seemingly attractive concept.

Our recent study in isolated canine ventricles loaded with computer-simulated arterial impedance [18] also indicated that when the arterial property expressed by an effective elastance was matched to the ventricular end-systolic elastance the ventricle produced maximal stroke work. The area of the pressure-volume loop trajectory of a ventricular contraction (the hatched area in the 2nd left panel of Fig. 23-6) accurately represents stroke work, i.e. mechanical energy transferred from the cardiac pump to the arterial vasculature during each beat. Given an end-diastolic volume (V_{ed}), two major determinants of stroke work are ventricular contractility, defined by the slope (E_{es}) of the end-systolic pressure-volume relationship (Fig. 23-6, 3rd lefthand panel), and the arterial effective elastance (E_a), defined by the slope of the relationship between stroke volume and arterial end-systolic pressure (see the 2nd, 3rd and 4th righthand panels of Fig. 23-6). If arterial input impedance, free from wave reflection, is represented by the three-element Windkessel model with arterial resistance R, compliance C, and characteristic impedance R_c, the arterial elastance can be approximated by:

$$E_a = \frac{R + R_c}{t_s + T[1 - \exp(-t_d/T)]} \tag{2}$$

where t_s and t_d are durations of systole and diastole, and $T = RC$. Roughly speaking, E_a was shown to equal total peripheral resistance divided by the duration of the cardiac cycle [18]. As suggested by the bottom panel of Fig. 23-6, we can describe ventricular stroke work (SW) as a function of preload V_{ed}, arterial effective elastance E_a, and ventricular contractility E_{es}:

$$SW = (V_{ed} - V_o)^2 \frac{E_a}{(1 + E_a/E_{es})^2} \tag{3}$$

This equation reveals that, given an E_{es}, the optimal E_a for maximal SW is equal to E_{es}. This conclusion can also be reached by geometric intuition as one looks at the bottom panel of Fig. 23-6. Obviously this is another version of the same physical principle of impedance matching, based on the beat-to-beat analysis. As Hunter [19] showed, this representation can be converted into the equilibrium diagram between cardiac output, mean arterial pressure, and total peripheral resistance.

The coupling conditions for maximal mechanical efficiency (in terms of E_{es} and E_a) are different from the above condition. Again, this difference was shown earlier by Elzinga and Westerhof [20].

We [21] have analyzed ventricular mechanical efficiency utilizing the data by Suga and co-workers [22] who demonstrated that ventricular O_2 consumption (MVO_2) linearly correlated with the total pressure-volume area (PVA) defined as the area bounded by the ventricular end-systolic and end-diastolic P-V relationship curves and the systolic segment of the P-V loop (i.e. the sum of the hatched and dotted areas in the 2nd lefthand panel in Fig. 23-6). Thus,

$$MVO_2 = aPVA + b, \tag{4}$$

where a is the slope coefficient and b the MVO_2 axis intercept parameter. The coefficient a is independent of contractility, whereas b varies linearly with contractility [23, 24]. Thus, PVA can be approximated by:

$$PVA = \frac{(V_{ed} - V_o)^2 E_a}{(1 + E_a/E_{es})^2} [1 + E_a/2E_{es}]. \tag{5}$$

Utilizing these experimental findings, we calculated the ventricular mechanical efficiency (Eff = SW/MVO_2) by the following formula:

$$Eff = \frac{1}{a\,(1 + E_a/2E_{es}) + \dfrac{b(1 + E_a/E_{es})^2}{E_a\,(V_{ed} - V_o)_2}} \tag{6}$$

The values of parameters such as E_a, V_o, V_{ed}, and a were varied independently of each other over a physiologic range for a 20 kg dog. The parameter b was considered to vary with E_{es} according to the formula$_{23}$:

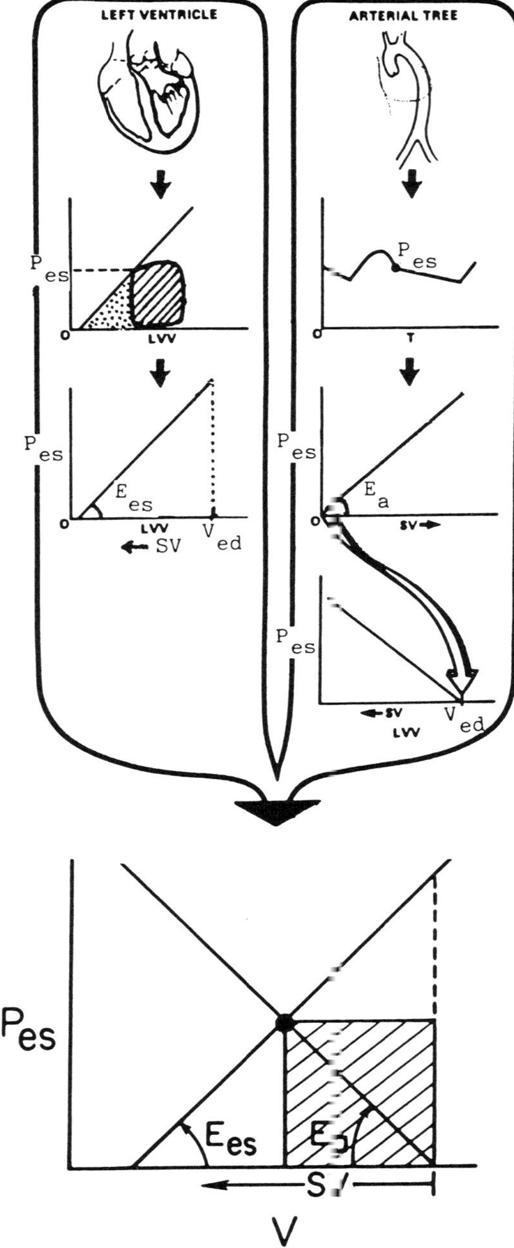

Figure 23-6. Schematic explanation of graphical analysis of ventriculo-arterial coupling. See text for further explanation. Reproduced after modification from Sunagawa et al. [18], with the permission of the American Heart Association.

$$b \text{ (ml } O_2/\text{beat)} = 0.0032\,E_{es} + 0.0104 \qquad (7)$$

To convert PVA and O_2 consumption into the same units, $1\,\text{mm Hg} \cdot \text{ml} = 1.33 \cdot 10^4\,J$, and the conventional equivalence of $1\,\text{ml}\,O_2 = 20$ joules were used. The effect of changing E_a and E_{es} on SW (Panel A), MVO_2 (Panel B), and Eff (Panel C) are shown in Fig. 23-7. As discussed above SW is maximal when $E_a = E_{es}$, whereas the efficiency is maximal when $E_a = E_{es}/2$. Note that when $E_a = E_{es}/2$, the ejection fraction is significantly greater than in the maximal stroke work condition.

In a more extensive theoretical analysis of the left ventricular mechanical efficiency, Suga et al. showed the combined effect of end-diastolic volume (preload) [24] and arterial pressure (afterload) as an efficiency surface. The surface indicated an approximately monotonic increase of efficiency with increasing preload while contractility caused a shift of the optimal arterial pressure.

The above studies led us to a hypothesis that the physiologic controller of the circulation may economize cardiac energy consumption by loading it with an arterial load which maximizes the mechanical efficiency in the resting condition, but, during stress, the controller may shift the optimization criterion to maximizing energy tranfer from the ventricle to the artery. This hypothesis seems worthy of pursuit in order to understand not only what the physiologic controller of the cardiovascular system is, but also the pathophysiology of cardiovascular control in patients with compromised cardiac function.

Relative importance of various factors on cardiac output

As a conclusion of this brief review, we will discuss the relative magnitude of the effects of ventricular contractility, heart rate, total vascular resistance, and total effective blood volume on cardiac output (Fig. 23-8). K plotted on the abscissa is E_a/E_{es}, normal. The data were obtained by a simple model of the entire circulatory system for a 20 kg dog [12]. The graph shows that, with all the vascular parameters fixed at the normal values and total effective blood volume at 300 ml and heart rate at 80 beats/min, the normal ventricular contractility ($K = 1$) gives rise to a cardiac output (large solid circle) which is as much as 90% of the maximal value that is possible at greatly enhanced contractility.

This is evidently the consequence of the strikingly shallow slope of the relation between cardiac output and contractility when K exceeds 0.5. Furthermore, even a decrease of contractility to 50% of control decreases cardiac output only by 8%. An increase of the heart rate (Fig. 23-8, triangles) from 80 to 160 beats/min increases cardiac output less than 20% above the control value at all levels of contractility. Halving the total systemic resistance (inverted triangles) increases cardiac output about 50% irrespective of ventricular contractility. Doubling the total effective blood volume increases cardiac output by approximately 100%.

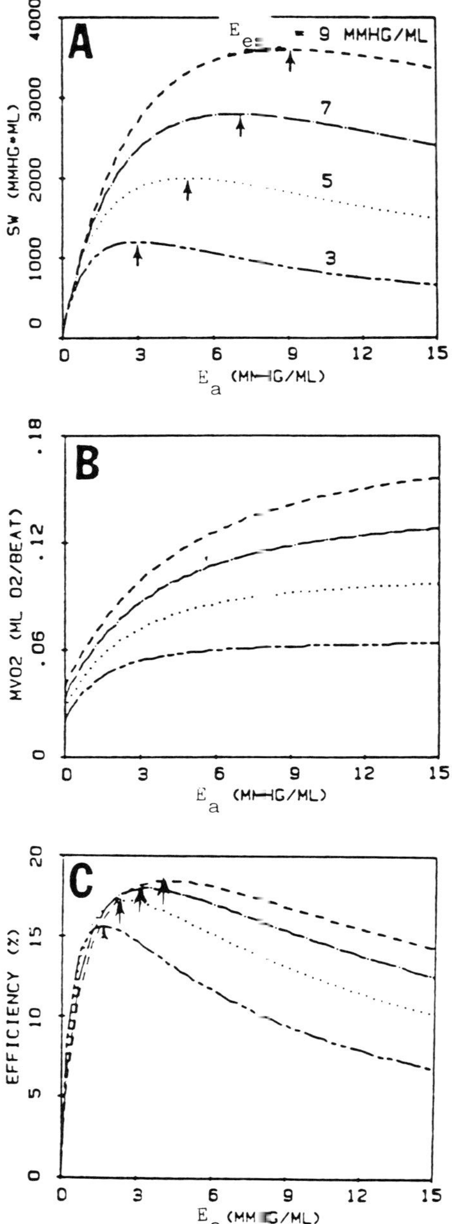

Figure 23-7. Effect of effective arterial elastance E_a (see Equation 2) on left ventricular stroke work (top panel), oxygen consumption (mid panel), and mechanical efficiency (bottom panel). Three curves in each panel are for three different ventricular contractility levels represented by E_{es} = 3, 5, 7 and 9 mm Hg/ml. Arrows indicate points of maximal stroke work (A) and maximal efficiency (C). Reproduced from Burkhoff and Sagawa [21], with the permission of the American Physiological Society.

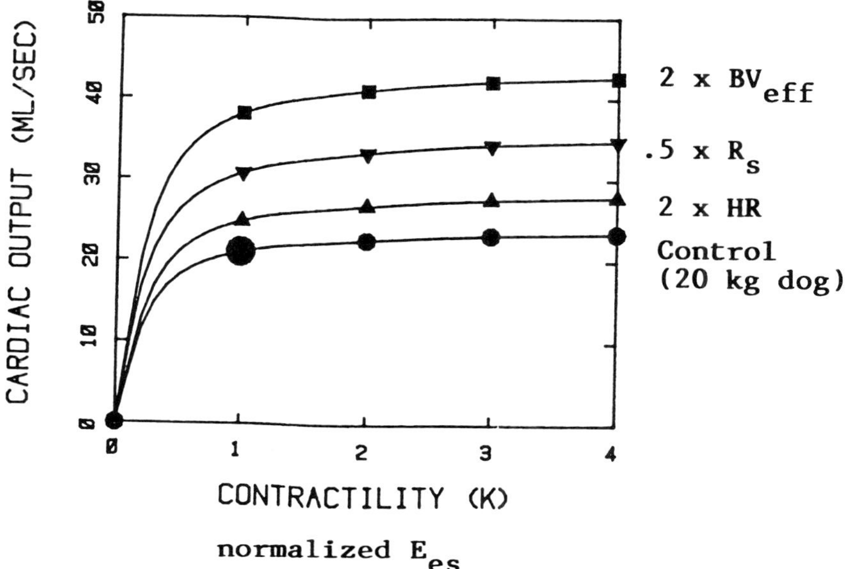

Figure 23-8. Effect of cardiac contractility (abscissa) on cardiac output predicted by a model of the entire circulatory system under control conditions (circles), when systemic resistance is reduced by 50% (inverted triangles), when heart rate is doubled (triangles), or the effective blood volume doubled (squares). Reproduced from Sunagawa et al. [12] after modification with the permission from the Biomedical Engineering Society.

Under all these different loading conditions, cardiac output at the control contractility was again about 90% of the maximal possible value. These results suggest that under normal loading conditions even considerable changes in ventricular contractility (50–400%) do not markedly affect cardiac output. In short, cardiac output is determined predominantly by the vascular properties and total effective blood volume. Therefore, when the cardiac contractile state is in the normal or supernormal range, cardiac output can be described in a further simplified form. On the other hand, changes in ventricular contractility are expected to play a much more important role when the ventricular function is greatly impaired (i.e. when K is less than 50% of normal).

Acknowledgements

Supported in part by USPHS NHLBI Research Grant HL14903.

References

1. Sagawa, K.: Baroreflex control of systemic arterial pressure and vascular bed. In: Handbook of Physiology: The Cardiovascular System III, Am. Physiol. Soc.; Washington, D.C., p 453–496, 1984.

2. Alexander, J., Jr. and Sagawa, K.: Insensitivity of the left atrial end-systolic pressure-volume relationship line to loading conditions. Circulation 68: III–372, 1983.

3. Alexander, J., Jr.: Instantaneous pressure-volume relationship of the impedance loaded canine left atrium: A. Ph.D. thesis submitted to The Johns Hopkins University, 1986.

4. Coutteney, M.M., De Clerck, N.M., Goethals, M.A., Brutsaert, D.L.: Relaxation property of mammalian atrial muscle. Circ. Res. 48: 352–356, 1981.

5. Brutsaert, D.L., Rademakers, F.E., Sys, S.U.: Triple control of relaxation: implications in cardiac disease. (Editorial) Circulation 69: 190–196, 1984.

6. Guyton, A.C.: Venous return. In Handbook of Physiology, Section 2, Volume 2, Ed. by W.F. Hamilton, Washington, D.C.; American Physiological Society, p 1099–1133, 1963.

7. Shoukas, A.A. and Sagawa, K.: Control of total systemic vascular capacity by the carotid sinus baroreflex. Circ. Res. 33: 22–23, 1973.

8. Shoukas, A.A.: Carotid sinus baroreceptor reflex control and epinephrine influence on capacitive and resistive properties of total pulmonary vascular bed of the dog. Circ. Res. 51: 95–101, 1982.

9. Levy, M.N.: The cardiac and vascular factors that determine systemic blood flow. Circ. Res. 44: 739–746, 1979.

10. Sylvester, J., Gilbert, J.R., Traystman, R., Permut, S.: Effect of hypoxia on the closing pressure of the canine systemic arterial circulation. Circ. Res. 49: 980–987, 1981.

11. Brunner, M.I., Greene, A.S., Sagawa, K. and Shoukas, A.A.: Determinants of systemic zero-flow arterial pressure. Am. J. Physiol. 245: H453–H460, 1983.

12. Sunagawa, K., Sagawa, K. and Maughan, W.L.: Ventricular interactions with the loading system. Ann. Biomed. Eng. 12: 163–189, 1984.

13. Yamashiro, S.M., et al.: Optimal control analysis of left ventricular ejection. In: Cardiovascular System Dynamics, Baan, J., Noordergraaf, A., Raines, J. (eds) Cambridge: MIT Press, p 427–431, 1978.

14. Kenner, T. and Pfeiffer, K.P.: Studies on the optimal matching between heart and arterial system. In: Cardiac Dynamics, Baan, J., Arntzenius, A.C., Yellin, E.L. (eds) Boston; Martinus Nijhoff, 1980, p 261–270.

15. Milnor, W.R.: Aortic wavelength as a determinant of the relation between heart rate and body size in mammals. Am. J. Physiol. 237: R3–R6, 1979.

16. Van der Horn, G.N., Westerhof, N. and Elzinga, G.: Optimal power generation by the left ventricle: A study in the anesthetized open thorax cat. Circ. Res. 56: 252–261, 1985.

17. Piene, H., Sund, T.: Does normal pulmonary impedance constitute the optimum load for the right ventricle? Am. J. Physiol. 242: H154–H160, 1982.

18. Sunagawa, K., Maughan, W.L. and Sagawa, K.: Optimal arterial resistance for the maximal stroke work studied in isolated canine left ventricle. Circ. Res. 56: 586–595, 1985.

19. Hunter, W.C.: Analysis of the net pulsatile effect of load on cardiac output. Proc. 35th Ann. Conf. Eng. Med. Biol., p 59, 1982.

20. Elzinga, G. and Westerhof, N.: Pump function of the feline left heart: Changes with heart rate and its bearing on the energy balance. Cardiovasc. Res. 14: 81–92, 1980.

21. Burkhoff, D. and Sagawa, K.: Ventricular efficiency predicted by an analytical model. Am. J. Physiol. 250: R1021–R1027, 1986.

22. Suga, H., et al.: Effect of positive inotropic agents on the relation between oxygen consumption and systolic pressure-volume area in canine left ventricle. Circ. Res. 53: 306–381, 1983.

23. Burkhoff, D., Yue, D.T., Oikawa, R.Y., Franz, M.R., Schaeffer, J. and Sagawa, K.: Influence of contractility on ventricular oxygen consumption. Circulation 72: III–298, 1985.

24. Suga, H., Igarashi, Y., Yamada, O. and Goto, Y.: Mechanical efficiency of the left ventricle as a function of preload, afterload, and contractility. Heart and Vessels 1: 3–8, 1986.

Index